Balancing the self

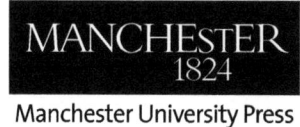
Manchester University Press

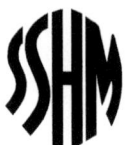

SOCIAL HISTORIES OF MEDICINE

Series editors: *David Cantor, Elaine Leong* and *Keir Waddington*

Social Histories of Medicine is concerned with all aspects of health, illness and medicine, from prehistory to the present, in every part of the world. The series covers the circumstances that promote health or illness, the ways in which people experience and explain such conditions and what, practically, they do about them. Practitioners of all approaches to health and healing come within its scope, as do their ideas, beliefs and practices, and the social, economic and cultural contexts in which they operate. Methodologically, the series welcomes relevant studies in social, economic, cultural and intellectual history, as well as approaches derived from other disciplines in the arts, sciences, social sciences and humanities. The series is a collaboration between Manchester University Press and the Society for the Social History of Medicine.

Previously published

The metamorphosis of autism *Bonnie Evans*

Payment and philanthropy in British healthcare, 1918–48 *George Campbell Gosling*

The politics of vaccination *Edited by Christine Holmberg, Stuart Blume and Paul Greenough*

Leprosy and colonialism *Stephen Snelders*

Medical misadventure in an age of professionalisation, 1780–1890 *Alannah Tomkins*

Conserving health in early modern culture *Edited by Sandra Cavallo and Tessa Storey*

Migrant architects of the NHS *Julian M. Simpson*

Mediterranean quarantines, 1750–1914 *Edited by John Chircop and Francisco Javier Martínez*

Sickness, medical welfare and the English poor, 1750–1834 *Steven King*

Medical societies and scientific culture in nineteenth-century Belgium *Joris Vandendriessche*

Managing diabetes, managing medicine *Martin D. Moore*

Vaccinating Britain *Gareth Millward*

Madness on trial *James E. Moran*

Early Modern Ireland and the world of medicine *Edited by John Cunningham*

Feeling the strain *Jill Kirby*

Rhinoplasty and the nose in early modern British medicine and culture *Emily Cock*

Communicating the history of medicine *Edited by Solveig Jülich and Sven Widmalm*

Progress and pathology *Edited by Melissa Dickson, Emilie Taylor-Brown and Sally Shuttleworth*

Balancing the self

Medicine, politics and the regulation of health in the twentieth century

Edited by Mark Jackson and Martin D. Moore

Manchester University Press

Copyright © Manchester University Press 2020

While copyright in the volume as a whole is vested in Manchester University Press, copyright in individual chapters belongs to their respective authors.

An electronic version of this book is also available under a Creative Commons (CC-BY-NC-ND) licence, thanks to the support of the Wellcome Trust, which permits non-commercial use, distribution and reproduction provided the editors, chapter authors and Manchester University Press are fully cited and no modifications or adaptations are made. Details of the licence can be viewed at https://creativecommons.org/licenses/by-nc-nd/4.0/

Published by Manchester University Press
Altrincham Street, Manchester M1 7JA

www.manchesteruniversitypress.co.uk

British Library Cataloguing-in-Publication Data
A catalogue record for this book is available from the British Library

ISBN   978 1 5261 3213 0   hardback
ISBN   978 1 5261 3212 3   open access

First published 2020

The publisher has no responsibility for the persistence or accuracy of URLs for any external or third-party internet websites referred to in this book, and does not guarantee that any content on such websites is, or will remain, accurate or appropriate.

Typeset
by Toppan Best-set Premedia Limited

Contents

List of figures and tables	*page* vii
List of contributors	ix
Acknowledgements	xiii
List of abbreviations	xv

1. Introduction: balancing the self in the twentieth century   1
   Mark Jackson and Martin D. Moore

Part I   Configuring balance   31

2. Balance and the 'good' diabetic in Britain, c.1900–60   33
   Martin D. Moore

3. From the alcoholic to the sensible drinker: alcohol health education campaigns in England   64
   Alex Mold

4. 'Look After Yourself': visualising obesity as a public health concern in 1970s and 1980s Britain   95
   Jane Hand

Part II   Regulating imbalance   125

5. Self-help and self-promotion: dietary advice and agency in North America and Britain   127
   Nicos Kefalas

6. Your life in your hands: teaching 'relaxed living' in post-war Britain 158
Ayesha Nathoo

7. Pilot fatigue and the regulation of airline schedules in post-war Britain 190
Natasha Feiner

Part III Reconfiguring balance 217

8. Extreme acts: narratives of balance and moderation at the limits of human performance 219
Vanessa Heggie

9. Self-help, marriage guidance and the making of the midlife crisis 250
Mark Jackson

10. Balancing contested meanings of creativity and pathology in Parkinson's Disease 286
Dorothy Porter

11. Conclusion: balance, malleability and anthropology: historical contexts 314
Chris Millard

Index 340

List of figures and tables

Figures

3.1	'Everybody likes a drink. Nobody likes a drunk.' Saatchi & Saatchi for the Health Education Council, 1974	page 72
3.2	'If you drink too much there's one part that every beer can reach.' Saatchi & Saatchi for the Health Education Council, 1979	74
3.3	'Eight pints of beer and four large whiskies a day aren't doing her any good.' Saatchi & Saatchi for the Health Education Council, 1979	75
3.4	'If you're drinking five pints of beer or more everyday …' Redlands for the Health Education Council, 1981	78
4.1	Is your body coming between you and the opposite sex? (Poster, Science & Society Picture Library, 10411400), 1978–80	102
4.2	'Do you hold your breath when a man looks at you?' (Poster, Science & Society Picture Library, 10411688), 1980	105
4.3–4.6	(clockwise from top left): Stills from *A Way of Life* (S. Clarkhall, Central Office of Information, 1976)	109

9.1	'Forty-phobia (fear of the forties)', *The Times*, 28 April 1938, p. 19	256
9.2	Divorces in the United States, 1867–1967 (Source: US Department of Health, Education and Welfare, *100 years of Marriage and Divorce Statistics: United States, 1867–1967* (Rockville, MD: Health Resource Administration, HRA 74-1902, 1973), p. 8	266

Tables

7.1	The basic limiting of flying duty periods for scheduling purposes, *Report of the Committee on Flight Time Limitations*, p. 8	203
7.2	Flying duty period commencing at 'base'. *Report of the Committee on Flight Time Limitations*, p. 18	206
9.1	Number of divorcing couples in England and Wales, 1945–85 (Source: Office for National Statistics)	265

List of contributors

Natasha Feiner is a Policy Officer at the British Heart Foundation. Prior to this post, Dr Feiner completed a PhD at the University of Exeter. Her doctoral dissertation (2018) examined fatigue and the politics of work in post-war Britain, particularly in the context of civil aviation.

Jane Hand is a Research Fellow for the Wellcome Trust Senior Investigator Award 'The Cultural History of the NHS', at the Centre for the History of Medicine, University of Warwick. Prior to this post, Dr Hand completed her PhD at the University of Warwick in 2014, titled 'Visualising Food as Modern Medicine: Gender, the Body, and Health Education in England, c.1940–1990'.

Vanessa Heggie is a Lecturer in the History of Medicine and Science at the University of Birmingham. Along with her work with the *Guardian*, she is author of *Higher and Colder: A History of Extreme Physiology and Exploration* (University of Chicago Press, 2019) and *A History of British Sports Medicine* (Manchester University Press, 2011). Dr Heggie has also published widely in *Isis* (2014), *British Journal of the History of Science* (2013), *Women's History Review* (2011), *Medical History* (2010) and *Social History of Medicine* (2010).

Mark Jackson is Professor of the History of Medicine and Director of the Wellcome Centre for Cultures and Environments of Health at the University of Exeter. He is the author of numerous monographs, including *New-Born Child Murder* (Manchester University Press, 1996), *Allergy: The History of Modern Medicine* (Reaktion, 2006), *The Age of Stress: Science and the Search for Stability* (Oxford University Press, 2013) and *The History of Medicine: A Beginner's Guide* (Oneworld, 2014). He has also edited a number of volumes, including *The Oxford Handbook of the History of Medicine* (Oxford University Press, 2011), *Stress in Post-War Britain, 1945–85* (Routledge, 2015) and *The Routledge History of Disease* (Routledge, 2016). His study of the history of the midlife crisis will be published by Reaktion in 2020.

Nicos Kefalas received his PhD in the History of Medicine from the University of Exeter in 2019 for his thesis 'Healthmania: Diet, Supplements and The Pursuit of Health in America and Britain, c.1945–80'. His research interests revolve around the history of healthy eating, gender and dietary practices, and the history of supplements in popular culture.

Chris Millard is Lecturer in the History of Medicine and Medical Humanities at the University of Sheffield. He is the author of *A History of Self-Harm in Britain: A Genealogy of Cutting and Overdosing* (Palgrave Macmillan, 2015), has another monograph – *Munchausen Syndrome: Illness and Deception in the Modern World* – under contract with Polity Press and has published in a wide range of academic journals, including *Medical History* (2015), the *British Medical Journal* (2014) and *History of the Human Sciences* (2013).

Alex Mold is Associate Professor in History at the London School of Hygiene and Tropical Medicine, where she is also currently the Director of the Centre for History in Public Health. Dr Mold is the author of *Making the Patient Consumer: Patient Organisations and Health Consumerism in Britain* (Manchester University Press, 2015) and *Heroin: The Treatment of Addiction in Twentieth-Century Britain* (Northern Illinois University Press, 2008), and co-editor (with Virginia Berridge) of *Voluntary Action and Illegal Drugs: Health and Society in Britain since the 1960s* (Palgrave Macmillan, 2010) and (with Virginia Berridge and Martin Gorsky) of *Public Health in History* (Open University Press, 2011).

Martin D. Moore is a Research Fellow in the Wellcome Centre for Cultures and Environments of Health at the University of Exeter. He is the author of *Managing Diabetes, Managing Medicine* (Manchester University Press, 2019) and has publications in *Social History of Medicine* (2015), *The Routledge History of Disease* (Routledge, 2016) and *Journal for the History of Medicine and Allied Sciences* (2018).

Ayesha Nathoo recently completed a Wellcome Trust Research Fellowship in the Centre for Medical History, University of Exeter. She has previously held research fellowships at Clare Hall, University of Cambridge, and the Science Museum, London, and was a collaborator with the Hubbub group, the first residents of the Hub at Wellcome Collection, London (2014–16). She is the author of *Hearts Exposed: Transplants and the Media in 1960s Britain* (Palgrave Macmillan, 2009), and has published numerous articles and chapters, most recently in the *Oxford Handbook of Meditation* (Oxford University Press, 2019).

Dorothy Porter is Professor in the History of Health Sciences at the University of California, San Francisco. Professor Porter is the author of numerous monographs, including *Health Citizenship: Essays on Social Medicine and Bio-medical Politics* (University of California Press, 2012) and *Health, Civilisation and the State: A History of Public Health from Ancient to Modern Times* (Routledge, 2nd edition, 2005). Professor Porter has also edited *The History of Health and the Modern State* (Rodopi, 2nd edition, 2006), and (with Galen Joseph) *Health Rights at the Crossroads: Women, New Science and Institutional Violence* (Special Edition, *Western Humanities Review*, 66:3, 2012).

Acknowledgements

The idea for this volume emerged from a conference held at the University of Exeter in 2016 as part of a broader research project investigating histories of concepts of balance in medicine. The papers presented, and subsequent discussion, developed our thinking about the relationships between contemporary discourses of balance and individual responsibility in the regulation of health in new directions, and we would like to thank the participants for their engagement and insight. Both were crucial in the genesis of this collection. Likewise, neither the conference nor this volume would have been possible without the generous support of the Wellcome Trust (Grant Reference 100601/Z/12/Z) and the broader Balance project team of Fred Cooper, Natasha Feiner, Ali Haggett, Nicos Kefalas, Ayesha Nathoo and Claire Keyte, to whom we are deeply grateful.

Collaboration with the scholars whose work appears in these pages has been a thoroughly enjoyable and intellectually enriching endeavour. We would like to thank them for their enthusiasm and engagement, which has not waned over the years it takes to get a volume like this to print. Equally, a great debt is owed to our series editor, David Cantor, for his encouragement and feedback on the manuscript at crucial stages, as well as to the team at Manchester University Press for their constant assistance throughout the production process. We would also like to thank colleagues at the Centre for Medical History and Wellcome Centre for Cultures and Environments of Health for providing such open and collegiate atmospheres, from which volumes like these can emerge.

Finally, both editors would like to thank their families for their limitless understanding and support during the editing of this volume. It is to Siobhán, Ciara, Riordan, Conall and Lucy that we would like to dedicate the following work.

The editors and author would like to acknowledge that sections of Alex Mold's chapter were previously published in Alex Mold, '"Everybody likes a drink. Nobody likes a drunk": Alcohol, Health Education and the Public in 1970s Britain', *Social History of Medicine*, 30:3 (2017), 612–36.

List of abbreviations

AAIB	Air Accidents Investigation Branch
ACA	Advisory Committee on Alcoholism
AMA	American Medical Association
ANO	Air Navigation Order
BALPA	British Airline Pilots Association
BBC	British Broadcasting Corporation
BDA	British Diabetic Association
BEA	British European Airways
BOAC	British Overseas Airways Corporation
CAA	Civil Aviation Authority
Caltech	California Institute of Technology
CAP	Civil Aviation Publication
CHD	coronary heart disease
CHIRP	Confidential Human Factors Incident Reporting Programme
COI	Central Office of Information
COMA	Committee on Medical and Nutritional Aspects of Food Policy
DHSS	Department of Health and Social Security
DOPA	L-amino acid decarboxylase
EASA	European Aviation Safety Agency
EEG	electroencephalogram
FDA	Food and Drug Agency
FPRC	Flying Personnel Research Committee

FTLB	Flight Time Limitations Board
HEC	Health Education Council
HMWC	Health of Munition Workers Committee
HSWA	Health and Safety at Work Act 1974
ICAO	International Civil Aviation Organization
IFRB	Industrial Fatigue Research Board
INPHEXAN	International Physiological Expedition to Antarctica
IUBS	International Union of Biological Sciences
IUPS	International Union of Physiological Sciences
L-DOPA	L-dihydroxyphenylalanine: L-isomer of the amino acid D
MAFF	Ministry of Agriculture, Fisheries and Food
MAOI	monoamine oxidase inhibitor
MOH	Medical Officer of Health
NACNE	National Advisory Committee on Nutrition Education
NCT	National Childbirth Trust
NHS	National Health Service
PE	physical education
PET	positron emission tomography
RAF	Royal Air Force
RAWP	Resource Allocation Working Party
RDA	recommended daily allowance
RGS	Royal Geographical Society
SCAR	Scientific Committee on Antarctic Research
SNC	substantia nigra compactica
TCI	Tridimensional Character Inventory
TNA	The National Archives
TPQ	Tridimensional Personality Questionnaire
UCSD	University of California San Diego
VTA	ventral tegmental area
WHO	World Health Organization

1

Introduction: balancing the self in the twentieth century

Mark Jackson and Martin D. Moore

Introduction

Writing in the early 1990s, the prominent British historian Eric Hobsbawm labelled the twentieth century – or at least the period between 1914 and 1991 – 'the age of extremes'.[1] Having witnessed a series of global economic disasters, ethnic cleansing, two world wars, the foundation and fall of the Soviet Union and the dismantling of pernicious empires – which were often replaced by insular and inequitable nation-states – Hobsbawm saw the twentieth century as devoid of balance, ravaged instead by the failed ideologies of nationalism, imperialism, communism, capitalism, fascism and liberalism. Following previous historical periods that Hobsbawm had referred to in turn as the age of revolution (1789–1848), the age of capital (1848–75) and the age of empire (1875–1914), the short twentieth century was extreme in two ways.[2] On the one hand, it was marked by oscillating moods and events ranging from early twentieth-century catastrophe, through a golden age in the decades after the Second World War, to a period of global crisis and collapse between 1973 and 1991. On the other hand, the twentieth century was characterised by a tendency to classify people, practices, and political systems in simple binary terms, an approach to knowledge and experience that had first gained legitimacy during the Enlightenment. Contrasts were established between seemingly oppositional categories such as: reason and emotion; sanity and insanity; self and other; normal and pathological; capitalist and communist; public and private;

female and male; creativity and conformity; individualism and incorporation; static and dynamic; and, as Hobsbawm pointed out, losers and winners.[3]

Hobsbawm recognised that extreme social conditions or political positions were not necessarily unbalanced or labile. Opposing forces – such as capitalism and communism during the Cold War – could be inherently stabilising, serving to preserve a precarious balance of power.[4] According to some post-war Western commentators, for example, global stability in a 'post-crisis world' could be achieved not only (or even primarily) through political negotiation, but also through the 'inhibiting nuclear balance of terror'.[5] However, experiences and representations of crises were not necessarily as uniform or universal as Hobsbawm imagined. Republican China, for example, regarded itself differently from the Western world; while European countries might be 'nations of extreme', China by contrast was, in its own eyes, a 'nation of moderation'.[6] Equally, the process of balancing competing interests was neither static nor predetermined, but always dynamic and emergent: the tipping point between seemingly polarised positions was forever shifting in ways that were dictated by socio-economic, cultural, political and environmental conditions. Although disturbances in equilibrium were often catastrophic, they could also be self-correcting. According to Hobsbawm, it was the social and moral crises of the second half of the twentieth century that provided momentum for the regeneration of communities and civil society, or at least for addressing more directly a growing sense of alienation from the modern mechanised world.[7]

If preoccupations with moderating extremism and mitigating conflict – or what Greg Eghigian, Andreas Killen and Christine Leuenberger have referred to as being 'obsessed with the enemy' – constituted a key aspect of military manoeuvres, political systems and economic theories, they also featured in twentieth-century articulations of personal identity and psychological conflict, although in these circumstances they were often subject to more critical appraisal.[8] In *The Divided Self*, first published in 1959, the Scottish psychiatrist R. D. Laing suggested that schizoid and schizophrenic individuals were split in two ways: 'in the first place, there is a rent in his relation to the world and, in the second, there is a disruption of his relation with himself', leading to 'despairing aloneness and isolation'.[9] According to Laing, the 'technical vocabulary' of psychiatry, which focused on abstract oppositional

Introduction

and divisive concepts such as mind-body and psyche-soma, was unable to account for the complexity or relationality of experience and illness, that is – in Laing's deliberate borrowing from Heidegger – of being in the world.[10] Contemporary fixations with achieving a normal, adjusted state – through medication or lobotomy, for example – were dangerous precisely because they suppressed the human capacity to experience extreme or transcendent emotions. From the perspective of antipsychiatrists such as Laing, David Cooper and Thomas Szasz, the pursuit of balance or equilibrium constituted not an effective pathway to integration and freedom, but merely a means of 'acquiring a false self to adapt to false realities'.[11]

Laing's position did not hold. In the midst of the global upheavals that characterised Hobsbawm's 'age of extremes', personal health and political stability were to be achieved through conformity rather than transgression, by regulating rather than expressing emotions, and by harmonising the interests of the self with those of the state through what Elisabeth Hsu has referred to, in the context of older humoral theories of balance, as the 'medico-moral nexus of moderation'.[12] In an increasingly individualised, liquid society in which self-interest and self-fulfilment – however desirable – might disrupt social order, balance operated as a 'catchall term',[13] one that expressed the need for stability and equilibrium within bodies, families, communities, societies, political systems and global relations.[14] The seemingly distinct domains of enquiry within which balance emerged as a concept were not disconnected: biological models of balance and homeostasis, for example, were employed to justify political arguments for the equitable distribution of resources and information; and political allegiances inflected physiological accounts of adaptation and health.[15] Similarly, although advice to balance marriages or to ensure work-life balance was framed explicitly in terms of enabling personal and family health, individualised techniques for achieving 'balance', or at least the illusion of balance, represented another manifestation of contemporary political economy and the disciplinary effects of 'empowerment' typical of the neoliberalisation of everyday life.[16]

This collection of essays argues that concepts of balance provided a central – though often diverse and contested – organising motif for a wide spectrum of medical and political projects in the twentieth century. More than this, it proposes that programmes dependent on, and designed to achieve or maintain, balance regularly sought to cultivate specific types of individuals and enrol them in various ways. Even when balance was seen to derive from collective enterprise, 'balance' and 'self' were closely intertwined. By focusing on health and the body, this volume explores the multiple ways in which institutions, actors and networks mobilised divergent concepts of balance for various ends, investigates how individuals were constituted and convinced to pursue bodily, psychological, emotional, spiritual, social and political equilibrium, and examines the challenges to – and reconfigurations of – conceptions of balance in an age of extremes. Together, the following chapters historicise and complicate assumptions about the links between individualised balance and forms of production or political regimes, and highlight the malleability and multi-valence of balance as a concept. Through its investigations into the diverse life of 'balance', therefore, the volume not only contributes to the cultural history of an everyday concept, but also generates insights into the history of health governance and subjectivity and into the close connections between medicine, politics and the regulation of social life.

Balancing acts

In her address to the 61st World Health Assembly in May 2008, the Director-General of the World Health Organization (WHO), Dr Margaret Chan, concluded her analysis of current threats to global health with the following words: 'A world that is out of balance in matters of health is neither stable nor secure.'[17] Dr Chan was not alone in conceiving patterns of health and illness, the delivery of healthcare services and the maintenance of global security in terms of balance. During the twentieth century it became customary to mobilise concepts of balance and imbalance to capture the multiple dimensions of human, non-human and planetary health. As a growing scholarly literature attests, the language of balance – as well its various synonyms and antonyms – permeated accounts of political stability, the cost-effectiveness of healthcare systems, the distribution of women and men in medicine and other professions, Eastern and Western approaches to the pursuit of happiness and well-being, the diversity and sustainability of ecosystems, and shifting patterns of infectious and non-infectious diseases.[18]

In modern Western medicine, balance has been applied quite literally to the capacity of bodies to remain upright and stable in the face of fluctuating internal and external demands. In conditions such as Parkinson's Disease, multiple sclerosis, strokes and Ménière's disease, an inability to maintain or restore physical balance – sometimes configured in terms of hidden physiological disturbances of a vital 'sixth sense' – has been regarded as the principal mechanism driving impaired function and the risk of physical injury.[19] Physiologically grounded accounts of balance, or the need to regulate the relationship between the inhibition and stimulation of biological processes, were evident elsewhere across the twentieth century: in studies of homeostasis, which emphasised the importance of the neuroendocrine system in maintaining vital functions;[20] in clinical formulations of the causes and symptoms of asthma, epilepsy and sexual dysfunction;[21] in pharmacological models of conditions such as manic depression (more recently bipolar disorder), which were understood in the interwar period as the product of dysregulation of acid-base equilibrium and subsequently in terms of 'chemical imbalances' in the brain;[22] and in approaches to monitoring blood sugar in patients with diabetes, exemplified by the official journal of the British Diabetic Association being renamed *Balance* from 1961.[23] Although these conditions were often portrayed in terms of natural biological processes, it is important to recognise that the concept of balance in these domains of medicine was imbued with emotional and political significance: as Martin Moore argues, patients who managed to balance their blood sugar levels were regarded (and rewarded) as 'good diabetics'; and holistic and organismic models of the regulatory processes that maintained physiological balance – or what Walter Cannon referred to as the 'wisdom of the body' – provided blueprints for social organisation.[24]

While balance helped to constitute modern biomedical understandings of health and disease, it also served to structure treatments. Balance helped to configure practices and treatments designed to reduce pain, improve posture and mobility, and promote health by strengthening or restoring bodily and emotional stability. Some therapies, such as yoga, meditation, herbalism and certain forms of massage, originated in Indian, Chinese and Islamic medical cultures that foregrounded the attainment of balance or harmony as a pathway to health.[25] Others, such as Pilates (pioneered by the German gymnast Joseph Pilates), the Alexander technique (developed in the 1890s), physiotherapy, osteopathy, chiropractic, the use of balance boards, and 'zero balancing' (a technique introduced by Dr Fritz Smith in 1973), were rooted in European and North American interest in the capacity for remedial gymnastics and massage therapy to rehabilitate injured servicemen and disabled workers.[26] Although sometimes dismissed as 'alternative therapies', or as practices merely supplementary to medicine, such approaches to physical, mental and spiritual health, in conjunction with health education advice to follow balanced diets, drink less and exercise more, were increasingly advocated – and purchased – as part of a healthy lifestyle: improving balance through movement and manipulation was thought to release energy, enhance resilience, promote endurance and productivity, combat obesity and increase a sense of 'wellness'.[27]

Balance also figured strongly in treatments of mental illness. From the 1920s, when Sigmund Freud emphasised the instinctive drive to maintain psychological stability, working through personal crises in order to balance and integrate competing facets of personality became a feature of psychological approaches to restoring emotional well-being, particularly at key transition points in the life course.[28] After the Second World War, clinical and pharmaceutical interest in the biochemical determinants of mental health led to the development and increasing consumption of antidepressants, which were thought to improve mood by restoring the balance of neurotransmitters. Similarly, 'mood stabilisers', a term applied initially to lithium but also later used to describe a range of anti-epileptic drugs, such as lamotrigine and sodium valproate, were prescribed to reduce the dramatic mood swings associated with manic depression.[29] Of course, these approaches to mental health have not been uncontested. Clinicians and historians such as David Healy and Joanna Moncrieff have critiqued the manner in which popular notions of balance and stability were exploited by pharmaceutical companies in order to broaden the boundaries of mental illness and create a lucrative market for psychoactive substances.[30] Yet, in spite of opposition to the commercialisation of the language of balance, such explanations for mental illness have persisted, allowing patients and their clinicians to articulate the anxieties and distress generated not merely by physiological changes, but also partly by economic uncertainty, professional insecurity, social turmoil and political instability – that is, by a world that is itself seemingly out of balance.[31]

Although they often rejected claims made by proponents of biological psychiatry, psychiatrists interested in the psychosocial determinants of mental illness also embraced a model of mood disorders that mobilised the concept of balance, or what the American psychiatrist Karl Menninger referred to in 1963 as 'the vital balance'.[32] Menninger's position is particularly instructive. Although he regarded 'balance' as a 'pretty metaphor',[33] he recognised its power to capture post-war concerns about personal adaptation and social adjustment, about the tensions between conformity and creativity, and about the necessity of ensuring and enabling regulatory mechanisms at psychological, physiological and social levels in order to maintain health and stability. His work also demonstrates the diversity and malleability of notions of balance. Regulation need not mean stagnation, adherence to a fixed norm, or a smooth, untroubled pattern of adjustment, Menninger insisted, but instead encompassed complex processes that oscillated and varied, not necessarily returning to the same steady state, but establishing a new relatively steady state generated by growth, learning and fulfilment. Indeed, for Menninger unbending stability compromised and trivialised life: 'Life cannot be without stability', he wrote, 'but is a completely stable life human?'[34] In the 'open systems' characteristic of living organisms, Menninger argued, the need to adapt in order to survive demanded flexibility and mobility in physiological and psychological systems: 'A system, to perform work, however, must not *be* in equilibrium but continually on the way toward attaining it.'[35]

Maintaining some measure of functional balance was regarded primarily as a problem of regulation. According to Georges Canguilhem, physiological regulation was the 'supreme biological fact'.[36] Regulation also emerged as a key mechanism of adaptation and health promotion in psychosocial and psychosomatic medicine. In both realms, an emphasis on regulation carried political overtones, related to how responsibility for stability was apportioned either to individuals or the state. During the twentieth century, at least in the Western world, it was increasingly individuals who became liable for regulating their behaviour and health, even in countries with state-funded welfare systems. Psychological illness in response to stress, for example, was interpreted as a failure on the part of individuals to effectively manage work-life balance or to cope with fluctuating environmental and economic pressures. Research on both sides of the Atlantic highlighting links between stressful life events, behaviour and illness or between migration and health,[37] as well as studies stressing the importance of perception and coping to the appearance of psychological disturbances,[38] encouraged psychiatrists and patients to regard mental illness as the product of an unbalanced – perhaps decadent or indulgent – lifestyle, in which effective adaptation to the stress of life was compromised.[39] In this paradigm, treatment focused primarily not on restoring biochemical balance in the brain, but on promoting self-help, that is by empowering people to balance their own lives through purchased programmes of cognitive behavioural therapy,[40] biofeedback and relaxation techniques,[41] or mindful meditation.[42]

The potency of balance as a normalising concept was not limited to debates about health. In a speech to the Royal Society delivered in 1988, the British Prime Minister, Margaret Thatcher, claimed that 'stable prosperity' could only be achieved 'throughout the world provided the environment is nurtured and safeguarded'. 'Protecting the balance of nature', she concluded, 'is therefore one of the great challenges of the late twentieth century.'[43] Although Thatcher's commitment to environmental preservation was politically expedient, since she had shown little interest in such issues until the emergence of a global green movement in the late 1980s, her comments testify to growing scientific, public and political interest in reducing environmental degradation, protecting ecological balance, ensuring the harmony and sustainability of the cosmos and preserving human health – interest that had been stimulated in the post-war years by Rachel Carson, James Lovelock and others.[44] While the precise meaning of the term 'balance of nature' was rarely explicated and often dismissed as a myth,[45] the notion served to structure political arguments for greater regulation of environmental hazards, improved mobilisation of economic resources, and more integrated, cross-sectoral approaches to global health and well-being.[46]

Emphasis on the benefits of preserving the balance of nature was not new. Drawing explicitly on Hippocratic notions of the 'healing power of nature', late nineteenth- and early twentieth-century clinicians and their patients increasingly regarded nature as an antidote to the perils of industrialisation and urbanisation. As a number of historical studies have suggested, city-dwellers seeking healthier environments to cure or relieve the symptoms of tuberculosis, asthma, hay fever, bronchitis, rickets and neurasthenia flocked to the mountains and coasts, where the air was supposedly cleaner and lifestyles healthier.[47] During the twentieth century, concerns about the impact of human patterns of consumption of fuel and food sources on environmental sustainability and anxieties about the health consequences of climate change deepened in the light of evidence that global variations in population growth and density were also adversely affecting ecological balance and human health. After the Second World War, researchers such as Paul Ehrlich, Lennart Levi and Lars Andersson insisted that uncontrolled population expansion was significantly reducing the quality of life for people in many regions of the world, largely through rising unemployment, poverty and famine.[48] According to Levi and Andersson, such evidence constituted an important argument for developing an integrated 'world plan of action' to redress inequalities in health, reduce the spread of infectious diseases and restore health and happiness to human populations.[49]

Similar arguments were evident in debates about global – and indeed cosmic – ecological stability. In the late 1960s, the English scientist James Lovelock suggested that the earth should be regarded as a 'superorganism', referred to as Gaia. Lovelock's hypothesis, which emerged initially from the recognition that 'a stable planet' was composed of 'unstable parts', postulated that the earth and its atmosphere operated as a complex entity that, like individual organisms, sought to maintain the optimal physical and chemical environment for life through the activation of homeostatic or cybernetic feedback mechanisms.[50] Lovelock's approach was predicated, like contemporary accounts of diseases of adaptation, on a belief that dynamic feedback systems intended to maintain functional stability constituted a characteristic feature of all living organisms. The capacity of the earth to adapt to ecological disturbances generated by the production of pollutants, toxins, radiation and waste materials, like the capacity of humans to cope with stressful life events, was dependent on effective self-regulation (or 'planetary homeostasis') and the ability to attain new points of equilibrium.[51] Although the Gaia hypothesis was initially received with some scepticism, Lovelock's adoption of a physiological framework began to appeal to scientists, politicians and policy-makers keen to stem the impact of human profligacy on the environment and to reduce the effects of environmental change on human and animal health. The challenge for modern populations, Lovelock insisted, was to raise awareness of human contributions to the balance of nature, to identify the regions of the world (like vital organs in the body) that were most critical to the health of Gaia and to devise strategies for facilitating ecological balance.

Lovelock's formulation of ecological homeostasis, like Cannon's model of homeostasis or Hans Selye's account of stress, represented the reincarnation of ancient notions of balance. The American historian of ecology Frank N. Egerton pointed out in 1973 that the origins of modern preoccupations with the 'balance of nature' could be traced to the providential ecology of ancient and medieval cultures, to influential analogies between microcosm and macrocosm, and to long-standing scientific and medical preoccupations with flux, equilibrium and harmony. From the eighteenth century, the work of the Swedish botanist Carl Linnaeus (1707–78) on the 'economy of nature' encouraged references to the notion of balance or proportion as a regulatory principle. Although evolutionary evidence of adaptation and diversity among species served to undermine belief in the primacy of stability in nature, early twentieth-century studies of homeostasis, nascent ecological formulations of the relationship between animals, societies and the environment, and United Nations and WHO initiatives to protect the biosphere collectively reinvigorated debates about the balance of nature and its translation into the social sphere.[52] By reconstituting beliefs in the potential for ecological and social systems to maintain functional stability, proponents of the Gaia hypothesis were endeavouring to restore a sense of order and control to a world that, according to many scientists, clinicians, social commentators and environmental activists, appeared to be accelerating towards self-destruction. Attempts to preserve the harmony of the cosmos were another manifestation of the late twentieth-century enthusiasm for regulating behaviour and promoting health in a dangerous and precariously unbalanced world.

Balanced selves

Whether restoring balance to the planet or physiological equilibrium to bodies, efforts to regulate social activity in the twentieth century frequently deputed responsibility for action to individuals. Actors as diverse as self-help authors, public health practitioners, patients' organisations, health and safety regulators and food and pharmaceutical companies all positioned individual subjects as the locus of imbalance and agent for change. To achieve or maintain balance, these actors suggested that individual citizens, consumers or patients needed to develop new relations to their minds and bodies, to how they perceived, represented and conducted themselves. Such ministrations were only partially altruistic, only partially aimed at soothing the inhabitants of a troubled world; they also offered authors, industries and state organisations opportunities to profit from widespread fears about personal and political instability.

According to Eghigian, Killen and Leuenberger, this proliferation of enterprises designed to 'turn the self' – the inner lives and self-representations of individual human subjects – 'into a project' provided one of the distinctive features of the twentieth century. 'Individuals across a range of regimes', they argue, 'became, in effect, sites for public projects and, at the same time, were encouraged to treat their own lives as projects to be fulfilled.'[53] But belief in, and practices of, self-reflection and self-regulation were not unique to the twentieth century. In pioneering work, Michel Foucault traced as far back as classical antiquity what he termed 'technologies of the self' – ways that individuals 'effect by their own means or with the help of others a certain number of operations on their own bodies and souls, thoughts, conduct and way of being, so as to transform themselves in order to attain a certain state of happiness, purity, wisdom, perfection or immortality'.[54] Though warning against any teleological story of the Western self, other scholars have outlined how attendance to the self in Europe was slowly disentangled from an understanding of divine or pre-ordained truths from the seventeenth century onwards.[55] Informed by racial, imperial, gender and class hierarchies, 'modern' philosophers, political theorists, religious thinkers and artists discussed one's identity, one's perceptions and perspectives, as well as one's station in life, as more malleable than their classical counterparts, subject to both external social and cultural forces and conscious self-directed transformation.[56]

Nonetheless, though building on such antecedents, it seems clear that selfhood and subjectivity became objectified in new ways and new settings over the twentieth century, not least in medicine and a proliferation of academic disciplines.[57] Similarly, the self became tied to new political projects, which, as recent scholarship has suggested, often searched for balance as a response to the age of extremes. In *The War Inside*, for example, Michal Shapira has explored how psychoanalysis provided important perspectives on welfare, the family and democracy in public and political discourse. With particular emphasis on children and the maternal relationship in the formation of reasonable, well-adjusted selves, psychoanalysts argued that state involvement in the well-being of the next generation was essential if democracy, with its checks and balances, could be secured against the extremes of totalitarianism.[58] Similarly, Martin Francis has outlined the limits of emotional economy in post-war British political life.[59] The performance of emotional balance, self-restraint and rationality was particularly important in the Labour Party during the early post-war years, given political and popular connections between a lack of emotional control and the destructive tyranny of Nazism and Socialism.[60]

The connection between politics and selfhood has thus been central to recent scholarship. Explorations of selfhood in the twentieth century debated the extent to which the construction of new types of subjectivity, and the cultivation of new views on the self, have been produced through state power, or been connected to programmes for surveillance and control. As Eghigian, Killen and Leuenberger suggest, the human sciences were certainly integrated closely with European state infrastructures over the twentieth century, and both Fascist and communist regimes keenly promoted visions for 'new men and women' and sought to root out deviancy in their nascent states.[61] By contrast, recent work on the German Democratic Republic has sought to complicate assessments of the power dynamics and success of state programmes, and to explore the ways in which subjects of new states negotiated projects and shaped their own 'becoming'.[62] Moreover, as recent sociological and critical theoretical reflections on subjectivity and selfhood in Europe (and its empires) have pointed out, critiques of subjectivity and gender, race, (dis)ability, sexuality, class and intersectionality emerged from – and provided the basis for – new political and social movements with international focus, most notably feminism.[63] Such movements explored how social, linguistic and cultural structures, often supported by the state, shaped experiences and subjectivities, and used reflection as the basis for radical fashioning of the self and progressive collective action.[64]

Similar debates about the role of the state have arisen with regard to Britain, particularly in relation to discussions of the 'psy' sciences and government of the self.[65] A central aim of the governmentality studies literature has been to move away from traditional state-centric analyses, and instead trace the multitude of ways in which individual conduct has been managed through technologies that link diverse political centres with sites of regulation.[66] By examining the ways that psychological disciplines came to reshape self-understanding during the post-war period, works like Nikolas Rose's *Governing the Soul* have illuminated the ways in which subjectivities have been historically constructed through the development of new techniques and languages of self.[67] Such accounts have also provided insight into the complex ways that political rationalities of liberalism have become entangled with the lay internalisation of psychological government as well as state efforts to manage the population.[68] However, though this literature has broadened our understandings of the political, as Grace Huxford has suggested, the state has nonetheless retained an important place in analyses of governmentality.[69] Critics such as Mathew Thomson, moreover, have also argued that studies of the 'psy' sciences have too often presumed the totalising effects of psychological disciplines, highlighting how a focus on 'governing at a distance' has reproduced narratives of control and regulation.[70]

In part, at stake in discussions of state and professional power are questions of individual agency that have recurred throughout debates on the formation of the self. Reflections on these questions during the first half of the twentieth century often mobilised concepts of conflict in their explorations. Freud's ego, for instance, was constantly assailed with drives from the id, and the development of other 'depth' psychologies fuelled a proliferation of beliefs about the role of the unconscious in shaping and motivating activity.[71] Outside of psychoanalytic discourses, however, concepts of balance and self intersected in interesting ways. In marginal economics, for instance, the rational consumer was one who consciously weighed options and risks in their pursuit of utility maximisation and self-benefit.[72] As Alex Mold suggests in this volume (see Chapter 3), similar autonomous selves were imagined in post-war public health initiatives, where health education came to provide the basis for self-directed action. Of course, twentieth-century economics, like post-war medicine, also incorporated sociological and psychological thinking into understandings of self and agency.[73] John Maynard Keynes, for instance, noted the importance of investors' 'animal spirits' and a 'delicate balance of spontaneous optimism' in shaping decision-making, and suggested that 'in estimating the prospects of investment, we must have regard, therefore, to the nerves and hysteria and even the digestions and reactions to the weather of those upon whose spontaneous activity it largely depends'.[74] Comparable considerations were found in public health programmes, which, as Jane Hand makes clear, incorporated marketing techniques to target the desires of patient consumers. Yet, in neither economic nor public health discourse were actors considered unable to exercise rational decision-making or incapable of self-direction.

By contrast, sociological, historical, philosophical, literary and psychoanalytical researchers have taken different approaches to exploring agency and selfhood in the post-war period.[75] Whether referring to social and economic institutions, discourse or other cultural forms of signification, much of this scholarship has emphasised the importance of external forces imposing on, and constituting, subjects. According to critics, at its most extreme this literature has framed the decentred self as the irresistible product of power, with subjects determined through discourse, ideology or socialisation, and learning to see and relate to themselves and others within the boundaries set for them by political and cultural systems.[76] Yet, as Hall suggests, more optimistic readings are possible.[77] The very categorisation and constitution of subjects that form the grounds for regulation also provide a point of resistance, reshaping and redefinition. Though 'made up', in Ian Hacking's phrase, the subject's new existence provides some foundation for self-directed action in ways that might exceed the role and identity afforded to them.[78] Indeed, Dorothy Porter's discussion of Parkinson's Disease in this volume (see Chapter 10) highlights the ways in which newly constituted selves negotiate agency and contest regulation. Whereas scientific and clinical understandings of 'Parkinson's personality' have framed creativity in patients as a pathological, iatrogenic symptom resulting from imbalanced treatment, patients have contested this meaning. Instead, they have described their artistic endeavours as establishing calm and transcendence, and some even exceed their recommended drug dosage to enhance their experiences.[79]

Contributions to this volume, then, have taken a diverse set of approaches to the question of self and balance, as well as issues of agency and regulation. Nonetheless, a common thread through all the chapters, often (though not always) drawn from a Foucauldian-inspired literature, is an understanding that subjectivities oriented to balance were produced relationally. The 'self'/'non-self' divide – which figured most strikingly as a means of articulating immunological integrity[80]

– was constantly permeated; even though they were accorded new forms of responsibility for balance, individuals were rarely left to act alone in projects for balanced selfhoods. A multiplicity of state and non-state agencies were involved in constructing self-balancing individuals, and searches for balanced selves enrolled subjects into new relations not only with themselves and their bodies, but also with a constellation of experts, service providers, family members and likeminded subjects, thus serving as the basis for entering individuals into new forms of sociality. As several chapters demonstrate, relationality stretched to non-human actants. Self-help books, audio equipment and exercise apparatus were just as important to projects of balanced selfhoods as life-writing and records were to the emergence of new forms of self-formation in medicine and the military.[81] Balancing the self in the twentieth century, therefore, did not mean exercising autonomy alone.

Structure and themes

Each chapter in this volume examines a novel instance of the ways in which selves became the objects of technical expertise and political projects for balance, predominantly in twentieth-century Britain. This shared interest in Britain provides a powerful methodological approach for articulating the heterogeneity of balance and its relationship to new understandings and parameters of selfhood. A common geopolitical focus, that is, provides a sense of contextual continuity, enabling each contribution to draw out the ways in which different selves were constituted in relation to balance according to specific constellations of disciplines, techniques of investigation, professional interests, institutional arrangements and subject populations. Conversely, given Britain's broad political shifts from Edwardian liberalism to neo-liberalism over the twentieth century, notably via distinctive blends of conservatism and social democracy, a stable focus also makes it possible to assess the influence of political rationalities on histories of balance when actors and subjects remain broadly similar. Comparative consideration of balance and self in the US – particularly in Chapters 5, 9 and 10 – enhances these reflections, offering the opportunity to examine what was distinct about Britain by contrasting fortunes and tracing connections between sites. Indeed, in this sense, the predominant interest in

British developments enables the volume to contribute meaningfully to the social and cultural history of a specific time and place.

In its exploration of efforts to balance the self, the volume is organised in three parts. The first explores the manner in which notions of balance informed public health education campaigns and clinical management strategies that enabled self-regulation in the context of diabetes, alcohol consumption and obesity. At the same time, it examines the ways in which these conditions served to configure and reinforce particular models of the body in balance. The second section reflects on debates about how to address and redress imbalances in diet, levels of stress and work that appeared to impact negatively on health, examining in turn the advice offered to the public by authors of self-help books, the scope of practical guides for relaxation aimed at ensuring balanced lives and the industrial regulation of fatigue in the workplace. The final section explores how experiences and understandings of physical and emotional imbalance and their impacts on both selves and others – in the context of extreme physiological exertion, midlife transitions and emergent neurological disease – served to challenge and reconfigure earlier notions of balance and to provide new tools for managing unregulated bodies and minds. The concluding chapter critically reflects on the methodological and moral dilemmas raised by even attempting to write histories of 'balanced selves'. As Millard notes, if historians conceptualise balanced selfhoods as historically and culturally situated constructions – subjectivities created (and contested) through power and for political purposes – then we must be ready to historicise our own knowledge, our own subject positions and epistemological foundations so as not to blind ourselves to the gaps and politics of our own work.

In the opening chapter of the first section, Martin Moore explores the ways in which balance was configured in diabetes care between the 1900s and 1960s. Self-care, Moore suggests, was considered an essential element of diabetes management during the twentieth century, and the careful balance of diet and insulin sat at the heart of therapeutic efforts to stabilise blood sugars. However, the chapter argues, glycaemia was by no means the only target of clinical intervention, and self-care formed only one part in a broader constellation of interventions by healthcare professionals, state and patients. Amid growing political and popular interest in affective life, clinicians and a novel patient organisation quickly connected bodily balance with psychological and emotional stability in new ways. Depression, complacency, denial, fear and optimism soon became subject to management in clinical spaces, mutual aid publications and long-term professional–patient interactions, in response to changing notions of health citizenship and self-discipline, and as certain states came to be considered dangerous or beneficial to physiological and political balance. Though focusing primarily on the work of the British Diabetic Association in the first half of the twentieth century, this chapter thus begins to map out the extensive array of tools and agencies involved in constructing selves oriented towards balance, as well as exploring the ways in which the pursuit of balance connected with ideas of gender, empire and shifting political regimes.

Chapter 3 by Alex Mold moves the focus from diabetes to alcohol consumption, and to political and public health efforts to cultivate the 'sensible drinker'. Focusing on a set of local health education campaigns, an expert committee report on alcohol prevention and a public consultation exercise on alcohol, the chapter highlights how the calculus of balance in relation to individual responsibility and public well-being has consistently been complex. Post-war changes in public health philosophy and practice had constructed individual behaviour as both cause and cure for public health problems. A vision of individual selves as responsive to expert advice was embedded in early Health Education Council campaigns around drinking in moderation. However, Mold argues, policy-makers disagreed on whether education alone could encourage individuals to moderate their alcohol consumption. Though rejected at the time, other approaches – most notably increasing the price of alcohol – were put forward as ways to reduce drinking at the population level. At issue was not simply the capacity of individuals to achieve healthy balance. Policy-makers weighed potential for improved health outcomes alongside individual rights, the social equity of reforms, effects on industrial and employment fortunes, Treasury income and electoral considerations. A growing focus on moderation may have expanded public health's target population, but a reliance on health education and ill-defined concepts like the 'sensible drinker' also reflected the ways that disciplinary power could be counterbalanced by political and economic concerns. As Mold concludes, 'exhortations towards self-regulation were not necessarily a tool of social or political control but could also operate as a way to balance competing interests'.

Jane Hand continues the focus on public health by exploring in Chapter 4 how obesity was visualised and communicated in health promotion campaigns; in doing so, she extends Mold's analysis of contested political programmes to cultivate balanced lifestyles in Britain's populace. Statistical concepts of risk became a central feature of post-war public health, with individual behaviour and consumer choices linked with a diverse array of negative (or potentially negative) health outcomes. As risk was internalised and invisible, Hand argues, health educators turned to obesity as an explicit marker for discussing a variety of 'hidden' risk factors and chronic diseases, though especially heart disease. As such, nutrition education campaigns came to use visual images of overweight bodies to redraw the boundaries of what constituted a balanced diet, and therefore what produced the healthy, balanced self. Messages about obesity, dietary moderation and exercise went beyond health, however, often being framed in terms of gendered bodily beauty. By coding disease risk in relation to culturally admonished visual attributes (the obese body) and specific practical preventive measures (such as eating less and exercising more), images thus functioned to articulate specific social ideologies and to promote the idea that individualised health risks could be overcome (at least in part) by complying with health advice. As Hand concludes, though, such official constructions of personal responsibility for balance were consistently disputed and reinterpreted. Personalised health advice was often consumed in disparate ways, with poorer citizens consciously trading health against financial risks. Likewise, by the end of the century mainstream documentaries had begun to connect personal risk with structural imbalances of wealth, and counter-discourses of health reasserted themselves in visually striking terms.

Chapter 5, by Nicos Kefalas, which begins the second section, turns from state-sponsored health education to the contested world of self-help experts. As Kefalas notes, there is a substantial literature considering the emergence of the 'healthy diet' as an object of political and medical interest in the late twentieth century. Historians have explored the impact of new food technologies, the rise of consumer culture and the globalisation of food consumption. Yet many of the sources from which lay people obtained information about 'healthy eating', including the notion of balanced diets, have not been fully explored in terms of either authorship or readership. This chapter traces the history of healthy eating in the second half of the twentieth century in terms of the advice offered by the authors of self-help books in the USA and the UK. By including American authors, the chapter examines the transatlantic nature of programmes for balance, comparing advice about obesity and dieting, exploring the cultural authority of celebrity dietitians and assessing the degree of knowledge exchange between the two countries. In doing so, it investigates the ways in which readers learned about 'healthy eating' on a day-to-day level, generating a more detailed historical analysis of the 'healthy diet' ideal and the ways in which the self-help genre contributed to the 'health manufacturing' process. Mobilising persuasive motivational language alongside scientific jargon, self-help authors were able to simultaneously promote their own status and appeal to readers' sense of agency. Analysis of self-help also reveals, however, the controversies associated with self-help and the promotion of healthy balanced diets.

Extending the methodological and conceptual scope of the discussion about regulation and balance, in Chapter 6 Ayesha Nathoo's exploration of 'relaxed living' in post-war Britain explores the multi-faceted nature of therapies for bodily balance and the material culture through which they were taken up and incorporated into individual lives. Therapeutic relaxation techniques proliferated in the twentieth century, designed to counteract the myriad maladies popularly associated with the pace and pressures of modern Western living. Practitioners advocated forms of neuromuscular relaxation as safe, effective, drug-free therapies for conditions ranging from high blood pressure to migraine, labour pain and anxiety. However, the therapeutic efficacy of relaxation techniques relied on them being expertly taught, conscientiously learned and persistently practised. This chapter focuses on the pedagogy of twentieth-century therapeutic relaxation methods in Britain, paying particular attention to their material and audio-visual culture. Relaxation instruction and ideology were communicated through numerous channels including self-help books, group classes, correspondence courses, the mass media, teacher training forums, cassettes and biofeedback equipment. As Nathoo notes, the specific techniques of relaxation were embedded in, and contributed to, a larger framework of debates about 'healthy lifestyles' that rested on individuals taking responsibility for and managing their own health and wellbeing. Nonetheless, the chapter makes clear that efforts to construct the self-balancing individual were deeply enmeshed with specific modes, processes and networks of communication. By considering the localised, socio-cultural specificities of relaxation therapies, it is possible to move beyond governmentality frameworks in our considerations of health education, health management and expertise of balance in the post-war period.

In Chapter 7, Natasha Feiner focuses on another dimension of the political tale about regulating health, examining efforts to regulate fatigue among airline pilots in post-war Britain. In the middle decades of the twentieth century fatigue was increasingly understood in terms of balance. If the dynamic equilibrium of the body was upset – by ill health, emotional stress or intensive working practices – fatigue would result. The notion that an imbalance between work and leisure time might cause fatigue (or what later became known as 'burnout') was commonplace in a number of industries by 1950. Complaints of fatigue resulting from long working hours and insufficient opportunities for rest were endemic among factory workers, teachers, doctors and pilots. With a specific focus on civil aviation, this chapter explores how fatigue in the workplace was managed and regulated in the twentieth century and evaluates who was considered responsible for monitoring and minimising worker fatigue. In Britain – as in America – civil aviation was one of the only industries to attempt to regulate fatigue after it was implicated in a number of aircraft accidents in the 1950s. As this chapter demonstrates, however, programmes to manage imbalance did not neatly map onto broader changes in British politics. Although regulations limiting working hours and attempting to balance the duty cycle were introduced in the middle and late twentieth century, responsibility for fatigue management ultimately remained with individual pilots. Despite supposed shifts from social democratic to neo-liberal governments in Britain, a liberal, gentlemanly professionalism provided a consistent frame for the regulation of work and fatigue.

Opening the final section of the volume, in Chapter 8 Vanessa Heggie traces discourses about balance in extreme social and physical environments, once more highlighting how considerations of physiological and social balance intersected with empire, race and gender. Human beings arrived at all three 'poles' – north, south and the so-called 'third pole' on the summit of Everest – in the twentieth century. The medical sciences that enabled and explained such performances were part of a long conversation rooted in mid-nineteenth-century concepts of the *milieu intérieur*, in which disruption, moderation and rebalance were the crucial functions of living bodies attempting to survive in challenging circumstances. But such activities also called into question other meanings of 'moderate' and 'balanced', requiring extremely risky human participation and drawing on research – often ethically challenging – conducted through the two world wars. For British and Anglophile participants, balance was also a contested part of their national identity – and extreme performances, whether caused by the environment or the pressure of increasingly competitive and high-stakes international sporting events, could be a mark of both the hero and the foreign 'Other'. Linking with Natasha Feiner's discussion of dangerous fatigue in the unregulated workplace, this chapter considers the many tensions between balance and imbalance in the context of extreme physiology – in exploration and sport – in the long twentieth century.

Mark Jackson's essay on the making of the midlife crisis in Chapter 9 considers how new subject positions were formed – and imbalances were regulated – through the different modalities of text and counselling in twentieth-century Britain and America. It became commonplace during the twentieth century to regard the age of 40 (or later 50) as a tipping point in the life cycle, a moment when many people could begin to shed the financial, domestic, parental and occupational worries of youth and early middle age and look forward to a more serene and comfortable period of their lives. The belief that life after 40 might present opportunities for, rather than obstacles to, health and happiness was given legitimacy by a post-Second World War popular culture that considered increased consumption and economic growth, at least in the West, as the primary route to self-realisation and emotional fulfilment. Made possible partly by increased life expectancy, the crisis of middle age was recast as an epiphany, a moment of temporary imbalance that was necessary if age-related cognitive and economic decline were to be effectively reversed and individuals inspired to achieve the highest levels of personal satisfaction and emotional well-being. By juxtaposing advice literature on healthy ageing in America, the work of marriage guidance counsellors in Britain, as well as cinematic and literary representations of the 'emotional typhoon' experienced during midlife transitions, Jackson argues that the popularity of the term 'midlife crisis' lay in its resonance with growing concerns about the collapse of the

American dream and post-Second World War anxieties about threats to the stability of the nuclear family. In both cases, notions of emotional balance were reconfigured by obsessions with the ways in which the autonomous individual and the gospel of consumption would effectively restabilise a seemingly unbalanced Western capitalist economy.

In Chapter 10, Dorothy Porter opens up the world of disease categorisation itself to examine how the construction of a specific 'Parkinson's personality' not only turned on physiological and therapeutic balances, but also on the balance of patient experience and medical expertise. Parkinson's Disease is often regarded as a condition marked primarily by imbalance and dysregulation, especially in terms of impaired physical balance and reduced dopamine production. However, there are other features of the disease that also reveal much about modern understandings of emotional balance, creativity and agency. This chapter explores the historical construction of a biopsychological model of a pre-diagnostic Parkinson's personality in the late twentieth and early twenty-first centuries. It interrogates historically situated assumptions about character traits that were correlated with neuromolecular variations measured in the brain, exploring these relationships within the history of neuromolecular and biopsychological research on creativity from the late 1980s. The epistemological security of the pathologisation of creativity (as a form of impulsiveness or dysregulation) in the biopsychological model of the Parkinson's personality is examined in the light of patients' own interpretations of their cognitive experiences and their feelings of dynamic and emergent, rather than static, dimensions of being human. Drawing on specific examples, Porter argues that there was an alternative narrative to the neuromolecular and essentialist notions of disability adopted by scientists and clinicians, one that was articulated by patients in terms of health and creativity, rather than in terms of pathological imbalances in neurotransmitters.

In the concluding contribution to the volume, Chapter 11, Chris Millard provocatively returns to the themes and questions that have been sketched out in this introduction. As the chapters in the volume make clear, histories of notions of 'balanced selves' are diverse. Ideas of balance differ across time and cultural space, as do the ways in which balance might be regulated, controlled and incentivised. Among all this variety, Millard's conclusion asks a more general question for those writing histories of balance: how is it possible to historicise balanced selfhood at all? What is the basis for the assumption that human selves might be differently realised, socially or culturally constructed, according to the norms of different times and places? This chapter raises and addresses two challenges. First, it argues that a significant part of the notion of 'malleable humanity' comes from early twentieth-century anthropology, especially from work in the tradition of Franz Boas and Margaret Mead. Second, it demonstrates how these assumptions have become visible as a result of a resurgence of neurological, neurochemical and genomic visions of humanity since the late 1990s. If the malleable selves that populate our histories of balance are significantly anthropological, then their relationship with imperialism must be clarified. In addition, as the visibility of malleable selves is related to the resurgence of a new biological vision of humanity, historians also need to clarify and contextualise their own position in this contested terrain.

Notes

1. E. Hobsbawm, *The Age of Extremes: The Short Twentieth Century, 1914–1991* (London: Michael Joseph, 1994).
2. E. Hobsbawm, *The Age of Revolution: Europe 1789–1848* (London: Abacus, 1962); E. Hobsbawm, *The Age of Capital, 1848–1875* (London: Weidenfeld and Nicolson, 1985); E. Hobsbawm, *The Age of Empire, 1870–1914* (London: Weidenfeld and Nicolson, 1987).
3. Hobsbawm, *The Age of Extremes*, p. 5.
4. Ibid., p. 8.
5. W. G. Carleton, 'Our post-crisis world', *American Scholar*, 33:1 (Winter 1963–4), 27–44.
6. Tze-ki Hon, *The Allure of the Nation: The Cultural and Historical Debates in Late Qing and Republican China* (Leiden: Brill, 2015), p. 91.
7. Hobsbawm, *The Age of Extremes*, p. 11.
8. G. Eghigian, A. Killen and C. Leuenberger, 'Introduction: the self as project: politics and the human sciences in the twentieth century', *Osiris*, 22 (2007), 1–25, at p. 12.
9. R. D. Laing, *The Divided Self: An Existential Study in Sanity and Madness* (London: Pelican Books, [1959] 1982), pp. 17–18. Laing pursued the distinctions and conflicts further in R. D. Laing, *Self and Others: Further Studies in Sanity and Madness* (London: Tavistock Publications, 1961).
10. Laing, *The Divided Self*, pp. 19–20.
11. Ibid., p. 12.

12 E. Hsu, 'What next? Balance in medical practice and the medico-moral nexus of moderation', in P. Horden and E. Hsu (eds), *The Body in Balance: Humoral Medicines in Practice* (New York: Berghahn, 2013), pp. 259–80. On the regulation and expression of emotions in the twentieth century, see M. Jackson, 'Medical and scientific understandings', in J. Davidson and J. Damousi (eds), *A Cultural History of the Emotions in the Modern and Post-Modern Age* (London: Bloomsbury Academic, 2018), pp. 19–36.

13 Hsu, 'What next?', p. 259.

14 For provocative discussion of the notions of individualised, liquid societies, see: Z. Bauman, *The Individualized Society* (Cambridge: Polity Press, 2001); Z. Bauman, *Liquid Modernity*, 2nd edition (Cambridge: Polity Press, 2012).

15 For discussion of the exchange between physiological and political accounts of balance, or the use of the 'organic analogy', see: M. Jackson, *The Age of Stress: Science and the Search for Stability* (Oxford: Oxford University Press, 2013), pp. 94–5, 161–2, 256–8; S. J. Cross and W. R. Albury, 'Walter B. Cannon, L. J. Henderson and the organic analogy', *Osiris*, 3 (1987), 165–92; C. E. Russett, *The Concept of Equilibrium in American Social Thought* (New Haven, CT: Yale University Press, 1966).

16 On the need to 'maintain the balance' in marriage, see R. P. Travis and P. Y. Travis, 'Preparing couples for mid-life and the later years', in D. Mace (ed.), *Prevention in Family Services: Approaches to Family Wellness* (Beverley Hills, CA: Sage, 1983), pp. 87–97.

17 Dr M. Chan, 'Address to the 61st World Health Assembly', Geneva, Switzerland, 19 May 2008, available at www.who.int/dg/speeches/2008/20080519/en/, accessed 28 April 2009.

18 For examples of these uses of balance, see: W. S. Churchill, *In the Balance: Speeches 1949–1950* (London: Cassell, 1951); J. C. Campbell and N. Ikegami, *The Art of Balance in Health Policy: Maintaining Japan's Low-Cost, Egalitarian System* (Cambridge: Cambridge University Press, 1998); E. S. More, *Restoring the Balance: Women Physicians and the Profession of Medicine, 1850–1995* (Cambridge, MA: Harvard University Press, 1999); E. de Bono, *The Happiness Purpose* (London: Maurice Temple Smith, 1977); L. Garrett, *The Coming Plague: Newly Emerging Diseases in a World Out of Balance* (London: Penguin, 1994).

19 S. McCredie, *Balance: In Search of the Lost Sense* (New York: Little, Brown and Company, 2007). See also Chapter 10 on Parkinson's Disease.

20 L. J. Henderson, 'The theory of neutrality regulation in the animal organism', *American Journal of Physiology*, 21:4 (1908), 427–48; L. J. Henderson, 'The regulation of neutrality in the animal body', *Science*, 37:950 (1913),

389–95; W. B. Cannon, 'Organization for physiological homeostasis', *Physiological Reviews*, 9:3 (1929), 399–431; W. B. Cannon, 'Stresses and strains of homeostasis', *American Journal of the Medical Sciences*, 189:1 (1935), 1–14.
21 For example, M. Sakel, *Epilepsy* (New York: Philosophical Library, 1958), p. 104.
22 K. E. Appel, 'The acid-base equilibrium of the blood in psychotic patients', in K. E. Appel, C. B. Farr and P. J. Hodes, *Manic-Depressive Psychosis* (Oxford: Williams and Wilkins, 1932), pp. 203–16; M. Harris, S. Chandran, N. Chakraborty and D. Healy, 'Mood-stabilizers: the archaeology of the concept', *Bipolar Disorders*, 5:6 (2003), 446–52; M. Harris, S. Chandran, N. Chakraborty and D. Healy, 'The impact of mood stabilizers on bipolar disorder: the 1890s and 1990s compared', *History of Psychiatry*, 16:4 (2005), 423–34.
23 See Chapter 2.
24 W. B. Cannon, *The Wisdom of the Body* (New York: W. W. Norton and Company, [1932] 1939). For historical discussion of the political resonance of physiological equilibrium, see: G. E. Allen, 'J. S. Haldane: the development of the idea of control mechanisms in respiration', *Journal of the History of Medicine and Allied Sciences*, 22:4 (1967), 392–412; Cross and Albury, 'Walter B. Cannon, L. J. Henderson and the organic analogy', pp. 165–92; Russett, *The Concept of Equilibrium*; J. Parascandola, 'Organismic and holistic concepts in the thought of L. J. Henderson', *Journal of the History of Biology*, 4:1 (1971), 63–113.
25 See the wonderfully diverse collection of essays in P. Horden and E. Hsu (eds), *The Body in Balance: Humoral Medicines in Practice* (New York: Berghahn, 2013). On the history of yoga, see: M. Singleton and J. Byrne (eds), *Yoga in the Modern World: Contemporary Perspectives* (London: Routledge, 2008), pp. 49–74; S. Newcombe, 'Stretching for health and well-being: yoga and women in Britain, 1960–1980', *Asian Medicine*, 3:1 (2007), 37–63.
26 For fuller discussion of the history of massage, remedial gymnastics and physiotherapy, see K. Nias, 'Negotiating intimacies: gender, rehabilitation and the professionalisation of massage in Britain, c.1880–1920' (PhD thesis, Exeter, 2018).
27 A. Phillips, *On Balance* (London: Penguin, 2011). The concept of 'wellness' was introduced in the 1950s by the American biostatistician Halbert L. Dunn (1896–1975): H. L. Dunn, *High-Level Wellness* (Arlington, VA: Beatty Press, 1961).
28 S. Freud, *Beyond the Pleasure Principle and Other Writings*, trans. J. Reddick (London: Penguin Books, [1922] 2003).

29 Echoing earlier work on the autonomic nervous system and physiological function, neuroendocrine and immunological imbalances have also recently been implicated in the pathogenesis of manic depression: A. Duffy, U. Lewitzka, S. Doucette, A. Andreazza and P. Grof, 'Biological indicators of illness risk in offspring of bipolar parents: targeting the hypothalamic-pituitary-adrenal axis and immune system', *Early Intervention in Psychiatry*, 6:2 (2012), 128–37.

30 D. Healy, *Mania: A Short History of Bipolar Disorder* (Baltimore: Johns Hopkins University Press, 2008); D. Healy, 'The latest mania: selling bipolar disorder', *PLoS Medicine*, 3:4 (2006), e185; F. Baughman, 'There is no such thing as a psychiatric disorder/disease/chemical imbalance', *PLoS Medicine*, 3:7 (2006), e318; S. N. Ghaemi, 'The newest mania: seeing disease mongering everywhere', *PLoS Medicine*, 3:7 (2006), e319; D. Healy, 'The best hysterias: author's response to Ghaemi', *PLoS Medicine*, 3:7 (2006), e320; J. R. Lacasse and J. Leo, 'Questionable advertising of psychotropic medications and disease mongering', *PLoS Medicine*, 3:7 (2006), e321; J. Moncrieff, *The Myth of the Chemical Cure: A Critique of Psychiatric Drug Treatment* (Basingstoke: Palgrave Macmillan, 2009).

31 For a discussion of some of these issues in North America, see: A. Scull, 'The mental health sector and the social sciences in post-World War II USA. Part 1: total war and its aftermath', *History of Psychiatry*, 22:1 (2011), 3–19; A. Scull, 'The mental health sector and the social sciences in post-World War II USA. Part 2: the impact of federal research funding and the drugs revolution', *History of Psychiatry*, 22:3 (2011), 268–84.

32 K. Menninger, *The Vital Balance: The Life Processes in Mental Health and Illness* (New York: Viking Press, 1963).

33 Ibid., p. 84.

34 Ibid., pp. 88–9.

35 Ibid., p. 93.

36 G. Canguilhem, 'Régulation (épistémologie)', in *Encyclopaedia Universalis*, p. 3, cited and discussed in M. Arminjon, 'Birth of the allostatic model: from Cannon's biocracy to critical physiology', *Journal of the History of Biology* (2015), doi: 10.1007/s10739-015-9420-9.

37 B. S. Dohrenwend and B. P. Dohrenwend (eds), *Stressful Life Events: Their Nature and Effects* (New York: John Wiley, 1974); B. P. Dohrenwend and B. S. Dohrenwend, *Social Status and Psychological Disorder: A Causal Inquiry* (New York: Wiley-Interscience, 1969); A. McCarthy and C. Coleborne (eds), *Migration, Ethnicity, and Mental Health: International Perspectives* (London: Routledge, 2012).

38 R. S. Lazarus, *Psychological Stress and the Coping Process* (New York: McGraw-Hill, 1966).

39 For a discussion of Hans Selye's theories of stress and coping, see Jackson, *The Age of Stress*, pp. 181–223.
40 A. T. Beck, *Cognitive Therapy and the Emotional Disorders* (New York: Meridian, 1976); A. T. Beck, 'The past and future of cognitive therapy', *Journal of Psychotherapy Practice and Research*, 6:4 (1997), 276–84.
41 H. Benson, *The Relaxation Response* (New York: Avon Books, 1975). See also Chapter 6 on relaxation.
42 J. Kabat-Zinn, *Full Catastrophe Living: How to Cope with Stress, Pain and Illness Using Mindfulness Meditation*, 2nd edition (London: Piatkus, 2004).
43 M. Thatcher, 'Speech to the Royal Society', 27 September 1988, available at www.margaretthatcher.org/document/107346, accessed August 2019.
44 R. Carson, *Silent Spring* (Boston, MA: Riverside Press, 1962); J. Lovelock, *Gaia: A New Look at Life on Earth* (Oxford: Oxford University Press, [1979] 1995).
45 F. N. Egerton, 'Changing concepts of the balance of nature', *Quarterly Review of Biology*, 48:2 (1973), 322–50; J. Kricher, *The Balance of Nature: Ecology's Enduring Myth* (Princeton: Princeton University Press, 2009).
46 A. Gore, *Earth in the Balance: Ecology and the Human Spirit* (New York: Penguin, 1993).
47 G. Mitman, *Breathing Space: How Allergies Shape Our Lives and Landscapes* (New Haven, CT: Yale University Press, 2007); M. Jackson, *Allergy: The History of a Modern Malady* (London: Reaktion Books, 2006); D. G. Schuster, *Neurasthenic Nation: America's Search for Health, Happiness, and Comfort, 1869–1920* (New Brunswick, NJ: Rutgers University Press, 2011).
48 P. Ehrlich, *The Population Bomb* (London: Ballantine Books, 1968); L. Levi and L. Andersson, *Psychosocial Stress: Population, Environment and Quality of Life* (New York: Spectrum Books, 1975).
49 Levi and Andersson, *Psychosocial Stress*, pp. xiv, 96.
50 Lovelock, *Gaia*, pp. ix–x, 10.
51 Ibid., pp. 44–58, 100–14, 119.
52 Egerton, 'Changing concepts of the balance of nature'. See also: G. Mitman, 'In search of health: landscape and disease in American environmental history', *Environmental History*, 10:2 (2005), 184–210; S. Müller-Wille, 'The economy of nature in classical natural history', *Studies in the History of Biology*, 4:4 (2012), 38–49.
53 Eghigian, Killen and Leuenberger, 'Self as project', pp. 3–4.
54 M. Foucault, 'Technologies of the self', in L. H. Martin, H. Gutman and P. H. Hutton (eds), *Technologies of the Self: A Seminar with Michel Foucault* (London: Tavistock Press, 1988), pp. 16–49.

55 For warnings against teleology: R. Porter, 'Introduction', in R. Porter (ed.), *Rewriting the Self: Histories from the Renaissance to the Present* (London: Routledge, 1997), pp. 1–14; P. Burke, 'Representations of the self from Petrarch to Descartes', in Porter (ed.), *Rewriting the Self*, pp. 17–28. Though not mentioned in these texts, it is enough to recall how *fin de siècle* theories of eugenics and social Darwinism offered much more cynical and deterministic visions of the self than earlier periods: N. Stepan, *The Idea of Race in Science: Great Britain, 1800–1960* (Basingstoke: Macmillan, 1982); D. Porter, *Health, Civilisation, and the State: A History of Public Health from Ancient to Modern Times* (London: Routledge, 1999).

56 S. Greenblatt, *Renaissance Self-Fashioning: From More to Shakespeare* (Chicago: University of Chicago Press, [1980] 2005); C. Taylor, *Sources of the Self: The Making of Modern Identity* (Cambridge: Cambridge University Press, [1989] 2004); D. E. Hall, *Subjectivity* (London: Routledge, 2004); J. Seigel, *The Idea of the Self: Thought and Experience in Western Europe Since the Seventeenth Century* (Cambridge: Cambridge University Press, 2005). On the policing of boundaries of individuality and selfhood along lines of race, gender, sexuality and status, despite (or perhaps because of) a rhetoric of universality: U. S. Mehta, *Liberalism and Empire: A Study in Nineteenth Century British Liberal Thought* (Chicago: University of Chicago Press, 1999); N. L. Stepan, 'Race, gender, science and citizenship', in C. Hall (ed.), *Cultures of Empire: Colonisers in Britain and the Empire in the Nineteenth and Twentieth Centuries* (Manchester: Manchester University Press, 2000), pp. 61–86.

57 D. Armstrong, *A New History of Identity: A Sociology of Medical Knowledge* (Basingstoke: Palgrave, 2002); M. Thomson, *Psychological Subjects: Identity, Culture and Health in Twentieth-Century Britain* (Oxford: Oxford University Press, 2006); R. Hayward, *The Transformation of the Psyche in British Primary Care, 1870–1970* (London: Bloomsbury Academic, 2014). See also the discussions below on social movements, 'psy' sciences and post-war academic work.

58 M. Shapira, *The War Inside: Psychoanalysis, Total War, and the Making of the Democratic Self in Postwar Britain* (Cambridge: Cambridge University Press, 2013).

59 M. Francis, 'Tears, tantrums, and bared teeth: the emotional economy of three Conservative prime ministers, 1951–1963', *Journal of British Studies*, 41:3 (2002), 354–87.

60 M. Francis, 'The Labour Party: modernisation and the politics of restraint', in B. Conekin, F. Mort and C. Waters (eds), *Moments of Modernity: Reconstructing Britain, 1945–1964* (London: Rivers Oram Press, 1999), pp. 152–70.

Introduction

61 Eghigian, Killen and Leuenberger, 'Self as project', pp. 12–13.
62 M. Fulbrook and A. I. Port (eds), *Becoming East German: Socialist Structures and Sensibilities after Hitler* (New York: Berghahn Books, 2013).
63 Hall, *Subjectivity*; A. Elliott, *Concepts of the Self*, 2nd edition (Bristol: Polity Press, 2007).
64 For instance: F. Fanon, *Black Skin, White Masks*, trans. C. L. Markmann (London: Pluto Press, [1952] 1986); S. de Beauvoir, *The Second Sex* (London: Vintage Classic, [1949] 2015); D. Riley, *Am I That Name?: Feminism and the Category of 'Women' in History* (Basingstoke: Macmillan, 1988); bell hooks, *Ain't I a Woman: Black Women and Feminism* (Oxford: Routledge, [1981] 2015).
65 For an overview of the role of 'psy' practices and knowledges in shaping the modern self: N. Rose, 'Assembling the modern self', in Porter (ed.), *Rewriting the Self*, pp. 224–48.
66 N. Rose and P. Miller, 'Political power beyond the state: problematics of government', *British Journal of Sociology*, 43:2 (1992), 173–205; M. Dean, *Governmentality: Power and Rule in Modern Society*, 2nd edition (London: Sage, 2010).
67 N. Rose, *Governing the Soul: The Shaping of the Private Self*, 2nd edition (London: Free Association Books, 1999). Though from a different perspective, similar arguments have been made for the sociological encounter: M. Savage, *Identities and Social Change in Britain since 1940: The Politics of Method* (Oxford: Oxford University Press, 2010).
68 Rose, *Governing the Soul*; H. M. Rimke, 'Governing citizens through self-help literature', *Cultural Studies*, 14:1 (2000), 61–78.
69 G. Huxford, *The Korean War in Britain: Citizenship, Selfhood and Forgetting* (Manchester: Manchester University Press, 2018), p. 6. For instance: P. Joyce, 'Governmentality and risk: setting priorities in the new NHS', *Sociology of Health and Illness*, 23:5 (2001), 594–614.
70 Thomson, *Psychological Subjects*.
71 S. Freud, 'The question of lay analysis', in A. Freud (ed.), *The Essentials of Psycho-Analysis* (London: Penguin, 1991), pp. 7–65. As Hayward notes, the concept of the unconscious has a rich history beyond Freud: Hayward, *The Transformation of the Psyche*. On the influence of such 'depth' psychologies, see: T. Chettiar, '"More than a contract?": The emergence of a state-supported marriage welfare service and the politics of emotional life in post-1945 Britain', *Journal of British Studies*, 55:3 (2016), 566–91. Also see Chapter 2.
72 A. Marshall, *Principles of Economics*, 8th edition (Basingstoke: Palgrave Macmillan, [1920] 2013). See particularly Book III on 'wants and their satisfactions'. Concepts of balance were also central to understanding the

working of firms and markets, such as life cycles of business and dynamic price equilibrium (see Books IV and V). Even here, however, although modelling markets depended on assumptions of rationality, not all consumers were considered rational, and exclusions again fell on race and class lines: ibid., p. 100.

73 D. Armstrong, 'The patient's view', *Social Science and Medicine*, 18:9 (1984), 737–44.
74 J. M. Keynes, *The General Theory of Employment, Interest and Money* (Cham: Palgrave Macmillan, [1935] 2018), pp. 141–2.
75 For twentieth-century academic objectifications of the self: E. Goffman, *The Presentation of Self in Everyday Life* (Edinburgh: University of Edinburgh Press, 1956); P. Bourdieu, *Distinction: A Social Critique of the Judgement of Taste* (London: Routledge, [1979] 2010); Foucault, 'Technologies of the self', pp. 16–49; J. Lacan, *The Language of the Self: The Function of Language in Psychoanalysis*, trans. A. Wilden (Baltimore: Johns Hopkins University Press, 1997); D. Moran, 'Lived body, intersubjectivity, and intercorporeality: the body in phenomenology', in L. Dolezal and D. Petherbridge (eds), *Body/Self/Other: The Phenomenology of Social Encounters* (Albany, NY: SUNY Press, 2017), pp. 269–309; Elliott, *Concepts of the Self*.
76 Hall, *Subjectivity*, pp. 87–8, 90–1. For a history of this decentering: C. J. Dean, *The Self and Its Pleasures: Bataille, Lacan, and the History of the Decentered Subject* (New York: Cornell University Press, 1992).
77 Hall, *Subjectivity*, pp. 94–109.
78 I. Hacking, 'Making up people', in H. C. Heller, M. Sosna and D. E. Wellbery (eds), *Reconstructing Individualism: Autonomy, Individuality and the Self in Western Thought* (Stanford: Stanford University Press, 1986), pp. 222–36.
79 Similar ideas are discussed in, for instance: M. D. Moore, 'Food as medicine: diet, diabetes management, and the patient in twentieth century Britain', *Journal of the History of Medicine and Allied Sciences*, 73:2 (2018), 150–67.
80 A. I. Tauber, *The Immune Self: Theory or Metaphor?* (Cambridge: Cambridge University Press, 1994).
81 See also: Huxford, *The Korean War in Britain*. On the importance of material objects to new ideas of selfhood, see: Hayward, *The Transformation of the Psyche*; A. Withey, *Technology, Self-Fashioning and Politeness in Eighteenth-Century Britain: Refined Bodies* (Basingstoke: Palgrave Macmillan, 2015).

Part I
Configuring balance

2

Balance and the 'good' diabetic in Britain, c.1900–60

Martin D. Moore

Introduction

Reporting on the performance of a notable debutant at the Wimbledon tennis championship of 1951, the *Diabetic Journal*, a magazine produced for patients by the Diabetic Association, set the scene for a dramatic underdog story. 'When Hamilton Richardson stepped on to Wimbledon's No.1 Court on June 27th last, scarcely any of the spectators ... could have believed he had any chance against his opponent, Budge Patty.' Patty 'was the world's singles champion of the year before', whereas Richardson 'was only eighteen years of age, and far less experienced'. Most importantly, 'to cap his disadvantages', Richardson 'was a chronic diabetic'. Against all such odds, Richardson triumphed.

Success, the *Journal* keenly pointed out, was founded on Richardson learning 'how to control his diabetes' and restoring short-term physiological balance to his body. 'As every "good" diabetic on insulin knows', the article explained, 'violent exercise rapidly burns up sugar in the blood, and, when playing games, great care must be taken to keep up the blood sugar to its right level and so avoid an insulin reaction.' To win, Richardson needed to 'study thoroughly the likely effect on his blood sugar of a series of hard games and take precautions'. It was this action that 'enabled him to maintain a diabetic balance throughout'.[1]

This chapter explores how clinicians and Britain's first patient organisation – the Diabetic (later, British Diabetic) Association (BDA) – constituted the 'good diabetic' as one able to undertake considerable self-care in line with medical advice during the first half of the twentieth century. Following the work of David Armstrong among others, it suggests that the self-caring 'diabetic' was not a given entity. Instead, through medical innovation, training and collective action, the 'good diabetic' was a figure who had to be made in relation to the shifting institutional and political structures of interwar and early post-war Britain.[2]

As the Richardson article suggests, concepts of balance were integral to visions of the 'good diabetic' during this period. Clinical and lay texts framed diabetes as a disease of physiological imbalance, a metabolic disturbance caused by an insufficient supply of endogenous insulin, and marked by biochemical deviations, most notably elevated blood sugar (hyperglycaemia) and, in the worst cases, acid bodies (ketones) in the blood. Treatment, moreover, was predicated on restoring normal function through a balance of diet and insulin supply. Although the boundaries of physiological balance were debated over this period, all practitioners subscribed to longitudinal disease management by professionals and patients, and good patients were those who undertook the quotidian actions necessary to keep their body in both short- and long-term equilibrium.

The discussion of Richardson's 'diabetic victory' also highlights how concerns about emotional and psychological stability permeated British medical and lay discussion of diabetes over the first half of the twentieth century. During the 1900s and 1910s, doctors framed mental and emotional balance as directly connected to physiological processes. Trauma or upset was believed to provoke or worsen diabetes via the nervous system, and clinicians prescribed tranquillity and moderation as part of their treatment.[3] By the 1920s and 1930s, clinical and lay articles also noted the emotional and psychological problems that patients with long-term diseases could face. They outlined the need to negotiate the Scylla of anxiety and depression that could follow diagnosis and constant (self-)surveillance, and the Charybdis of complacency that might accompany reassurance. Such a challenge assumed individualised and public forms, as an alliance of patients and practitioners sought to challenge discrimination and negative perceptions of diabetes. Offering self-care advice, idealising 'the diabetic life', and celebrating achievements of public figures with diabetes were key strategies designed to promote emotional and psychological balance and well-being.[4]

In discussing the plurality of balances involved in diabetes management during the first half of the twentieth century, this chapter extends recent discussion of how political, medical and popular lay agencies came to reread wide areas of governance and everyday life in psychological and emotional terms during the interwar and early post-war period.[5] Though efforts to constitute the 'good diabetic' were rarely based on systematic or academic models of 'depth psychology' such as psychoanalysis, they nonetheless constituted affective relations as central to human behaviour, and sought to subject psychological life to management in the name of health.[6] Indeed, even when programmes of balance were coded in classic masculine values of rational self-control, they operated as forms of psychological management; the suggestion that health could be secured through knowledge and individual will offered the reassurance of control to people whose bodily integrity had seemingly been compromised.[7]

This medical and lay interest in the emotional and psychological life of people with diabetes was thus central to efforts to constitute new subject positions for patients, organised around physiological balance.[8] Self-care, it will be argued, was considered essential in light of the insufficiencies of British healthcare, and balanced selves were increasingly needed for effective production and civic life.[9] Yet, as this chapter will also highlight, balance was not solely deputed to individuals. Not only would self-care be supported by a range of other actors, but it formed only part of a broader constellation of interventions by healthcare professionals, the state and organised patients.[10] By examining the boundaries of balance and self in the specific confines of British diabetes care, therefore, it is hoped that this chapter will draw attention to the complex interplay of power, politics and medicine in the constitution of identity, and set out relations explored further in the chapters that follow.[11]

Physiological and therapeutic balance in diabetes, c.1900–50

Medical understandings of diabetes during the early decades of the twentieth century were permeated by concepts of balance and stability, owing to a growing influence of physiological perspectives on clinical medicine.[12] Gradually revitalising concepts of illness as disorder, textbooks and articles of the 1910s framed diabetes as a 'disturbance' of metabolic function.[13] In health, physiological perspectives suggested, ingested food would be broken down into constituent parts, and would either be used immediately as energy or be stored for later use. In diabetes, however, impaired processes meant that the body was unable to 'properly utilise carbohydrate', resulting in a characteristic elevation of blood glucose levels that would pass into the urine.[14] Moreover, without effective carbohydrate metabolism 'the incomplete combustion of fats' would produce dangerous acid bodies that heralded the onset of coma.[15]

Building on these insights, one London specialist declared in 1912 that 'the aim of modern treatment in diabetes' was 'to balance the diet in such a way that nutrition is as perfect as possible without … unnecessary strain on the organs of metabolism in any direction'.[16] During this period, practitioners devised managerial frameworks of ongoing surveillance and therapeutic adjustment to achieve this balance.[17] Doctors and physiologists with a special interest in diabetes disagreed on the exact composition of diets, and whether periods of fasting were necessary.[18] They nonetheless recommended strict limits on dietary intake, and that the quantifiable effects on glycosuria (sugar in urine) and ketonuria (acid in urine) be monitored.[19] Although not completely disregarding a patient's subjective assessment – nor marginalising the classic symptoms of extreme thirst, hunger, urination and wasting – experts suggested that changes in biochemical metrics should strongly influence prescriptions and the subsequent longer-term 'titration' of dietary therapy.[20]

The isolation of insulin, and the development of insulin therapy, cemented these managerial practices and extended equilibrium-centred frameworks for understanding diabetes.[21] By the mid-1920s, practitioners were describing insulin as the regulatory agent for the body's self-correcting metabolism. 'The normal pancreas', wrote the pre-eminent British diabetes specialist R. D. Lawrence (King's College Hospital, London), 'produces amounts of insulin which vary naturally with the carbohydrate intake, and normal metabolism is maintained by a balance between the carbohydrate of the food and the endogenous insulin of the body'.[22] Insulin, Lawrence suggested, was the 'hand that holds the reins' of the carbohydrate metabolism, 'the ignition spark which controls and regulates the combustion'.[23] Treatment once more focused on restoring order: 'In diabetes, where insulin is deficient, the diet and insulin have to be balanced artificially to produce normal metabolism', either by controlling diet, or 'if this balance cannot be achieved without too great [a] restriction', then through dietary control and insulin 'added by injection'.[24]

These balance-oriented explanations of causation and treatment were broadly accepted by practitioners throughout the interwar and post-war decades, although they were gradually challenged and adjusted. For example, Harold Himsworth (Professor of Medicine, University College Hospital, London) proposed in 1949 that diabetes was a syndrome. Unlike a disease, the syndrome had 'its philosophical basis ... in a chain of physiological processes, interference with which at any point produces the same impairment of bodily function'.[25] This suggestion emerged from Himsworth's earlier experimental work, in which he hypothesised that two clinical types of diabetes arose from different impairments.[26] Insulin insensitivity was considered a cause of diabetes in generally older, overweight patients with insidious onsets and who did not require injections for effective management; and deficiency of insulin was held as a cause of the condition in generally younger, thinner patients with acute onsets, and who were dependent on, and sensitive to, injected insulin. This plurality of possible mechanisms also found expression in neo-humoral frameworks that remained persistent throughout the century, with researchers and drug manufacturers also implicating an over- or undersupply of insulin antagonists and other hormones in glycaemic disorder.[27]

Despite clinicians agreeing over the importance of managerial approaches to care, the exact meaning of therapeutic balance – how it should be defined and monitored – was subject to dispute.[28] Initial controversies emerged during the 1920s in relation to blood testing, and the achievability of near-normal blood sugars. For many physiologically minded practitioners, normoglycaemia provided the ideal aim of treatment, believing it allowed the pancreas (and thus carbohydrate metabolism) to recover from the exhaustion underpinning diabetes.[29] However, this practice required regular blood sugar examinations, which were difficult to perform outside of sophisticated teaching hospitals. Furthermore, the required regulations on diet, insulin timing and physical activity could be punishing for patients.[30] Practitioners with more traditionally clinical backgrounds, therefore, tended to moderate their demands. They gradually adjusted dietary prescriptions to alleviate the distress of patients with acutely severe diabetes, and suggested that urinary monitoring – and thus the less demanding goal of minimising glycosuria – could provide the basis of effective treatment.[31]

More vigorous opposition to normoglycaemia arose, at least discursively, in the promotion of almost unrestricted 'free diets' between the 1930s and 1950s.[32] Unlike the majority of clinicians (and the Diabetic Association), proponents of free dieting confidently believed that 'it has never been shown that a high blood sugar *per se* did anybody any harm'.[33] As such, these practitioners rejected clinical approaches based on the most common parameters of therapeutic and physiological balance (hyperglycaemia and glycosuria) for imposing regulations that impinged unnecessarily on patient well-being. Instead, they argued for a robust rebalancing of clinical focus towards the subjective feelings of the patient. They recommended matching insulin intake to appetite in non-obese patients, and accepted only the appearance of ketonuria as indication that any resulting physiological imbalance might threaten patient health. Provided no physiological signs of acute, critical imbalance were present, free-diet clinicians were happy to forgo restrictions and assess health based on a patient's outlook, vigour and ability to happily live and work.[34]

Tensions between short-term and long-term physiological balance, and between the relative weight afforded to various clinical considerations in diabetes care, also manifested in intertwined debates around long-term complications. For advocates of free diets, the ever-growing list of complications noted from the 1930s onwards – such as blindness, kidney failure or cardiovascular disease – were an inevitable long-term outcome of diabetes.[35] Other doctors, by contrast, practised under the belief that 'the surest way to avoid such complications is to maintain the best blood-sugar control compatible with safety and a reasonably normal mode of life'.[36] This was despite admitting that the evidence for a relationship between persistent hyperglycaemia and complications was contentious, making it impossible to 'answer the question dogmatically'.[37] At the heart of the clinical dilemma, however, was the potential conflict between different temporalities of balance. For many patients, their errant bodies, social and financial obstacles, and competing priorities militated against daily maintenance of physiological balance, while control was impossible while they were asleep.[38] Relaxing an emphasis on metabolic control in treatment plans could alleviate the conflicts between social life and biological needs, but only at the cost of potentially serious problems in the long term. For methodological and epistemological purposes, researchers were unable to produce convincing evidence about the effects of control until the 1980s and 1990s, and clinical decisions were strongly guided by a doctor's beliefs and cultural values.[39] How to weigh the certainty of the present against the possibilities of the future, however, remained a persistent concern over the century.

Self-care in British diabetes management

For the most part, 'free diets' appeared to gain little support among British practitioners. Mid-century surveys indicated that some physicians might allow for mild hyperglycaemia (but not uncontrolled blood sugars), and they still imposed regulations for diet.[40] Whatever their goal, managerial frameworks and self-care practices remained an important element of long-term diabetes treatment. Self-care had been practised in diabetes care since ancient Greek physicians first used the term 'diabetes' to describe a symptomatic state of persistent urination, extreme thirst, and quick and painful wasting.[41] Followers of humoral traditions had prescribed a mixture of regimen changes, drug treatments and dietary plans in a bid to restore equilibrium, a broad outline that persisted through to the twentieth century despite radical changes in content and rationale.[42] With the development of the hospital system in Britain, and the spread of scientific dieting for diabetes in the early 1900s, initiating treatment could require lengthy institutionalisation, at least where patients received charitable admission to hospital or could afford private care. Doctors gradually placed less emphasis on hospital admission over the interwar period, even for starting insulin, but once admitted patients could stay for weeks to titrate dose and receive education about injections.[43]

Nonetheless, much as physicians praised the control achievable on the ward, patients could not be retained forever. In the absence of Soviet-style control and distribution of clinical facilities and expertise, Britain's mixed economy of healthcare meant that 'the exigencies' of practice made it 'impossible' for doctors to 'see a patient twice, or even once at a specified time' for injections, and 'the cost to the patient [of such an approach] would be prohibitive'.[44] Only workers whose income was low enough to be eligible for the government-backed National Insurance programme could routinely access medical expertise and prescriptions free at the point of use, and then coverage was only for community-based general practitioners. Of course, for these individuals, access to state-funded provision was tied to the capacity for work, which was often incompatible with rigidly timed oversight and treatment.

The institutional and cultural connections between work, healthy behaviour and citizenship also underpinned continued emphasis on self-care in the post-war period. The creation of the National Health Service in 1948 nationalised Britain's hospitals and secured universal coverage for primary care in general practice.[45] Healthcare would now be free for all at the point of use, and people with diabetes could either see their GP or be referred to specialist outpatient clinics that had emerged in major teaching hospitals during the 1920s.[46] Nonetheless, although some local innovations extended access to daily care to more vulnerable populations (such as the rural elderly), self-care remained an essential part of diabetes management.[47] Persistent resource shortages meant that there was an insufficient supply of labour to deliver personalised care without a substantial reworking of institutional arrangements. Politically, the impulse to self-care had also been built into Britain's universalist welfare state. Framed as a universal social right, post-war welfare was predicated on able-bodied citizens engaging in productive activity and paying taxes relative to their means.[48] Universal services in this instance would free the citizenry from inequitable obstacles to health, while simultaneously enabling them to practise the 'laws of health' in pursuit of national well-being.[49] Furthermore, as historians like Virginia Berridge and Gareth Millward have demonstrated, the state and various 'publics' placed extra expectations on the citizen with respect to healthcare, such as an expectation to follow medical instructions and health education advice.[50] Self-care in pursuit of physiological balance thus became an act of ongoing health citizenship, enabling patients to undertake productive activity and not 'drain' welfare resources.[51]

For institutional, political and cultural reasons, therefore, doctors and patients alike saw self-care as central to the longitudinal care of diabetes, and as in previous centuries patients were charged with following a prescribed regimen.[52] The tasks involved in self-care, however, expanded in managerial approaches to treatment, and with new technologies. By the 1920s, self-testing became essential. Writing on 'prognosis in diabetes' on the cusp of insulin treatment, an Edinburgh clinician suggested that 'regular weighing once a week is necessary; loss of weight usually means glycosuria'. As a precaution, 'the patient should also know how to recognise [urinary] sugar ... and he should examine a sample of the 24 hours urine daily'.[53] This procedure was not straightforward. Until at least the 1950s, patients testing for glycosuria or ketonuria were required to heat a test tube of their own urine, combined with a chemical reagent, for around three minutes (usually over a stove or Bunsen burner), and then compare the colour of the cooled sample with a coded strip. Accidents were rather unpleasant. Nevertheless, monitoring was designed to inform both quotidian care and medical oversight, with doctors using the data recorded at regular consultations.[54] Following the spread of insulin therapy, the daily work of self-care was also increased by the essential task of daily injections and equipment care, and some doctors reiterated the importance of self-testing (and even food weighing) for these patients.[55]

As clinicians noted, however, a patient's capacity for, and commitment to, self-management could not be presumed.[56] The 'self' dedicated to self-care had to be created.[57] Training patients on the wards was one direct way to reorient a patient's priorities towards long-term physiological and therapeutic balance, but there were others. Some clinicians believed that self-monitoring – both the practice of urinalysis and the recording of results – was essential for cultivating patient dedication, with self-care helping to constitute the self that cared. For instance, a Manchester-based clinician suggested that urine testing was important not only because it provided 'early and accurate information', but also because 'it keeps the patient interested in his progress, and provides a constant reminder of the need for care'.[58] Other practitioners echoed similar sentiments, only couched in more Christian, moralistic tones. A. C. Begg, a respected practitioner in Swansea, explained how testing 'impresses on patients the necessity of adhering to the prescribed diet' because 'the evil of any surreptitious addition to the diet is forcibly brought home to them [presumably by colour changes in the urine solution] and they do not offend again'.[59]

Another powerful approach to constituting the self-caring patient was through ongoing advice in the form of a patient handbook. This approach reached its most developed state in the work of Scottish physician R. D. Lawrence (b. 1892, d. 1968). Lawrence undertook his medical studies in Aberdeen before taking up a position at King's College Hospital in London. He was diagnosed with diabetes in 1920 (after an accident which left him nearly blind in one eye), and incorporated his own experiences with the disease and its treatment into his clinical practice.[60] Although preaching the gospel of 'normal blood sugars' as a therapeutic aim, Lawrence acknowledged that this would not be practical for all patients, and prescribed more moderate restraints on diet and insulin than many of his peers.[61] He introduced innovations in patient education, and his work underpinned self-care prescriptions for numerous practitioners and patients.[62]

Uniquely, Lawrence codified his ideas about patient self-management in his widely used and reprinted *The Diabetic Life* (first appearing in 1925, with a final edition in 1965), a manual of care for both practitioners and patients.[63] Through its changing list of essentials for 'diabetic education', dietary management and general health, Lawrence articulated a structured vision for patient activity, and provided patients with a legitimation for their self-care, as well as 'how-to' advice. For instance, according to the sixth edition of the handbook published in 1931, it was essential for a patient to be able to: 'work out and follow the prescribed diet'; 'examine his urine' for sugar and acids, and 'keep a note of the results'; 'if necessary … give insulin skilfully', observing 'the correct relation between the timing of the injection and meals'; 'never break the proper balance of diet and insulin', and understand the actions to take if insulin had been omitted or if illness strikes; and 'visit his doctor regularly, taking with him notes of his diet, weight, and the results of his tests, and of any questions he wants to ask'. Through these actions patients could achieve metabolic control, but it was also attendant on patients to look after their general health. They were therefore advised to 'have abundance of rest and sleep, and lead a life of moderation in all respects'; 'take as much mild exercise as he can without getting tired'; 'take great care of his teeth' and 'his skin' (the former by regular brushing and 'visits to the dentist', the latter by 'warm baths' with special attention paid to the 'feet'); and 'avoid constipation' and 'the risk of infection with influenza or tuberculosis or even common colds with a care which might savour of undue selfishness and timidity in a normal individual'.[64] Following this advice would ultimately have had considerable influence on a patient's daily life, often in unexpected ways.

Balance and the 'good' diabetic

In many respects, this was the distinguishing feature of Lawrence's work. Whereas other practitioners spoke of training, Lawrence articulated a new way of living. If they could 'accept the diabetic creed and follow it faithfully', Lawrence wrote in his first preface (included in every subsequent edition), patients would have 'enough energy for all the ordinary pursuits of life'. In exchange for 'self-control', 'a little intelligence' and 'some determination', this 'diabetic life' would give 'a full and active existence, with no real privations'.[65] There would be 'inconveniences', and rhythms of regulated diets, injections, self-testing and clinical oversight. But they would become 'second nature' and help to 'develop strength and independence of character'.[66] By learning about, and adjusting to, their difference, then, patients could almost become better after diagnosis and assume 'normal' life once more.[67]

Although framed as simple self-help tools, providing information to help patients rationally adjust their behaviour, Lawrence's handbooks did not only seek to inform patients: they were instruments for cultivating an active, risk-conscious self. Such efforts were notably coded in traditional values of masculine, Christian self-restraint, forged in the industrial and imperial context of Britain's nineteenth century, and which continued to provide the most prominent – if contested – signs of masculine character in interwar and early post-war Britain.[68]

There were likely epidemiological and cultural explanations for the dominance of gendered advice across the first half of the twentieth century. The invocation of white, male, middle-class values reflected not only the backgrounds of the leading British experts on diabetes, but also the historic and statistical associations between the prevalence of diabetes and upper- and middle-class male life.[69] The latter connection was particularly disconcerting given British anxieties around national efficiency and imperial rule during the interwar and early post-war period.[70] Indeed, in light of debates about masculinity emerging after two world wars, the impaired male body represented a cultural and political problem.[71] As well as reflecting his own formative experiences with Presbyterianism, medical school life and the military, Lawrence's strong rhetoric of 'mastery' over self and disease might thus be read as an attempt to ease cultural anxieties – to compensate for a potential threat to masculine governance among the supposedly natural ruling classes.[72] Equally, the persistence of such rhetoric into the early post-war period may be explained by the way in which the British welfare state had been predicated on a heteronormative male breadwinner model, and it is perhaps unsurprising that justifications for, and culture of, self-care thus remained gendered.[73]

In practice, where clinical staff offered training in self-care, discrimination did not take place along gender lines, with education delivered to all adult patients and the parents of children with diabetes.[74] Rather, the stress that some early-century clinicians placed on patient intelligence was often an indicator of class-based presumptions about capability, with these practitioners believing a patient's socio-economic status, education or ethnicity provided barriers to effective self-governance.[75] Describing an encounter with 'a young Irish soldier, who had escaped school in the past', one London physician wrote in 1917 of how he 'attempted to explain to [the patient] in simple language that he was suffering from a disease which would kill him very soon if he did not consent to undergo certain treatment'. 'After listening patiently', the patient allegedly 'said "Ma fayther never did belave in doctors"'. 'Patients of no education who have not been taught control are unsuitable' for strict dietary programmes, the author concluded, 'prov[ing] a trial to their physician' with their non-compliance after discharge.[76]

Such open disdain and 'othering' became rarer in British journals and textbooks over time, especially with regard to class.[77] In terms of race and ethnicity, despite the imperial whiteness coded in appeals to self-control, it tended to be in colonial contexts – where issues of self-governance had clear political overtones – that discussions of treatment and self-care overtly intersected with racialised discourses of masculinity.[78] Nonetheless, though rarely articulated, implicit cultural norms manifested in other ways. For instance, mid-century texts rarely considered the differing dietary requirements of Britain's increasingly diverse population. Such an absence was indicative of the way that white middle-class standards provided the basis of medical and dietary advice for self-care, despite the rising visibility of demographic change. Only local initiative seemingly provided a corrective until the politicisation of inequalities much later in the century.[79]

Self-care and emotional management

Historically, a key element of discourses about disciplined masculinity had been the capacity to control emotion, and to rise above irrational

Balance and the 'good' diabetic

responses through self-improvement. In this sense, an emotional economy had been central to concepts of masculinity even when supposedly excluded. Emotional and psychological management had also played a significant part in professional approaches to diabetes care during the early and mid-twentieth century, though the rationale for this management subtly shifted over time.[80] Texts in the 1900s and 1910s tended to couch discussions of cause and treatment of diabetes in traditions that linked overstimulation to bodily disturbance via the nervous system.[81] For instance, discussing the aetiology of diabetes in 1913, one textbook suggested that diabetes had 'been observed to follow ... traumatic and other lesions of the nervous centre' and had 'apparently been traceable occasionally to emotional shock, anxiety, and mental strain'.[82] Minimising such nervous disturbances became an important element of treatment. On the one hand, doctors recommended moderation of lifestyle, remarking how 'a moderate amount of work without any anxieties, excitements or worries suits best'.[83] On the other hand, knowledge of the possible effects of strain on diabetes also fed into clinical decision-making. As one London practitioner pointed out, doctors needed to know when to adjust dietary therapy and when to avoid intervention. 'The reappearance of sugar after some time without any alteration of the diet', he suggested, 'does not necessarily mean that a fresh period of alimentary rest need be prescribed, or even a modification in the diet is essential.' Rather, as 'exposure to cold, anxiety about catching a train, and many other minor things can lead to a return of sugar', other potential causes of disturbance 'should be inquired about before any alteration in the diet is ordered'.[84]

These frameworks of causation and management retained a long influence in British discussions of diabetes.[85] However, by the 1930s, clinical and lay discussions of emotional and psychological states in diabetes were increasingly devoid of models that physically connected mental or emotional duress and physiological balance. Instead, they were concerned with the importance of emotional and psychological management for effective self-care, and how the difficulties and temporal implications of a diagnosis provided specific challenges. It was feared that a changed sense of self following diagnosis, or the introspection and hard work of lifelong self-surveillance, would produce fatalism, while patients who appeared too optimistic might be complacent about their situation with devastating results not manifesting until years later.

As one article in the *Diabetic Journal* put it: 'the diabetic patient has to steer a course between that of being over-confident and that of undue anxiety'.[86] This meant that those charged with managing patients also had a difficult task: practitioners and agencies promoting patient interests sought to carefully manage patient outlooks, finding a useful balance between extremes, and harnessing and channelling negative and positive outlooks into health-promoting behaviours.

An important starting place for this work was once again the acts and instruments of self-testing, which were designed to elicit affective responses and to manage the mental lives of patients. A clinician in Hull, for example, noted that even negative responses to the longitudinal inscriptions of a patient-made glycosuria chart could prove useful in generating more positive reactions. He suggested that after 'mistakes' a patient might 'take pride in producing a chart without ... blemishes, and hence is more careful in his diet'. The graphic nature of the resulting data even enabled patients to cope with physically punishing experiences, for example providing 'reward [to a patient] visibly for his starvation days if they are imposed'.[87]

Affective management also took place during clinical encounters. In part due to the way insulin treatment became folded into emergent networks of British scientific medicine, clinicians and researchers in general medical hospitals created specialist outpatient clinics for the long-term management of patients with diabetes during the 1920s and 1930s.[88] Clinics proliferated in subsequent decades, especially after the creation of the NHS, and some practitioners sought to explicitly use their clinics to reinforce medical attempts at cultivating self-governing patients.[89] For instance, an article published in 1927 about a clinic in Salford reflected on the techniques applied in its communal spaces. Firstly, the author noted, 'considerable importance was attached to th[e] matter of "atmosphere"'. An 'informal' environment was fostered to carefully manage patients' emotional and psychological responses and harness them for optimal therapeutic results. 'It [the atmosphere] kept the patients cheerful and good-tempered', the article noted, 'enabled one to obtain their confidence, and kept them interested in their progress with the least possible tendency to depression.' Mirroring the discussion about urine testing, the doctor feared that introspection over an incurable condition might generate unhelpful psychological states. The clinic was designed, therefore, to ensure that patients were neither overly pessimistic nor dangerously complacent, and so to optimise effective disease management both within and outside the institution.[90]

Once established, this atmosphere provided the space for more classic disciplinary techniques.[91] The article detailed how 'patients were encouraged to compare notes of their progress, blood sugar content, and so forth'. Through such informal activity, strategies of examination and comparison could be deployed to encourage appropriate behaviours. Similarly, public punishment was dispensed to those 'convicted of dietary indiscretions', albeit delivered in a way that did not infringe on formal access to care. In line with the clinic's emphasis on psychological management through 'joviality', perpetrators were 'good-humouredly but roundly rated in front of their fellow patients', with the author noting that 'whilst these scoldings were always taken in good part, they seemed to have an excellent effect'.[92]

The semi-public management of early clinics seemingly faded over time, and may well not have been replicated elsewhere. Similarly, despite some clear reflection on psychological and emotional management in medical texts, systematic and extended reflection was often implicit rather than explicit. During the 1930s, however, a new source for constituting patient identity emerged and assumed the mantle of managing psychological outlook and emotional life: the Diabetic Association (later the British Diabetic Association, or BDA). Consciously formed in the 'mutual aid' tradition, the Association was a mixed professional–lay body created by R. D. Lawrence, his colleagues and patients during 1933–34.[93] Although predominantly run by medical and nursing professionals, the Association was funded by patients and their families, and lay people served on organisational committees.[94] The Association was not unique. Along with their families, medical practitioners and researchers, patients with other long-term conditions had created similar organisations throughout the interwar period.[95] During these years, clinical and public interest in degenerative and chronic conditions had begun to build, and charitable association provided a means to support research and treatment.[96] The BDA, however, was perhaps the most expansive in terms of its focus on the welfare of patients and its efforts to build an identity around a given disease.[97] Demonstrating the complex networks of medical institutions, state provision and professional surveillance in which self-care was embedded, the Association supplemented its advice literature and patient education efforts with lobbying the government and health services on a wide range of issues affecting people with diabetes. Access to clinics, provision of medications and staffing, the education and care of children with diabetes, rationing allowances and employment discrimination against people with diabetes were of considerable interest to the BDA during the first three decades of its existence, the latter of particular concern due to the connection between work, identity and pensions.[98]

The *Diabetic Journal* was the main public outlet for the Association's views, produced for subscribers. It was through this publication – renamed *Balance* in 1961 – that the Association sought to construct a new 'diabetic' identity for people with the condition, and to constitute selves oriented to maintaining physiological balance. Throughout the decades under discussion, the *Journal* used numerous genres and techniques to achieve this aim. Alongside appeals for, and news on, the Association itself, the periodical carried articles on the latest research into diabetes and therapeutic innovations. It revised food tables, produced 'diabetic recipes', and published regular correspondence sections with question and answer pages. It also carried frequent 'personal' stories about patient experiences, covering everything from receiving diagnosis and struggles with treatment, to experiences of holidays and other activities supposedly deemed unsuitable for patients with complex care needs. In later years, it also celebrated famous achievements of people with diabetes, partly extending the Association's historic – and very public – connections with figures like H. G. Wells.

Although rarely drawing on systematic psychological models, editorials and personal reflections were particularly important for the Association's efforts to manage psychological life and cultivate adherence to professional advice about physiological balance. As with Lawrence's ode to willpower, the *Journal*'s reportage and personal stories could be aspirational in tone. They suggested that patients should not be limited in their goals or activity, stressing that – with proper attention to self-care – patients could live a full life. Notably, the tone of articles could vary. Some, for instance, were keen to emphasise that self-care need not be a problematic, or even noticeable, part of a patient's existence. This was the case with certain reports on holidays, the frequency of which probably reflected the middle-class membership of the Association. One article, describing an author's lengthy cycling holiday with his wife, ran for fourteen pages but only detailed self-care practices during the final four paragraphs.[99] Despite self-management being a notable daily feature, the work of self-care was largely hidden from the reader, whose own temporal investment in the piece perhaps provided an opportunity for (vicarious) escape. The article offered rich descriptions of holiday pleasures – hotels, social interactions, physical exertion and 'the open rugged grandeur of the [Highlands] mountains' – a sense of what could be for patients, without puncturing the dream with the labour of self-care. Indeed, even when self-management appeared, the author acknowledged that he was 'unable to carry out my proper tests on tour', instead relying 'entirely on my very developed sense of balance'. This was not recommended as 'a good method in general practice', but perhaps such a relief from duty added to the allure.[100]

By contrast, other material stressed the importance of firm regulation. For instance, the author of one reflection on diagnosis and years of treatment attributed their persistent good health to 'two things': 'firstly to refusing any article of foodstuffs not included in my very liberal diet chart, and, secondly, to taking plenty of exercise all year round'. Even here, however, self-care was downplayed as fitting within regular life. The author recalled how daily injections began as 'something I disliked very much', but soon became a matter of 'mere routine', with morning insulin fitting 'unconsciously into the usual round of shaving, bathing and dressing'. 'Normal life' remained undisturbed, with the author noting that they were able to work 'harder than ever' (being 'fully competent to meet the extra strain'), and recalling that they were able to successfully negotiate '16 days' holiday on the continent … despite considerable difficulties in the way of obtaining correct food'.[101] These personal stories found support in later editorials that emphasised how 'the diabetic routine need not intrude unduly on your activities', and could leave 'plenty of opportunity for the major and minor pleasures of life' if not followed with 'fanaticism'.[102] Similarly, even when acknowledging that there is 'not one of us who does not need to go on striving towards the perfect balance in diabetes, mentally, spiritually, and physically', such claims were motivational, promising that a renewed engagement with self-care routines could be 'rewarded by a happier and better state of health'.[103] Through such articles, the journal looked to ensure emotional balance by countering negative introspection and harnessing optimism for long-term motivation.

Modelling aspirational, 'good' behaviour was not the sole means that the Association deployed to manage public perceptions and facilitate self-care. Their advice literature could also mobilise the figure of a bad diabetic 'other' to this end, often through short references. For example, the author of one article, titled 'A young diabetic in business', concluded by declaring that 'whatever else I do, I shan't let the diabetic side down. They'll never find me in a coma or silly from an overdose of insulin and come to the conclusion that diabetics are unreliable employees.' Just as the invocation of 'the diabetic side' was designed to interpellate its readers with a positive 'diabetic' identity, the 'bad', imbalanced diabetic served as a warning to readers. The possible damage done to the collective by poor individual behaviour, the piece implied, should be enough to encourage adherence to medical norms.[104]

Extended personal reflections were also used to contextualise experiences. Outlining her own response to disease and treatment over nine years, one author wrote in 1938 about her life since diagnosis as a period of 'unhappy ups and downs ... and ... final satisfactory adjustment'. The author noted how her first response had been to 'withdraw from my usual activities, to keep myself safely alone where no contact emphasised my difference'.[105] Eventually, 'pride and necessity ended this withdrawal'. The author gained 'familiarity with the rules' that offered 'courage to disregard some of them', and 'associates' became used to her routine. From the outside – and judging from the norms of self-care advice – the author had 'apparently fitted diabetes into my life'. However, 'self-consciousness didn't end when the routine was set', and 'superficia[l]' adjustment couldn't stop the fact that 'subconsciously there remained a barrier'. The author tried to make her life like those of 'other people', but though she 'ate as I pleased and seldom bothered with the tests', she 'worried all the time': 'for all the fun I had', the author confessed, 'I might as well have gone to prison'. A worsening of her condition followed, as did a month-long hospital admission and stricter regime, and after another 'relapse' the author ended up back in hospital due to 'frequent insulin reactions'. This stay, however, helped her to 'thin[k] of myself as a diabetic'.[106] Whereas she had previously 'schooled myself to ignore what [the words] meant, because I disliked them', now she 'gradually ... admitted the handicap I had'.[107] She no longer 'required energy to pull against' her condition, and saw that 'a diabetic could live a well-rounded life, accepting the meaning of being a diabetic, realising his limitations and adjusting life accordingly'. 'Without knowing it … I was free … Suddenly … the future I wanted grew pleasantly possible, because I felt able to attempt it.' By psychologically accepting her condition and its limitations, she could let go of fear and resentment: 'when examined, it was no problem'.[108]

Articles like this had a dual importance for the *Journal*. In some respects, they served as warnings. The author acknowledged, for instance, that her experiences gave her 'the knowledge' and 'the desire to help all other diabetics to avoid bumps in the diabetic road of life'.[109] Indeed, by contrasting her superficial coping with inner turmoil, the author appeared to be encouraging patients to be honest with themselves, and to be constantly vigilant for any affective problems that might eventually lead to dangerous physiological imbalance. On the other hand, such articles could also be seen to provide insight for patients into what their psychological and emotional trajectory could be. The author characterised herself as a normal patient. She suggested that she encountered obstacles, despite the fact that 'I am supposed to be an intelligent, reasonable person, capable of adjusting myself to life'. Similarly, she noted how she had 'looked around at other members of the diabetic clan and talked to them', finding that 'too many of them have in one way or another had the complex, dishonest attitude I had'.[110] Such work thus normalised certain responses and states, and once again held out the hope to readers that their struggles can improve with reflection. In either scenario, articles such as this, published on the hinterland of medical discourse, made plain that emotional stability and psychological management were important to achieving effective self-care, and vice versa.

Conclusion

Armed with a talk titled 'how to be happy though diabetic', the Honorary Secretary of the British Diabetic Association, Mr J. P. McNulty, gave the principal address to the BDA's 1954 general meeting.[111] From the off, McNulty rejected the idea that 'happiness and diabetes are somehow inconsistent'.[112] Rather, he noted, 'happiness comes and goes', and he used his lecture to muse on the barriers to happiness that individuals faced, and the ways that these barriers might be reduced.[113] Though McNulty had no formal medical or psychiatric training – he spent most of his working life in procurement and advertising – his address mobilised psychological terminology, such as references to 'the struggle between ... opposing desires' and the danger of 'a fixed immaturity'.[114] Such allusions did not draw on a particular system of thought, so much as reflect a growing psychologisation of everyday life in postwar Britain, which McNulty freely mixed with a Christian morality and Bible citation.[115]

McNulty's talk, though, was indicative of the shifting ways in which emotional and psychological balance had come to inform discussion of diabetes and self-care by the 1950s. It proposed that happiness came to those who adjusted themselves to the world and their own capacities. 'Might it not ... be better', McNulty suggested, 'to acknowledge one's limitations and accept them with good humour, making the best use we can of those faculties of hand and brain with which we have been endowed, claiming nothing beyond our merits, rejoicing in good fortune and foregoing pride'? By eschewing 'vanities' and 'fears', individuals could reduce 'the barriers to happiness'.[116] Such a call might have been informed by middle-class anxieties around a decline of deference and rising working-class affluence, but the message would certainly have had special significance for people with diabetes.[117] Following the *Diabetic Journal*'s example, McNulty implied that patients who accepted their disease required management would be less liable to dangerous complacency. Indeed, McNulty spent a considerable portion of his talk reminding his audience about self-care regimes and the importance of readjusting 'our nutritional balance' to bodily capabilities.[118]

In part, masculine self-control held the key to both physiological and emotional balance. 'Whether on insulin or not', McNulty claimed, 'the diabetic who wishes to remain healthy must maintain a constant self-discipline.' This self-discipline, though, was not a 'source of unhappiness' for 'it can in fact develop a self-reassurance which resists fear'. So long as 'it does not generate pride', McNulty suggested, 'self-discipline strengthens the moral as well as the physical fibre of man'.[119] Despite his insistence on control, McNulty admitted that there were times when 'despite our care, our diabetes gets out of control'. Whether as the result of illness, or 'emotional disturbances' such as 'a domestic loss, a financial setback, an affront, real or imagined, to our dignity', hyperglycaemia could return. Perhaps worse, integrating discourses on the somatic effects of emotional trauma with newer concerns on mental health,

McNulty suggested that 'unless we check it, depression takes hold of us and joins the prime saboteurs of our health and our peace of mind'. It was only, McNulty concluded, by recognising that misfortune ebbs and flows, and that death is the 'natural destiny of all living things', that patients could either regain control or find peace.[120]

Given McNulty's role in both the BDA and the *Diabetic Journal*, it was unsurprising that his address was reprinted in the *Journal* for members not in the room. Indeed, the talk chimed with McNulty's vision for the publication, which had for years been dedicated to addressing the 'strong momentum of fear' around diabetes inherited 'from the pre-insulin days'. Although also connecting members, giving advice and 'spread[ing] enlightenment', the creators of the *Journal* – like McNulty – saw it as having 'an important role to play' in 'raising diabetic morale', something which was crucial given the 'natural tendency for the "new" diabetic ... to feel unduly depressed' by their diagnosis.[121]

One notable part of McNulty's speech was his quotation of Donne's 'no man is an islande [sic] unto himself'.[122] McNulty used it to encourage patients not to withdraw from society, but its invocation of the relationality of care also usefully highlighted the dynamics of self-care within broader institutional and social arrangements. Discussions of self-care often marginalised an integral part of this relationality, that important elements of self-management – for instance, eating at regular periods or preventing hypoglycaemia – often relied on unacknowledged labour of friends and family. This chapter, however, has sought to show other sides to self-care's relationality. Firstly, it has suggested that healthcare professionals, innovative practices and instruments of care, and new patient organisations were central to the constitution of the self oriented to physiological balance. Patients and their families or friends may have performed the labour, but their new identities and activities were constructed from new social relations and interactions with 'external' sources.[123] Secondly, it has highlighted how these same agencies sought to regulate patients' affective lives. Though such regulation initially emerged from beliefs that emotional shocks could physically manifest in physiological disturbance, clinicians and institutions of the interwar and post-war period increasingly justified attempts to manage psychological life with claims that depressed, complacent or emotionally unstable patients could fail to care for themselves effectively.

Finally, this chapter has indicated how self-care was itself embedded within broader relations of care. As references to medical professionals, special outpatient clinics and a prominent patient association have made clear, responsibility for balance was by no means individualised during this period. Not only did networks of patients and professionals mobilise in new forms of social and political activism, but by 1948 the British state had also assumed a central role in diabetes care by securing access to services, technologies and expertise.[124] There was, moreover, a further balance of interests and reciprocity in these arrangements. Though initially only supporting the care of a minority of the population, the British state increasingly required balanced citizens to engage in productive activity, pay taxes, avoid unnecessary claims and engage with democratic decision-making without turning to extreme alternatives.[125] Even as an individualising 'neoliberal' political philosophy gained greater influence on British policy-making and governance after the mid-1970s, neither the state nor the BDA withdrew support from patients who failed to comply with their interests.[126]

Concepts of balance – political, physiological, psychological and emotional – were thus central to ideas of the 'good diabetic' in the first half of the twentieth century. Although discursively this ideal patient was a self-governing individual, in control of their emotions and bodies, self-care only ever formed one part of treatment for diabetes. Equally, in practice, efforts to constitute the self-balancing subject came from numerous directions, and depended on a range of practices, instruments and social relations. Patients rarely reacted to state, professional or collective efforts to cultivate self-governance in the ways intended.[127] Nonetheless, such efforts were indicative of the complex relations, motivations and politics involved in balancing the self in twentieth-century Britain.

Acknowledgements

The research on which this chapter is based was generously funded by a Wellcome Trust Senior Investigator Award, 'Lifestyle, health and disease: changing concepts of balance in modern medicine', Grant No. 100601/Z/12Z. I would also like to thank Mark Jackson, Laura Salisbury, Lisa Baraitser, Harriet Palfreyman and Gareth Millward for their incisive comments on earlier drafts.

Notes

1 Anon., 'A diabetic's great feat', *Diabetic Journal*, 6:7 (1951), 89.
2 D. Armstrong, 'Actors, patients and agency: a recent history', *Sociology of Health and Illness*, 36:2 (2014), 163–74; Ian Hacking, 'Making up people', in H. C. Heller, M. Sosna and D. E. Wellbery (eds), *Reconstructing Individualism: Autonomy, Individuality and the Self in Western Thought* (Stanford: Stanford University Press, 1986), pp. 222–36.
3 On the development and contestation of such ideas beyond diabetes, see M. Jackson, *The Age of Stress: Science and the Search for Stability* (Oxford: Oxford University Press, 2013), pp. 56–62.
4 Anon., 'A diabetic's great feat', p. 89.
5 M. Thomson, *Psychological Subjects: Identity, Culture and Health in Twentieth-Century Britain* (Oxford: Oxford University Press, 2006); M. Shapira, *The War Inside: Psychoanalysis, Total War, and the Making of the Democratic Self in Postwar Britain* (Cambridge: Cambridge University Press, 2013); C. Langhamer, 'An archive of feeling? Mass Observation and the mid-century moment', *Insights*, 9:0 (2016), 1–12; T. Chettiar, '"More than a contract?": The emergence of a state-supported marriage welfare service and the politics of emotional life in post-1945 Britain', *Journal of British Studies*, 55:3 (2016), 566–91.
6 Chettiar refers to 'depth psychology' as all forms of psychological knowledge predicated on the existence of an unconscious: Chettiar, '"More than a contract?"', p. 567, n.6. For the history and variety of such models: Thomson, *Psychological Subjects*; R. Hayward, *The Transformation of the Psyche in British Primary Care, 1870–1970* (London: Bloomsbury Academic, 2014).
7 On 'will', information and psychological persuasion in public health campaigns, see Chapters 3 and 4. On the scientific status of emotions in response to perceived excess emotionality of Nazism, see M. Jackson, 'Medical and scientific understandings', in J. Davidson and J. Damousi (eds), *A Cultural History of the Emotions in the Modern and Post-Modern Age* (London: Bloomsbury Academic, 2019), pp. 19–36.
8 N. Rose, *Inventing Our Selves: Psychology, Power, and Personhood* (Cambridge: Cambridge University Press, 1996).
9 Shapira, *The War Inside*. On the relationship of balance to production, see Chapter 7.
10 On the politics of self-help, see Chapters 5, 6 and 9.
11 A. Peterson and D. Lupton, *The New Public Health: Health and Self in the Age of Risk* (London: Sage, 1997); D. Armstrong, *A New History of Identity: A Sociology of Medical Knowledge* (Basingstoke: Palgrave, 2002); and Chapter 10.

12 On the development and limits of physiological perspectives: Jackson, *The Age of Stress*, pp. 62–75; C. Lawrence, 'Moderns and ancients: the "new cardiology" in Britain, 1880–1930', *Medical History*, 29:5 (1985), 1–33; C. Lawrence, *Rockefeller Money, The Laboratory and Medicine in Edinburgh, 1919–1930: New Science in an Old Country* (New York: University of Rochester Press, 2005).
13 Anon., 'Treatment of diabetes', in I. Burney Yeo, Raymond Crawfurd and E. Farquhar Buzzard (eds), *A Manual of Medical Treatment and Clinical Therapeutics*, vol. 2, 5th edition (London: Cassell and Co., 1913), pp. 519–48, at p. 519. For ancient Greek conceptions of balance: L. I. Conrad, M. Neve, V. Nutton, R. Porter and A. Wear, *The Western Medical Tradition, 800 BC to AD 1800* (Cambridge: Cambridge University Press, 2003), pp. 23–31.
14 Anon., 'Modern views on diabetes', *Lancet*, 192:4950 (1918), 49.
15 Anon., 'Treatment of diabetes', pp. 525–6.
16 P. J. Cammidge, 'The dietetic treatment of diabetes', *Lancet*, 179:4621 (1912), 788–90, at p. 788.
17 C. Feudtner, 'Pathway to health: juvenile diabetes and the origins of managerial medicine', in A. M. Stern and H. Markel (eds), *Formative Years: Children's Health in the United States, 1880–2000* (Ann Arbor, MI: University of Michigan Press, 2002), pp. 208–32.
18 Anon., '"Cures" for diabetes', *Lancet*, 186:4813 (1915), 1207.
19 Anon., 'Modern views on diabetes', p. 49; O. Leyton, 'The modern treatment of diabetes mellitus', *British Medical Journal [BMJ]*, 1:2930 (1917), 252–4.
20 On the relative importance of clinical, subjective and biochemical indicators: Anon., 'Treatment of diabetes', pp. 519–20, 528–38.
21 M. Bliss, *The Discovery of Insulin*, 25th anniversary edition (Chicago: University of Chicago, 2007).
22 R. D. Lawrence, *The Diabetic Life: Its Control by Diet and Insulin: A Concise Practical Manual for Practitioners and Patients*, 1st edition (London: J. A. Churchill, 1925), p. 31.
23 Ibid., p. 4, p. 6 respectively.
24 Ibid., p. 31.
25 H. P. Himsworth, 'The syndrome of diabetes mellitus and its causes', *Lancet*, 253:6551 (1949), 465–73.
26 H. P. Himsworth, 'The mechanism of diabetes mellitus', *Lancet*, 234:6047 (1939), 171–6.
27 Anon., 'Diabetes and sanatogen', *Diabetic Journal*, 1:11 (1937), 5; Anon., 'Diabetes mellitus and hormone imbalance', *BMJ*, 2:5265 (1961), 1484. On neo-humoralism, see Jackson, *The Age of Stress*, pp. 63–4.

28 Lawrence, *Rockefeller Money*, pp. 276–85. Also: Feudtner, 'Pathway to health', pp. 217–23.
29 P. J. Cammidge, *The Insulin Treatment of Diabetes Mellitus* (Edinburgh: E&S Livingstone, 1924), pp. 152–3.
30 E. L. Furdell, *Fatal Thirst: Diabetes in Britain until Insulin* (Leiden: Brill, 2009), p. 154. In general, glycosuria only occurred once blood glucose levels were elevated above 'normal' levels, and ketones only when metabolism was seriously impaired beyond that. Practitioners considered 'normal' levels of glycaemia to vary during the day, between 80mg/100ml and 120mg/100ml 'fasting', and between 130mg/100ml and 170mg/100ml up to two hours post-eating. The level at which sugar passed from the blood to the urine was termed the 'leak point'. This point could vary in different individuals, though contemporary knowledge positioned leakage to occur when blood glucose levels reached 180mg/100ml: Lawrence, *The Diabetic Life*, 1st edition, pp. 19–22. The gap between these two points concerned some clinicians, as removing glucose from the urine alone might not correct metabolic problems. Blood sugar could remain above 120mg/100ml for much of the day without showing in the urine, and undermine attempts to restore pancreatic activity through physiological rest.
31 M. D. Moore, 'Food as medicine: diet, diabetes management, and the patient in twentieth century Britain', *Journal of the History of Medicine and Allied Sciences*, 73:2 (2018), 150–67, at pp. 155–9. On glycosuria monitoring: A. C. Begg, *Insulin in General Practice: A Concise Clinical Guide for Practitioners* (London: William Heinemann, 1924), pp. 82–3; H. P. Himsworth, 'Management of diabetes, part II', *BMJ*, 2:3942 (1936), 188–90. Some clinicians maintained the importance of blood sugar estimations during early treatment, and periodically thereafter, as a means to assess metabolic status, check for misleading 'leak points', and to make changes of regimen safer: R. D. Lawrence, *The Diabetic Life: Its Control by Diet and Insulin: A Concise Practical Manual for Practitioners and Patients*, 6th edition (London: J. A. Churchill, 1931), pp. 49–60, 164.
32 C. Sinding, 'Flexible norms? From patients' values to physicians' standards', in W. Ernst (ed.), *Histories of the Normal and the Abnormal: Social and Cultural Histories of Norms and Normativity* (London: Routledge, 2006), pp. 225–44, at pp. 232–5; R. B. Tattersall, *Diabetes: The Biography* (Oxford: Oxford University Press, 2009), pp. 85–9.
33 J. C. Prestwich, 'The diet in diabetes', *BMJ*, 1:4299 (1943), 676.
34 R. H. Micks, 'The diet in diabetes', *BMJ*, 1:4297 (1943), 598–600; G. Luntz, 'The diet in diabetes', *BMJ*, 2:4304 (1943), 21.

35 D. M. Dunlop, 'Are diabetic degenerative complications preventable?', *BMJ*, 2:4884 (1954), 383–5.
36 Anon., '"Free diet" in diabetes', *BMJ*, 1:4715 (1951), 1133–4.
37 R. D. Lawrence, *The Diabetic Life: Its Control by Diet and Insulin and Oral Treatment by Sulphonyl-Ureas: A Concise Practical Manual*, 16th edition (London: J. A. Churchill, 1960), p. 93.
38 Moore, 'Food as medicine'.
39 Sinding, 'Flexible norms?', pp. 235–6.
40 G. F. Walker, 'Reflections on diabetes mellitus: answers to a questionary', *Lancet*, 262:6800 (1953), 1329–32. Most respondents believed hyperglycaemia was connected to complications, yet half aimed for normoglycaemia, and half for mild hyperglycaemia.
41 Tattersall, *Diabetes*, p. 11. Self-care was probably performed by sufferers of similar symptomatic conditions not given the label 'diabetes' (most notably in non-Greek traditions). Discussion here is restricted to subjects classified as having 'diabetes' (however defined) to avoid retrospective and cross-cultural application of contemporary biomedical knowledge.
42 Furdell, *Fatal Thirst*, pp. 1–37.
43 It appears that some patients were even admitted for months, especially with co-morbidities – see Lawrence, *Rockefeller Money*, pp. 293–6, 300–2. Oral testimonies indicate two-week stays for children on wards in the 1930s: interview with M. Elliott conducted by the University of Oxford, 7 December 2004, available at www.diabetes-stories.com/interview.asp?UID=33, accessed July 2018. On admission, see Lawrence, *The Diabetic Life*, 6th edition, p. 38.
44 Begg, *Insulin in General Practice*, pp. 86–7. State-centric approaches to diabetes attracted some praise in Britain during the 1930s: E. A. Steele, 'The treatment of diabetics in the USSR', *Diabetic Journal*, 1:11 (1937), 16–18.
45 C. Webster, *The Health Services Since the War, Volume I: Problems of Health Care, The National Health Service Before 1957* (London: HMSO, 1988).
46 M. D. Moore, *Managing Diabetes, Managing Medicine: Chronic Disease and Clinical Bureaucracy in Post-War Britain* (Manchester: Manchester University Press, 2019), pp. 50–1.
47 Ibid.; J. B. Walker, 'Field work of a diabetic clinic', *Lancet*, 262:6783 (1953), 445–7.
48 T. H. Marshall, *Citizenship and Social Class and Other Essays* (Cambridge: Cambridge University Press, 1950).
49 Bevan quoted in '"Houses in great numbers"', *The Times*, 4 January 1946, p. 4.

50 G. Millward, *Vaccinating Britain: Mass Vaccination and the Public since the Second World War* (Manchester: Manchester University Press, 2019); V. Berridge, 'Medicine and the public: the 1962 report of the Royal College of Physicians and the new public health', *Bulletin of the History of Medicine*, 81:1 (2007), 286–311. See also Chapters 3 and 4.
51 Read in this light, appeals in one text for patients to take good care of themselves, adding 'no invalidism, please', take on new meaning: Lawrence, *The Diabetic Life*, 16th edition, p. 192.
52 D. M. Lyon, 'Prognosis in diabetes mellitus', *Lancet*, 199:5152 (1922), 1043–5, at p. 1045.
53 Ibid., p. 1045.
54 C. J. C. Earl, 'Treatment of diabetics as hospital out-patients', *BMJ*, 1:3461 (1927), 831–3, at p. 832; Begg, *Insulin in General Practice*, p. 86.
55 Lawrence, *The Diabetic Life*, 1st edition. On the labour of daily self-care: C. Feudtner, *Bittersweet: Diabetes, Insulin, and the Transformation of Illness* (Carolina: Carolina University Press, 2003), pp. 89–120.
56 Lyon, 'Prognosis in diabetes mellitus', p. 1045.
57 D. Willems, 'Managing one's body using self-management techniques: practicing autonomy', *Theoretical Medicine and Bioethics*, 21:1 (2000), 23–38.
58 Earl, 'Treatment of diabetics as hospital out-patients', p. 832.
59 Begg, *Insulin in General Practice*, p. 86.
60 J. G. L. Jackson, 'R. D. Lawrence and the formation of the Diabetic Association', *Diabetic Medicine*, 13:1 (1996), 9–21.
61 Lawrence, *The Diabetic Life*, 1st edition, pp. 59–60; Furdell, *Fatal Thirst*, p. 154.
62 Moore, 'Food as medicine', pp. 157–60.
63 Ibid., pp. 9–10.
64 Lawrence, *The Diabetic Life*, 6th edition, pp. 162–4.
65 Ibid., p. vii.
66 Ibid., p. 139.
67 Moore, 'Food as medicine', p. 9.
68 D. E. Hall, *Muscular Christianity: Embodying the Victorian Age* (Cambridge: Cambridge University Press, 1994); M. Sinha, *Colonial Masculinity: The 'Manly Englishman' and the 'Effeminate Bengali' in the Late Nineteenth Century* (Manchester: Manchester University Press, 1995); J. Tosh, *Manliness and Masculinities in Nineteenth-Century Britain: Essays on Gender, Family and Empire* (Harlow: Pearson Longman, 2005). On the contested after-lives of such constructions: M. Francis, 'The domestication of the male? Recent research on nineteenth and twentieth-century British masculinity', *The Historical Journal*, 45:3 (2002), 637–52;

A. McLaren, *Playboys and Mayfair Men: Crime, Class, Masculinity, and Fascism in 1930s London* (Baltimore: Johns Hopkins University Press, 2017). On masculinity and balance, see Chapter 5.

69 S. O'Donnell, 'Changing social and scientific discourses on type 2 diabetes between 1800 and 1950: a socio-historical analysis', *Sociology of Health and Illness*, 37:7 (2015), 1102–21; I. Sutherland, 'Variations in occupational mortality between and within the social classes', *British Journal of Social Medicine*, 1:2 (1947), 126–34. In 1931, Lawrence suggested that diabetes occurred 'in both sexes at any age, but is more common in middle and late life, and probably in men than in women': Lawrence, *The Diabetic Life*, 6th edition, p. 9.

70 I. Zweiniger-Bargielowska, 'Building a British superman: physical culture in interwar-Britain', *Journal of Contemporary History*, 41:4 (2006), 595–610; J. Tomlinson, *The Politics of Decline: Understanding Post-War Britain* (Harlow: Pearson, 2001); B. Harrison, *Seeking a Role: The United Kingdom, 1951–1970* (Oxford: Oxford University Press, 2009).

71 J. Bourke, 'Love and limblessness: male heterosexuality, disability, and the Great War', *Journal of War and Culture Studies*, 9:1 (2016), 3–19. The idea of 'mastering' one's body was also prominent in efforts to address a range of conditions during the mid-century, not least stress: Jackson, *The Age of Stress*, pp. 177–80.

72 J. Lawrence, *Diabetes, Insulin and the Life of RD Lawrence* (London: Royal Society of Medicine Press, 2012).

73 On the gendered welfare state: J. Clarke and J. Newman, *The Managerial State: Power, Politics and Ideology in the Remaking of Social Welfare* (London: Sage, 1997), pp. 2–4.

74 Interview with M. Winn conducted by the University of Oxford, 2 December 2004, available at www.diabetes-stories.com/transcript.asp?UID=31, accessed July 2018. Training could be patchy, however, and in some instances non-existent: interview with Grace conducted by the University of Oxford, 3 August 2004, available at www.diabetes-stories.com/interview.asp?UID=13, accessed July 2018; interview with Roy conducted by the University of Oxford, 29 October 2007, available at www.diabetes-stories.com/interview.asp?UID=85, accessed July 2018.

75 On discourses of intelligence and class: O'Donnell, 'Changing social and scientific discourses', pp. 1102–21. Public debate about 'ignorant' patients also hung over questions of insulin use: Furdell, *Fatal Thirst*, p. 155.

76 Leyton, 'The modern treatment of diabetes mellitus', p. 253.

77 On the importance of 'others' to self-identity: E. Said, *Orientalism* (London: Penguin, 2003).

78 D. Arnold, 'Diabetes in the tropics: race, place, and class in India, 1880–1965', *Social History of Medicine*, 22:2 (2009), 245–61, at p. 258.
79 Wellcome Library Archives, P9890, The British Diabetic Association, 'Healthy Asian cooking: a guide for people from the Indian subcontinent', 1996; R. Bivins, *Contagious Communities: Medicine, Migration, and the NHS in Post-war Britain* (Oxford: Oxford University Press, 2015).
80 See also Jackson, 'Medical and scientific understandings'.
81 Furdell, *Fatal Thirst*, pp. 135–6; O'Donnell, 'Changing social and scientific discourses', pp. 1108–11.
82 Anon., 'Treatment of diabetes', p. 527.
83 W. Hale White, 'An address on glycosuria', *Lancet*, 183:4719 (1914), 367–73, at p. 370.
84 Leyton, 'The modern treatment of diabetes mellitus', p. 254.
85 Lawrence, *The Diabetic Life*, 6th edition, p. 10.
86 Anon., 'Evening clinics for diabetics', *Diabetic Journal*, 2:14 (1938), 18.
87 F. C. Eve, 'Diabetic treatment simplified', *BMJ*, 1:3362 (1925), 1033–5, at p. 1033.
88 On insulin's introduction to Britain via the Medical Research Council: J. Liebenau, 'The MRC and the pharmaceutical industry: the model of insulin', in J. Austoker and L. Bryder (eds), *Historical Perspectives on the Roles of the MRC: Essays in the History of the Medical Research Council of the United Kingdom and its Predecessor, the Medical Research Committee, 1913–1953* (Oxford: Oxford University Press, 1989), pp. 163–80; Moore, *Managing Diabetes, Managing Medicine*, p. 22, n.115.
89 Ibid., pp. 50–1, 53–4, 63–6.
90 Earl, 'Treatment of diabetics', p. 832.
91 M. Foucault, *Discipline and Punish: The Birth of the Prison*, trans. A. Sheridan (London: Penguin, [1975] 1991).
92 Earl, 'Treatment of diabetics', p. 832.
93 Jackson, 'R. D. Lawrence', pp. 9–21. For mutual aid orientations: H. G. Wells, 'Diabetics in sympathy', *The Times*, 15 February 1934, p. 10.
94 Jackson, 'R. D. Lawrence', pp. 18–19.
95 M. Jackson, *Allergy: The History of a Modern Malady* (London: Reaktion Books, 2006), p. 81.
96 Such organisations were informed by the period's political concerns, such as industrial efficiency and imperial rule: D. Cantor, 'Cortisone and the politics of empire: imperialism and British medicine, 1918–1955', *Bulletin of the History of Medicine*, 67:3 (1993), 463–93.
97 By contrast with organisations for cancer, arthritis and asthma, research funding only slowly became a part of the Association's mission. On post-war single-disease organisations: M. Nicolson and G. Lowis, 'The early

history of the Multiple Sclerosis Society of Great Britain and Northern Ireland: a socio-historical study of lay/practitioner interaction in the context of medical charity', *Medical History*, 46:2 (2002), 141–74.
98 Anon., 'The employment of diabetics', *Diabetic Journal*, 2:17 (1939), 12–14; Moore, *Managing Diabetes, Managing Medicine*, pp. 26–8, 82.
99 Anon., 'Travels on a tandem – II', *Diabetic Journal*, 2:13 (1938), 32–46.
100 Ibid., p. 46.
101 Anon., 'A diabetic's life', *Diabetic Journal*, 1:11 (1937), 27–8, at p. 28.
102 Anon., 'Diabetic routine', *Diabetic Journal*, 6:7 (1951), 79.
103 Anon., 'New Year resolution', *Diabetic Journal*, 5:1 (1946), 8.
104 Anon., 'A young diabetic in business', *Diabetic Journal*, 7:5 (1954), 20.
105 E. Craven, 'With life injected', *Diabetic Journal*, 2:13 (1938), 14–16, at p. 14.
106 Ibid., p. 15.
107 Ibid., pp. 15–16.
108 Ibid., p. 16.
109 Ibid., p. 14.
110 Ibid.
111 Anon., 'How to be happy though diabetic', *Diabetic Journal*, 7:7 (1954), 83–7.
112 Ibid., p. 83.
113 Ibid., p. 84.
114 Ibid. McNulty's engagement in marketing may well have informed his thinking in terms of desires: S. Schwarzkopf, 'Discovering the consumer: market research, brand innovation, and the creation of brand loyalty in Britain and the United States in the interwar years', *Journal of Macromarketing*, 29:1 (2009), 8–20; J. G. L. Jackson, 'J. P. McNulty', *Diabetic Journal*, 9:1 (1959), 19–20.
115 McNulty had been educated by the Irish Christian Brothers as a child. Thomson, *Psychological Subjects*.
116 Anon., 'How to be happy though diabetic', p. 85.
117 J. Moran, 'Queuing up in post-war Britain', *Twentieth Century British History*, 16:3 (2005), 282–305.
118 Anon., 'How to be happy though diabetic', p. 86.
119 Ibid., pp. 86–7.
120 Ibid., p. 87.
121 J. McNulty, 'Twenty five years ago: the Honorary Secretary looks back', *Diabetic Journal*, 9:1 (1959), 9–10, at p. 10.
122 Anon., 'How to be happy though diabetic', p. 84.
123 Hacking, 'Making up people'. As Rose suggests, a division between 'internal' and 'external' is problematic once we question the coherence of the

self as a unified entity: Rose, *Inventing Our Selves*. It is nonetheless useful shorthand if used advisedly.
124 On forms of sociality forged from efforts to cultivate self-managing individuals: A. B. Rodrick, 'The importance of being an earnest improver: class, caste, and "self-help" in mid-Victorian England', *Victorian Literature and Culture*, 29:1 (2001), 39–50.
125 On the creation of the democratic self: Shapira, *The War Inside*.
126 D. Stedman Jones, *Masters of the Universe: Hayek, Friedman, and the Birth of Neoliberal Politics* (Princeton: Princeton University Press, 2014); N. Rollings, 'Cracks in the post-war Keynesian settlement? The role of organised business in Britain in the rise of neoliberalism before Margaret Thatcher', *Twentieth Century British History*, 24:4 (2013), 637–59.
127 Moore, 'Food as medicine'.

3

From the alcoholic to the sensible drinker: alcohol health education campaigns in England

Alex Mold

Introduction

For centuries, the consumption of alcohol has challenged contemporary notions of balance. From Galen and the impact of wine on the four humours, to twenty-first-century worries about 'binge drinking' and alcohol-related violence, too much alcohol upsets the equilibrium of the individual and the society which surrounds them. The question of how much is too much, what the consequences of excessive alcohol consumption might be, and how to deal with the results are, however, less stable. This chapter considers how the notion of balance figured in alcohol health education in England during the 1970s and 1980s. It suggests that the development of campaigns which aimed to promote 'sensible drinking' reflected a shift away from focusing on those already experiencing problems with alcohol, predominantly alcoholics and heavy drinkers. This move was underpinned by changes in the philosophy and practice of public health. During this period, individual behaviour was increasingly seen as both cause and cure for public health problems. The linking of practices like smoking, overeating and alcohol consumption to common conditions such as heart disease, diabetes and cancer meant that individuals and their actions became a legitimate target for public health authorities. Agreeing on the best method for promoting individual behaviour change was, however, much more problematic. Were individuals capable of taking a balanced approach to their health, or did they need to be manoeuvred into doing so?

These issues were underpinned by the evolving relationship between 'the public' and the 'self'. Focusing on a set of local health education campaigns, an expert committee report on alcohol prevention and a public consultation exercise on alcohol, the chapter highlights tensions between different approaches to dealing with drink. Health education efforts were intended to encourage individuals to moderate their alcohol consumption: to behave responsibly by becoming 'sensible drinkers'. Yet, at the same time, considerable scepticism was expressed (even by those involved in the campaigns) about the ability of health education to change behaviour. Other approaches, such as increasing the price of alcohol, were put forward as ways of reducing alcohol consumption at the population level. The apparent political and social unpalatability of such measures, however, forced a return to health education, and the 'sensible drinker' emerged as the cornerstone of alcohol health education policy.

Such an approach speaks to deeper tensions between 'the public' and the 'self' that continue to beset health education today. At first glance, the public and the self would appear to be diametrically opposed. The 'self' conjures up images of the individual: self-centred, selfish, selfie. As Michel Foucault and his followers suggested, the making of modern selves was a project concerned with individual subjectivity.[1] In contrast, 'the public' is more associated with the collective: public spirited, public good, public sphere, public services and so on. The meanings of 'the public' are multiple and contested, but these do tend to cohere around the group rather than the individual.[2] Publics and selves may well come into conflict, as illustrated by long-running debates in public health. In the case of vaccination, for instance, a parent's refusal to vaccinate their child may diminish herd immunity, thus placing the health of the public in jeopardy. But there are all sorts of other ways in which the self and the public intersect and even overlap. As the social epidemiologist Nancy Krieger points out, 'population' and 'individual' are not antonyms.[3] We are simultaneously individuals and populations; selves and publics. The interlocking nature of the self and the public was further reinforced by the added responsibility placed on individuals for their own well-being and public health more broadly during the latter part of the twentieth century.

Some of the ways in which 'the public' and the 'self' overlapped in post-war England can be observed in the public health approach to alcohol. There were tensions within alcohol policy between the supposed needs of the population and the individual, and the self and the public, but there were also ways in which these were mutually constitutive. The chapter will begin by considering the place of the self in post-war public health, particularly in the context of changing patterns of disease and its aetiology. The second section describes how alcohol came to be seen as a public health problem, rather than as a social order issue or purely medical concern. The chapter then moves on to look in more detail at the Health Education Council's (HEC) anti-alcohol campaign in the North East of England during the 1970s. It is suggested that a gradual change in the tactics and focus of the campaign was indicative of a shift towards focusing on the creation of 'sensible drinkers' rather than on alcoholics or heavy drinkers. This could be seen as a move away from concentrating on the imbalance associated with overconsumption and towards the promotion of moderation. The fourth section of the chapter details a contrasting approach to dealing with drink, one that focused not so much on individuals, but on the whole population. Getting everybody to drink less, it was suggested, would result in fewer alcohol problems at the population level. Yet this approach was politically controversial, and population-level measures to curb drinking were not introduced. Instead, as the final section of the chapter outlines, policy became directed towards encouraging the public to 'drink sensibly'. The production of such 'balanced selves' was riven with uncertainty and, despite many decades of policy initiatives, remains largely out of reach.

Public health, the self and individual behaviour

The post-war period was a time when the self seemed to matter in public health more than it had done in the past. Getting people to change their behaviour had long been part of health education, but in the UK and in other high-income countries the linking of lifestyle to disease prompted closer examination of individual ways of living.[4] In Britain, the work of Richard Doll and Austin Bradford Hill in the 1950s on smoking and lung cancer was especially important in connecting individual behaviour to disease. In his classic text of 1957, *Uses of Epidemiology*, the epidemiologist Jerry Morris asserted that 'prevention of disease in the future is likely to be increasingly a matter of individual action and personal responsibility.'[5] As the list of behaviours that were thought to bring about ill health expanded to encompass diet, exercise and alcohol, public health educators began to change their approach to communicating with the public about threats to their health. For instance, the 1964 Cohen report on health education recommended moving away from 'specific action campaigns', such as educating the public about vaccination, and towards areas of what it termed 'self-discipline', such as smoking, overeating and exercise.[6]

By the mid-1970s public health policy was increasingly orientated around the idea that individual behaviour was responsible for many public health problems, and the way to address these was through health education. As Jane Hand indicates in Chapter 4, one of the ways to deal with increasing levels of obesity was through health education. Just as with smoking, individuals could be encouraged, persuaded or frightened (depending on the tactics used) into changing their behaviour so as to improve their health.[7] Taken together, the prioritisation of health education, the focus on managing individual risk and a new emphasis on disease prevention at the personal level was part of what was called the 'new public health'.[8] Such a view was predicated on a particular kind of self – an autonomous individual capable of self-government in response to expert advice.[9] People could choose to respond to illness or maintain their health within a broader culture of 'healthism' that situated the problem of sickness at the individual level.[10] A focus on individual behaviour thus resulted in a conception of the public as a collection of self-governing rational actors able to respond to public health messages and change their behaviours accordingly. The role of the state, from a neo-liberal perspective, was to facilitate the entrepreneurial actions of individuals rather than to create the broader social, economic and political conditions for good health.[11]

Although individually focused health education designed to encourage personal prevention became the dominant method for dealing with public health problems, there was an alternative approach. During the 1970s and 1980s the social, economic and environmental determinants of health began to attract increased attention, especially at the global level through the World Health Organization.[12] Individual behaviour was still important as a factor in disease causation, but the proponents of a social determinants of health approach regarded behaviour as something shaped by wider political, economic, social and environmental factors over which the individual had little control. Placing emphasis on the deeper structural underpinnings of ill health would suggest that health education alone was not enough to combat public health problems. Indeed, if we take a look at one such problem in more detail, we can see that there were tensions between those who wanted to focus on reforming individual behaviour and those who wanted to change the social environment.

Alcohol: a public health problem?

The imbalanced consumption of alcoholic beverages and their effects on drinkers was not a new area of government concern in the 1970s. Alcohol had posed problems in terms of public order, and danger to health and morality for centuries. During the nineteenth century, the habitual consumption of alcohol came to be seen as the disease of 'alcoholism', comprising both medical and moral elements.[13] There were public health dimensions to the alcohol issue, especially around the impact drinking had on industrial production, but drink was not seen as a public health problem. The temperance movement, for instance, rarely intersected with those pressing for sanitarian reform.[14] It was not until the 1950s, when there was an apparent rise in the number of alcoholics, that the disease-based view of alcoholism was 're-discovered', prompting the establishment of dedicated treatment units for individuals with alcohol problems.[15]

A wider appreciation of the difficulties that alcohol could cause began to emerge in the 1960s. Initially, the focus was on drink driving. Measures such as the introduction of the breathalyser in 1967 were designed to protect the public from intoxicated drivers and reduce the number of car accidents.[16] Towards the end of the decade, a more distinct public health view of alcohol problems started to appear. This was prompted by a marked growth in alcohol consumption during the 1960s and 1970s, and with it an increase in alcohol-related illnesses such as cirrhosis of the liver.[17] Alcohol consumption almost doubled between 1950 and the mid-1970s, rising from 5.2 litres of pure alcohol per person to 9.3 litres.[18] Deaths from liver cirrhosis increased from just over 20 per million in 1950 to more than 40 per million by 1970.[19] Alcohol clearly posed a danger to public health, but it was not the established authorities and institutions in public health policy-making and practice that pushed alcohol onto the public health agenda. Instead, a distinct 'alcohol policy network', made up of doctors and researchers who specialised in alcohol and addictions, voluntary organisations and sympathetic civil servants, was instrumental in getting the government to take alcohol issues seriously.[20] This alcohol policy network was able to take the lead in defining alcohol as a public health issue because the traditional bastions of public health practice and policy-making were in disarray in this period. The key public health official, the Medical Officer of Health (MOH), had undergone a gradual diminution in status following the establishment of the NHS.[21] The position of MOH was abandoned altogether when public health services moved out of local government following the reorganisation of the health service in 1973, although it was later replaced with the Director of Public Health role when public health 'returned' to local government in 2012.[22] Academic public health was also undergoing significant change, most notably around the uses of epidemiology to demonstrate causal links between behaviour and disease.[23]

Indeed, it was an epidemiological view of alcohol consumption that helped redefine alcohol as a public health issue. Key members of the British alcohol policy network championed a thesis first put forward in 1956 by the French demographer Sully Ledermann.[24] Ledermann argued that the level of alcohol consumption in a population was related to the extent of alcohol problems in that population. As the total amount of alcohol consumed increased, so too did the number of individuals with alcohol problems such as alcoholism and cirrhosis of the liver. Reducing the amount of alcohol consumed by everyone, whether a problem drinker or not, would result in better health outcomes overall. Moderation was thus not only a desirable individual goal, but an important collective one too. This epidemiological approach to alcohol prompted a series of government reports and investigations by medical professional bodies throughout the late 1970s and early 1980s. As will be discussed further below, there was some support for the idea that tax should be used to increase the price of alcohol (or at least not let it decline further in real terms) so as to decrease population-level consumption, and therefore alcohol-related harms. Such an approach was controversial: a report produced by a government think tank that had suggested the use of taxation to control the price of drink was suppressed.[25] The government was reluctant to use tax policy in this way and fearful of the economic impact such measures would have on the drinks industry, tax revenue and jobs.

Nonetheless, something needed to be done about alcohol problems. The apparent solution was to focus on health education. Here was something that all parties, including health professionals, government and the alcohol industry, could agree on. Health education was unlikely to have a significant impact on the revenue generated from alcohol sales, nor would it be politically or publicly unpopular. Yet this supposed 'island of consensus' was really a mirage.[26] A close examination of the development of alcohol education in the 1970s demonstrates that there was a good deal of conflict, not only between the interested actors but also around the appropriate target: should this be the individual self or the wider public?

The HEC's North East campaigns on alcohol education, 1974–81

In the early 1970s, the newly established Health Education Council (HEC) decided to mount a health education campaign on alcohol. Such a move can be explained by the growing concern in government about alcohol problems, but was also rooted in the HEC's view of public health and its role in promoting it. The HEC saw health as 'more than bodily fitness – that ultimately our concern was to help people live in a state of harmony with themselves and with the community as a whole'.[27] Alcohol problems fitted within this balance-orientated approach. In November 1973, the HEC agreed to run a pilot anti-alcohol campaign in the North East of England.[28] The Council was tasked with delivering health education nationally and locally, although most of their work at the local level was restricted to providing information, leaflets and guidance to local authorities.[29] The North East campaigns on alcohol were different: they were intended to test the approach before rolling the programme out to other regions. Why the North East region was chosen for the pilot is unclear. The fact that the area had the highest alcohol consumption levels for men in the UK was later used to justify its selection, although this irritated local service workers who felt that problems in the North East were no worse than anywhere else in the country.[30] The selected region was also coterminous with the boundaries of the Area Health Authority and the Tyne Tees television area, facilitating the distribution of TV advertisements. The HEC's alcohol education programme in the North East was divided into three distinct phases. The first was in 1974; the second between 1977 and 1979; and the final phase occurred in 1981. Each campaign adopted a different approach, and the difficulties encountered reveal varied aspects of the problems underpinning alcohol health education.

'Everybody likes a drink. Nobody likes a drunk.', 1974

The first stage of the HEC's anti-alcohol programme began in October 1974. It aimed to increase professional awareness of alcohol problems and to establish the feasibility of health education about alcohol problems.[31] The campaign cost £88,000, with £60,000 being spent on TV, press and poster advertisements.[32] The campaign material was designed by the advertising agency, Saatchi & Saatchi. The HEC had used Saatchi & Saatchi previously to create health education material, including a controversial image of a naked pregnant woman smoking.[33] The advertisements that the agency designed for the anti-alcohol campaign were equally provocative. Based around the tag line 'Everybody likes a drink. Nobody likes a drunk.', the advertisements attempted to convey some of the dangers of heavy drinking; the signs and symptoms indicative of problems due to heavy drinking; and where to get help.[34] The posters used for the campaign were stark and simple, with no visual imagery beyond the slogan itself, and a further exhortation to 'Drink in moderation' and not 'let alcohol go to your head'. The HEC felt that the central slogan 'would be a powerful and positive message to adopt, without exposing the Council to accusations of being killjoys'.[35] Yet, not everyone agreed. Local psychiatrist Anthony Thorley argued that the slogan was 'criticised and misunderstood by many North-easterners. Not everybody does like a drink. People are not all agreed as to what a "drunk" is. One man's "sensible drinking" is another man's stupidity'.[36] The Medical Council on Alcoholism and the Alcohol Education Centre also objected to the tag line, preferring 'Almost everybody likes a drink'.[37]

Criticism of the campaign went beyond its tag line. The campaign was intended to be a piece of primary prevention – that is, it was designed to stop alcohol problems from developing. Yet the focus of the advertisements, and even the way that the agency and the HEC described the campaign, suggested that the target group was those already using alcohol excessively, such as alcoholics and heavy drinkers, rather than

Everybody likes a drink.

Nobody likes a drunk.

Drink in moderation. Don't let alcohol go to your head.

If you're worried about the amount you drink, see your doctor or contact:
The North East Council on Alcoholism, Mea House, Ellison Place, Newcastle upon Tyne. NE1 8XS Tel: Newcastle upon Tyne 20792

The Health Education Council

3.1 'Everybody likes a drink. Nobody likes a drunk.' Saatchi & Saatchi for the Health Education Council, 1974

the general population. The HEC tended to refer to their efforts as the 'anti-alcoholism campaign' and saw the fact that over 900 people contacted treatment services in the wake of the campaign as a sign of its success.[38] On the ground in the North East, local alcohol agency workers were less convinced. Services were overwhelmed and they lacked the capacity to assist everyone who came forward for help.[39] An evaluation of the campaign suggested that while penetration was high there was little lasting change in attitudes towards drinking or drinking behaviour.[40]

'It's always the boozer who's the loser', 1977–79

The HEC took on board some of the criticisms made of the 1974 campaign when designing a second phase, which ran between 1977 and 1979. This stage of the campaign had similar aims to the first phase, and initially used the same material, but later developed new resources under the slogan 'It's always the boozer who's the loser.' Fresh visual and audio-visual material was commissioned by the HEC, which again made use of Saatchi & Saatchi. The agency produced 'playlets' which were shown on Tyne Tees TV and in local cinemas. These advertisements were criticised by local agencies, which regarded them as still too focused on alcoholics rather than on everyday drinkers. Moreover, the campaign betrayed a lack of understanding of the local population. Voices of the actors in the advertisements had Yorkshire accents rather than those of people from the North East, and the content of the commercials was too geared to a 'middle class view of life'.[41] Thorley argued that one of the posters, which featured a picture of manicured female hand reaching for a bottle of vodka, was a 'jet-set' image that did not resonate in the North East. Another poster focused on the effect that alcohol could have on men's sexual performance. Making use of the universal symbol for male, the poster suggested that having too much to drink could result in erectile dysfunction, or 'brewer's droop'. The poster won an advertising prize, but not everyone viewing the poster understood the symbols.[42] Thorley suggested that 'in the North-east the vast majority of people had no idea at all what the symbols represented. One wit even queried whether it represented a crashed Volvo car!'[43]

Another poster featured an image of a crying child. Her dirty, bruised face was streaked with tears, and the strapline read: 'Eight pints of beer and four large whiskies a day aren't doing her any good.' Once again, Thorley felt that the image was misunderstood, and though the poster 'became well known throughout the region' a 'minority thought it was the *girl* who had been drinking!'[44]

Misunderstood or not, these posters indicated a change of tactics and focus. Both posters appealed to the emotions of the viewer in order

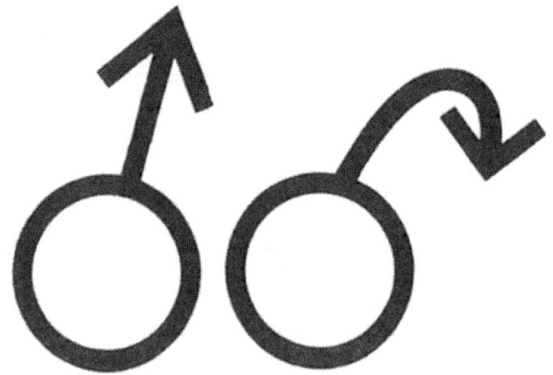

3.2 'If you drink too much there's one part that every beer can reach.' Saatchi & Saatchi for the Health Education Council, 1979

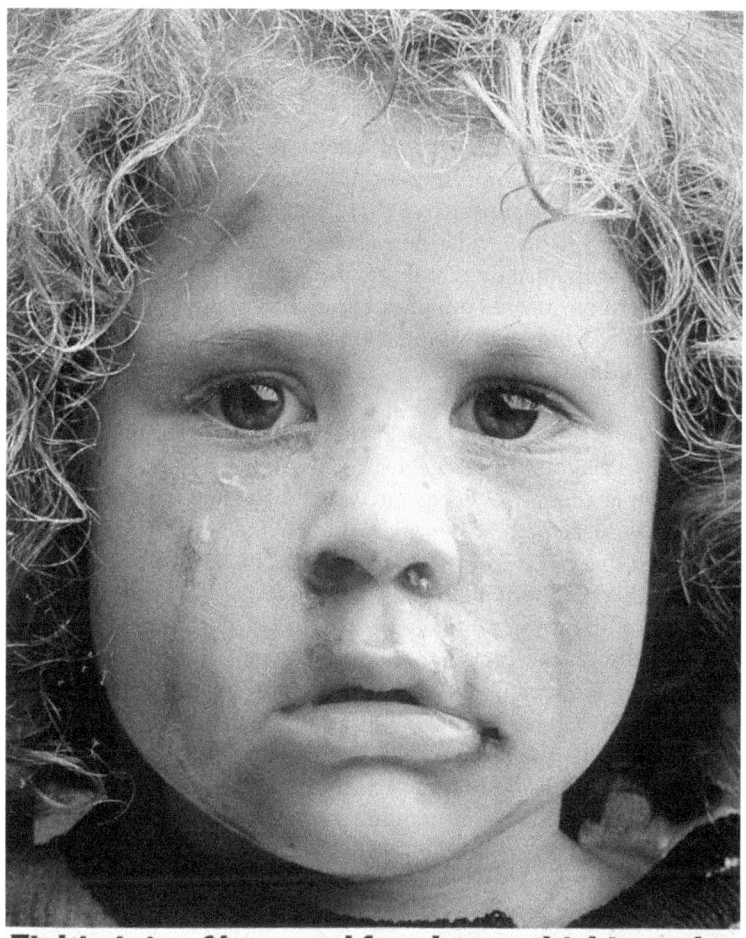

3.3 'Eight pints of beer and four large whiskies a day aren't doing her any good.' Saatchi & Saatchi for the Health Education Council, 1979

to provoke reflection on the amount of alcohol s/he consumed. The 'brewer's droop' poster made use of humour to encourage the viewer to think about the consequences of heavy drinking for themselves and for their sexual partner. The 'battered child' poster focused on the damage alcohol could cause to an 'innocent victim', a trope found in nineteenth-century temperance material and in more contemporary public health campaigns, such as those around smoking.[45] The posters drew attention to the wider consequences of alcohol consumption, beyond the individual drinker themselves, thus emphasising the social dimension to the alcohol problem, rather than purely the medical one. This was reinforced by the impression that the posters appeared to be aimed at ordinary (albeit 'heavy' or 'excessive') drinkers rather than alcoholics.

The second phase of the campaign came to an end in 1979. According to an evaluation of the campaign, the HEC reported that it had decided to abandon its efforts due to lack of action and coordination on the ground, something denied by those in the North East.[46] Thorley contended that by '1979 it was clear that the media work, now costing almost half a million pounds, was ineffective and increasingly embarrassing to all concerned'.[47] For their part, Saatchi & Saatchi were also dissatisfied with the campaign, finding the central brief, to focus on encouraging moderation in drinking, a difficult task to fulfil.[48] Indeed, the campaign material gave little indication as to what 'moderate' drinking consisted of. The 'battered child' poster did appear to suggest that eight pints of beer and four large whiskies a day was 'too much', but setting limits to alcohol consumption formed a more central part of the campaign's third phase, in 1981.

'Why spoil a good thing?', 1981

The final stage of the HEC's anti-alcohol campaign in the North East was framed around a desire to promote 'moderate drinking'. Those involved in devising the campaign wanted it to focus on heightening awareness of alcohol problems rather than cutting the consumption of alcohol *per se*.[49] The HEC dropped Saatchi & Saatchi, and instead made use of a Newcastle-based advertising agency, Redlands. The agency devised new campaign materials featuring local TV presenter and botanist, David Bellamy. Bellamy was chosen by Redlands because they felt that he would be seen by the public as intelligent and honest, but would also be able to connect with the intended audience as he was from the North East and a drinker himself.[50] The advertisements offered guidance on how much alcohol was 'too much' (five pints of beer or more) and also suggested a level of moderate consumption as being 'something like two or three pints two or three times a week'. Indeed, the benefits of moderate alcohol consumption were tacitly acknowledged by the campaign's tag line, 'Why spoil a good thing?'

The Bellamy campaign also offered a more precise sense of how balance in relation to alcohol could be calculated than the previous posters. Some saw the campaign's issuing of guidance on levels of alcohol consumption as more informative and less moralising than previous messages.[51] The promotion of moderation in consumption, whether it be of alcohol or other foodstuffs, was nothing new, but the setting of drinking limits was controversial.[52] There was little agreement among experts about what a 'safe' level of drinking consisted of. In their 1979 report, the Royal College of Psychiatrists suggested that four pints, four double whiskies or one bottle of wine a day 'constitute reasonable guidelines of the upper limit of drinking'.[53] Other experts were concerned that setting an upper limit would encourage people to drink up to that level in the belief that their behaviour could do no harm.[54] Yet others insisted that, although there was no clear evidence about what amount of alcohol increased the risk of particular conditions and by how much, guidelines were helpful as a way of changing attitudes to drinking.[55] Indeed, devising guidance around safe alcohol consumption limits became a feature of alcohol policy in the mid-1980s, but this campaign was one of the first to attempt to communicate information about 'sensible drinking' to the wider public.

A survey conducted in the North East following the Bellamy campaign suggested that the core message around moderate drinking did get through to the local population. More than two-thirds of the 750 people interviewed recalled the campaign, and all but four could remember something relevant when questioned about the main message of the campaign. When asked if the campaign had changed their behaviour, 12.7 per cent claimed that it had, but only three people said that they had tried to drink less.[56] As an evaluation of the campaign pointed out, it had not been designed to change behaviour and, based on its original goal of raising public awareness about moderate alcohol consumption, the campaign could be judged a modest success.[57] However, the HEC's

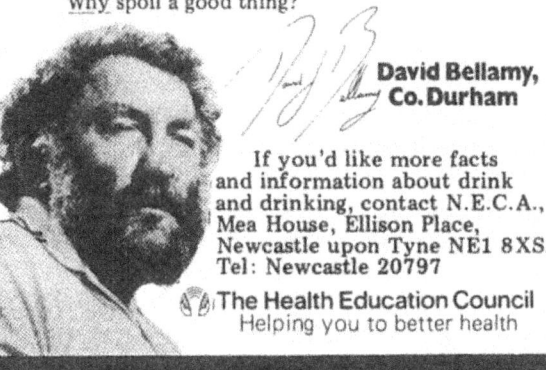

3.4 'If you're drinking five pints of beer or more everyday...' Redlands for the Health Education Council, 1981

paymasters, the Department of Health and Social Security (DHSS), were less convinced. The department and its ministers were aware that changing behaviour was challenging and time-consuming. In 1981, the Secretary of State for Social Services, Patrick Jenkin, told a meeting of the National Council on Alcoholism that it 'is difficult to modify social attitudes and difficult to measure what, if anything, has been achieved. Health education is a long haul.' But he also remarked that at 'a time when money is clearly limited, Ministers and all concerned need to be convinced that the available resources will be used to good effect'.[58] The HEC was under pressure to demonstrate the cost-effectiveness of its work but was unsure that alcohol health education would reduce alcohol consumption, at least directly. The Council's alcohol programme strategy for 1982–83 argued that many forces influenced alcohol consumption, and as a result 'health education **by itself** [original emphasis] has only a limited ability to reduce it'. Other measures, such as greater control of alcohol, and aiming to reduce per capita consumption, also had a part to play in dealing with alcohol-related harm.[59]

Taken together, the three phases of the HEC's alcohol education campaign in the North East point to an evolution in targets, techniques and tactics. In the first phase of the campaign, the target group seemed to be alcoholics, or the 'drunk'. In the second phase, the target group was the 'heavy drinker'. In the final phase, it appeared that a wider drinking public was the target, with the desire to promote 'sensible' or 'moderate' drinking. This represented a shift away from concentrating on what might be termed 'pathological' drinking and towards focusing on the health consequences of alcohol in the 'normal' population. Such an approach could be seen as a precursor to that advocated by the epidemiologist Geoffrey Rose a few years later.[60] Rose argued that the greatest amount of ill health was experienced not by those at high risk, but by those in low-risk groups, simply because there were more of them. Prevention strategies should therefore target the whole population, lowering the risk for everyone, not just those in high-risk groups.[61] This kind of approach could also be read in the changing techniques used in the campaigns, with humour and emotional entreaties giving way to a more 'rational' approach, appealing to the drinker as a 'sensible' individual able to moderate their behaviour. Such varying techniques spoke also to varying tactics, with a more specific sense of the kinds of behaviour that should be encouraged or discouraged emerging by the end of the period. These shifts reflected broader developments at the policy level that will be explored in the remainder of the chapter, but at the same time there was also a lack of confidence about health education itself. Significant doubts were expressed, not least by the HEC, about the ability of health education to shrink alcohol consumption. Other means, such as reducing drinking at the population level, seemed to offer a solution.

The report of the Advisory Committee on Alcoholism on *Prevention*, 1975–77

The best way to prevent the development of alcohol problems, including the role of population-level measures and health education, was examined by several expert committees in the 1970s. A key report, titled *Prevention*, was produced by the Advisory Committee on Alcoholism (ACA), which was established in 1975 to advise the government on the provision of services relating to alcoholism. According to Betsy Thom, its terms of reference were vague, allowing the Committee to interpret their brief widely, examining not only treatment services, but also the prevention of alcohol problems.[62] As a result, the ACA was interested not only in alcoholics and heavy drinkers, but also those who might develop drinking problems, and the consumption of alcohol in the population more broadly. In its report, the ACA argued that 'we have to consider not only the affected individual, those who come into contact with him, and vulnerable groups, but also deep rooted attitudes, assumptions and traditions which blind people to the wide range of problems caused by alcohol misuse.'[63]

The ACA's expansive interpretation of the potential damage that alcohol could cause led it towards a broad understanding of the ways in which such problems could be prevented. The Committee's decision to focus on prevention was, however, 'against the Chairman's wishes and our [the DHSS'] advice'. The DHSS was well aware that the ACA was likely to stray into areas that were the concern of other government departments, such as the Ministry of Agriculture, Fisheries and Food (MAFF), which it saw as 'the sponsoring department for the drinks industry'.[64] A particular flash point was the Ledermann thesis and the notion that introducing measures to decrease alcohol consumption throughout the population could reduce drink problems. At the ACA's first meeting, members accepted Ledermann's arguments, stating that 'the available facts pointed strongly towards the need for a reduction in per capita consumption of alcohol as one of the objectives of any preventive strategy'. But at the same time, the Committee was also aware of the potential political and social consequences of such an approach. It noted that 'Increasing the price of alcohol in real terms to a point where consumption was substantially affected would be difficult politically and might cause secondary poverty.'[65] Such a view implied that some drinkers were capable of responding to price increases in a rational manner by reducing their consumption, but others were thought likely to continue to drink at the same level, even if this resulted in poverty. As a result, the Committee did not suggest any changes to fiscal controls or the licensing laws; instead it recommended that 'alcohol should not be allowed to become cheaper in real terms'.[66]

Alongside this moderate form of price control, the Committee proposed that more effort be put into health education. In the final report, the ACA recommended that 'Health education designed to alert people to the dangers of alcohol and to discourage excessive drinking should be encouraged and expanded'.[67] In the discussions leading up to the publication of the report, however, health education had occupied a more controversial position. The psychiatrist and addiction researcher Griffith Edwards 'had considerable reservations about any campaign which attempted to change people's behaviour' as he was sceptical about the effectiveness of alcohol treatment and counselling services. Edwards was instead in favour of the introduction of greater controls on the price and availability of alcohol, and he suggested that 'any campaign which was mounted should attempt to educate the public about the need for controls over the availability of alcohol as a means of preventing alcoholism'.[68] Not everyone on the Committee agreed, and at a later meeting (where Edwards was absent) they moved towards an approach that emphasised 'safe' or 'healthy' drinking.[69] The Committee expressed some doubt about the 'value of referring to "healthy drinking" or "safe drinking levels"' as 'the message conveyed was so complex that it seemed likely to be misunderstood'.[70] Nonetheless, the ACA report did touch on the issue, suggesting that there was a need to 'define a level of heavy drinking and to discourage drinking above that level'. It even made a tentative suggestion as to what this level should consist of, noting that a daily intake of 15 cl of ethanol, equivalent to about half a bottle of spirits or 8–10 pints of beer, was 'generally regarded as unsafe'.[71]

The ACA's provisional approach, and reluctance to either offer firm guidelines on 'safe drinking' or wholly endorse stronger population-level control measures, was a result of its recognition that such issues were 'controversial' and 'sensitive'. The Committee was unsure about the extent to which it was 'justifiable to interfere with the activities of drinkers on account of those who may cause or come to harm'. Political concerns were just as, if not more, important than scientific uncertainty about 'safe' drinking levels or the Ledermann thesis. The issue was not 'thought to be one on which a Government could impose its will without paying the most careful regard to the views of the people'.[72] As a result, the ACA argued that 'stricter controls cannot and should not be introduced without informed public discussion'. Moreover, the 'problems resulting from alcohol misuse have not yet been widely enough discussed: we believe that the public should be given more information, including an estimate of the true cost of alcohol misuse to society so that it can reach a realistic view of the restraints that should be placed on drinking'.[73] This approach was also endorsed by the DHSS' booklet, *Prevention and Health: Everybody's Business*, which stated that 'The best combination of strategies for our society, and the attitudes to alcohol which should be encouraged in it, are matters which deserve public discussion.'[74]

Indeed, some level of public debate about alcohol health education campaigns was already taking place. Most of the broadsheet newspapers simply summarised the key findings of the ACA's report, but some of the more libertarian publications offered editorials on the wider issue of health education. An article by Colin Welch in the *Daily Telegraph* was highly critical of government-backed health education efforts against smoking and drinking, which he saw as a 'sinister step towards tyranny'. Taylor asserted that 'When the British people imposed on the State the duty of caring for all our ailments free of charge we forgot that wise adage – *there is no free lunch* … For the State at that very moment acquired the right to order us to live healthy lives – to eschew this or that substance or practice.'[75] 'Peter Simple', also writing in the *Daily Telegraph*, took a similar tack. He stated that government plans to put a health warning on the labels of alcoholic drinks was an 'idiotic message' and a 'symbol of bureaucratic welfarism'.[76] Others in the media, however, were less critical of such an approach. Reporting on a speech made by the Minister of Health and Social Services, David Ennals, where he had asked whether or not alcohol problems should be tackled more 'vigorously', *The Economist* responded: 'The answer surely is yes: and for a start his [Ennals'] advisory committee on alcoholism has suggested preventive measures that would not conflict with the enjoyment of normal drinking.'[77] It is impossible to know the extent to which the wider public shared the views expressed by 'Simple' and Taylor, but their presence suggested that there was some level of feeling that introducing stronger control measures on alcohol might be an unacceptable restriction of liberty, something the ACA itself had acknowledged. There was a perceived need for public debate about the approach to be taken to alcohol, and the extent to which individual drinking should be curbed for the public good.

Drinking Sensibly, 1977–81

An opportunity for dialogue about the response to alcohol was provided by a 'nationwide debate' initiated at the end of 1977. When launching the debate, Ennals said that there were questions about alcohol that 'we must all ask ourselves'. Was it the role of government, he wondered, 'to concern itself with personal behaviour – or do you believe the Government has a duty to represent the interests of the community and seek to contain a growing ill?' Should government, Ennals inquired, 'impose a much bigger tax on all intoxicating drink as a deterrent to drinking, or would this be unfair to the majority who are sensible drinkers'?[78] A 'consultative document', to be prepared by the DHSS, was intended to 'outline for discussion the arguments for and against various possible preventive measures' and it was hoped that 'the ensuing debate will assist the Government to draw up firm proposals for improvement.'[79] Work began on the document in 1977, with publication intended for the following year, but it took until 1981 for the final report, *Drinking Sensibly*, to appear.

The long gestation of *Drinking Sensibly* was the result of significant interdepartmental tension. The central difficulty surrounded the control of alcohol prices, the impact that this would have on consumption, and whether taxation should be used to increase the price of drink. Not everyone in the DHSS was convinced of the Ledermann thesis, but key officials and the Minister were of the opinion that 'there is sufficient evidence available to link price, consumption and damage as to make it desirable that drink in all its forms should not become *cheaper* [original emphasis]'.[80] Such views found their way into an early draft of the consultation document. The document stated that: 'There seems little doubt that lowering the price of alcoholic drink does tend to encourage greater consumption, while raising prices leads to a fall-off in the amount people drink.' The draft was equivocal on whether tax should be used to increase price – this was for the government and the wider public to decide – but the document implied that inexpensive alcohol meant that the problem would worsen: 'Cheaper and cheaper drink prices would severely hamper efforts through health education and other means to tackle the problem of alcohol misuse and perhaps make all such efforts abortive.'[81]

Other government departments did not share this view. In a similar way to the discussion of flight time limitations examined by Natasha Feiner in Chapter 7, economic and business concerns could trump public health. The Department of Trade, Customs and Excise, MAFF, the Home Office and the Treasury all had difficulties with aspects of the draft text on alcohol taxation and price disincentives. As a letter from an official at Customs and Excise noted, it 'is clear that this chapter [on tax and price control] raises issues about which there is considerable disagreement between Departments'.[82] The Department of Trade was concerned about 'the practicability and desirability of seeking to hold down the consumption of alcohol through action on prices, and the implications for competition and consumer choice of any more restrictive approach to licensing'.[83] MAFF wanted the document to recognise the importance of the drinks industry to the economy, and to 'avoid suggesting that there is one single problem that can be dealt with by general solutions'. Such 'general solutions would penalise unfairly the majority of sensible drinkers and without any guarantee that the number of problem drinkers would be reduced'.[84] The Treasury sought to delay release of the document, and possibly prevent it from being published at all. The change of government in May 1979 offered an opportunity to 'seek guidance from Ministers before a great deal of additional effort is put into revising the present draft'. Treasury officials noted that the 'first question is whether the present Government will wish to publish any document along these lines; and we for our part would want to recommend to our Ministers that they should consider carefully the policy implications before coming to a firm decision.'[85]

The consultative document survived, but in a significantly modified form, and only after it was approved at Cabinet level. The section on price and tax was rewritten substantially. No direct comment was made about the link between price and consumption; instead the final document summarised the recommendations made by other committees and reports, such as the ACA's *Prevention*.[86] The document was unequivocal, however, on the issue of taxation: 'Taking account of the economic as well as the health and social considerations, and bearing in mind the practical difficulties involved', it argued, 'the Government cannot accept recommendations that have been made for the systematic use of tax rates as a means of regulating consumption.'[87] The possibility of using taxation to control the price of drink was not up for discussion. Indeed, the overall tone of *Drinking Sensibly* was not as 'consultative' as originally intended. Although the text was billed as a 'discussion document', it was unclear how exchange would take place. Instead, *Drinking Sensibly* was intended to 'help clarify public views' and offer 'statements of the government's position'.[88]

In any case, it does not seem that *Drinking Sensibly* stimulated much public debate. The DHSS had intended the document to 'be aimed at the intelligent layman, in the hope that the Press and TV will be sufficiently interested to follow up some of the points and so reach a wider audience'.[89] Yet they decided to publish the document with a plain cover, since the anticipated readership was 'the influencers of opinion' rather than 'impulse buyers'.[90] The media did report on the publication of *Drinking Sensibly*, but most newspapers just summarised the document's key statements and highlighted the fact that the government was not recommending an increase in the tax on alcohol. The *Guardian* was alone in sounding a critical note: 'The Government is to take no direct action – either by tax increases on alcohol or by curbing drinks advertising – to halt a dramatic rise in the misuse of alcohol.' Instead, the 'drive to curb abuse would rely entirely on voluntary effort'.[91] The only other source of criticism came from the medical press. The psychiatrist and addiction expert Thomas Bewley, writing in the *British Medical Journal*, summed up his views as 'Drinking sensibly, perhaps. Thinking sensibly, no.'[92]

Although provoking little public debate at the time, the report, and especially the notion of 'drinking sensibly', was important. The DHSS pondered long and hard over the title of the document. Alternatives included 'Responsible Drinking', 'Sensible Drinking', 'Sensible Attitudes to Drinking', 'Preventing Alcohol Misuse' and 'Alcohol – The Right Balance'.[93] Other suggested titles were less than serious, perhaps because they were developed in the run-up to Christmas 1979. It seems unlikely that 'Not Only Mother's Ruin', 'Don't Trifle With Sherry', 'I Drink Therefore I Am' or 'Steady as she Flows' were ever in contention, but the debate over the title of the consultative document does draw attention to the way in which alcohol consumption was framed by the text.[94] Although 'Drinking Sensibly' emerged as the victor, this was not defined in the final document. The text referred to 'sensible attitudes towards the use of alcohol', but it was not at all clear what these were.[95] *Drinking Sensibly* mentioned the Royal College of Psychiatrists' suggestion that drinkers limit themselves to no more than four pints of beer, or four double spirits, or one bottle of wine a day, but the report also pointed out 'drawbacks' to such an approach, such as the varied effect of alcohol on different people. The 'sensible drinker' may have been synonymous with the 'responsible citizen', who 'must consider in the light of these facts what they themselves can do to limit the harm to their own health and the health of others'.[96] The rationality of the self was being appealed to, not only to protect his or her own health, but also that of the wider public.

Conclusion

At the time of publication of *Drinking Sensibly*, the concepts of 'moderate drinking' and the 'sensible drinker' seem to have been still in development, but they came to hold significance in the later evolution of alcohol policy and alcohol health education. On a practical level, a more specific notion of what sensible drinking consisted of in terms of the amount of alcohol consumed began to develop in the latter half of the 1980s. Suggested daily limits had already been proposed by the Royal College of Psychiatrists, but in 1984 the HEC issued a pamphlet setting out the 'safe limits', to which people should restrict their drinking. 'Safe limits' for drinking were defined as eighteen 'standard drinks' (equivalent to half a pint of beer, a small glass of wine or a single measure of spirits) a week for men and nine for women.[97] In 1986 and 1987 the Royal College of Psychiatrists, the Royal College of Physicians and the Royal College of General Practitioners each published reports on alcohol, and all recommended that 'sensible limits of drinking' consisted of not more than twenty-one 'units' of alcohol a week for men, and not more than fourteen units a week for women. A unit of alcohol was equal to 10 ml or 8 g of pure alcohol, or about half a pint of beer.[98] In January 2016, the recommended weekly limit for alcohol consumption for men (previously twenty-one units) was brought into line with that of women (fourteen units).

Fluctuations in the recommended levels of alcohol consumption over time, and the fact that many individuals continue to exceed these limits, suggests that 'sensible drinking' was a mutable concept not a fixed category.[99] Nonetheless, alcohol policy has continued to encourage individuals to strive for a sense of balance in their drinking. Population-level arguments about alcohol consumption have reappeared, but as disputes over the introduction of minimum unit pricing in England make clear, such measures are bitterly contested.[100] Public health policy and practice around alcohol continues to centre on health education – on persuading individuals to alter their drinking behaviour. Whether such measures 'work' is still open to question. There is evidence to indicate that health education can help push alcohol problems up the public and political agenda, but there is little to suggest that health education alone can change drinking behaviour.[101]

In a sense, however, the debate about whether health education works misses a more fundamental point. The promotion of such a strategy was the result not only of the activities of vested interests, like the alcohol industry, but part of a more complex negotiation over the question of balance between the 'public' and the 'self' and the relationship between them. On one level, the continued appeal to the drinker to consume alcohol 'sensibly' seems like a victory for the notion of a self-orientated approach to public health problems. The controversy around measures such as minimum unit pricing, designed to increase the cost of alcohol, also points to a reluctance to address the environmental and structural factors that facilitate overconsumption. Alcohol policy is thus another example of public health's focus on the individual and their behaviour as both cause of, and remedy for, public health problems. Sensible drinking, was not, however, solely about health, but about balancing public and private interests in other spheres too. The ability of the alcohol industry to produce and sell alcohol, and the liberty of the individual to consume it, needed to be taken into account even if there were health consequences. Exhortations towards self-regulation were not necessarily a tool of social or political control but could also operate as a way to balance competing interests, albeit imperfectly.

Indeed, there are all sorts of ways in which the self and the public continue to be mutually constitutive. In alcohol policy, as in so many areas of public health, the self being imagined is required to act for the public as well as individual good. As with any attempt to control behaviour, a moral element can be detected. Alcohol policy is not applied evenly, with women and young people tending to come off worse, despite consumption being the highest among middle-aged, middle-class men.[102] Yet alcohol does cause damage to health, and reducing individual consumption would have population-level benefits. An appeal to selves has become a necessary part of any public health strategy. That is not to say that public health should ignore the wider structural and environmental factors that underpin health and well-being. But here again the self makes an appearance: one of the reasons minimum unit pricing has been so contested is because of a concern that it would be seen to penalise individual drinkers by raising prices. It has now become difficult to think about public health problems without also thinking about the selves that experience them. The self and the public have become intertwined to such an extent that it is no longer always possible to separate them.

Elegies for the public, or rather a specific vision of it, are not hard to find. Ever since (and long before) Margaret Thatcher said that there is no such thing as society, 'the public' has been seen to be in decline.[103] This line of argument, however, can be pushed too far. After all, the public is an elastic concept: if it can be broadened from the elite white men of Habermas's public sphere to include women, the working classes and ethnic minorities, accommodating the self-governing individual should be possible.[104] And just as we can observe multiple signs of the hollowing out of the public, there are all sorts of ways in which it persists. Public health cannot exist without a public. Until public health becomes self-health, there will continue to be a place for both the public and the self.

Notes

1 M. Foucault, 'Technologies of the self', in L. H. Martin, H. Gutman and P. H. Hutton (eds), *Technologies of the Self: A Seminar with Michel Foucault* (London: Tavistock Press, 1988), pp. 16–49; N. Rose, *Governing the Soul: Shaping of the Private Self* (London: Free Association Books, 1999); N. Rose, *Inventing Our Selves: Psychology, Power, and Personhood*, revised edition (Cambridge: Cambridge University Press, 2010).
2 J. Habermas, *The Structural Transformation of the Public Sphere: An Inquiry into a Category of Bourgeois Society* (Cambridge, MA: MIT Press, 1989); J. Coggon, *What Makes Health Public? A Critical Evaluation of Moral, Legal and Political Claims in Public Health* (Cambridge: Cambridge University Press, 2011); D. Marquand, *Decline of the Public: The Hollowing Out of Citizenship* (Cambridge: Polity Press, 2004).
3 N. Krieger, 'Who and what is a "population"? Historical debates, current controversies, and implications for understanding "population health" and rectifying health inequities', *Milbank Quarterly*, 90:4 (2012), 634–81, at p. 651.
4 L. Berlivet, 'Uneasy prevention: the problematic modernisation of health education in France after 1975', in V. Berridge and K. Loughlin (eds), *Medicine, the Market and the Mass Media* (Abingdon: Routledge, 2005), pp. 95–122; W. G. Rothstein, *Public Health and the Risk Factor: A History of an Uneven Medical Revolution* (Rochester, NY: University of Rochester Press, 2003); E. Fee and R. M. Acheson (eds), *A History of Education in Public Health: Health That Mocks the Doctors' Rules* (Oxford and New York: Oxford University Press, 1991); C. Timmermann, 'Appropriating risk factors: the reception of an American approach to chronic disease in the two German states, c.1950–1990', *Social History of Medicine*, 25:1 (2012), 157–74.
5 J. N. Morris, *Uses of Epidemiology* (London: E&S Livingstone Ltd., 1957), p. 39.
6 Central Health Services Council and Scottish Health Services Council, *Health Education* (London: HMSO, 1964).
7 V. Berridge and K. Loughlin, 'Smoking and the new health education in Britain 1950s–1970s', *American Journal of Public Health*, 95:6 (2005), 956–64.
8 V. Berridge, *Marketing Health: Smoking and the Discourse of Public Health in Britain, 1945–2000* (Oxford: Oxford University Press, 2007); R. Baggott, *Public Health Policy and Politics* (Basingstoke: Palgrave Macmillan, 2000).
9 P. Miller and N. Rose, 'Governing economic life', *Economy and Society*, 19:1 (1990), 1–31.

10 D. Armstrong, 'Origins of the problem of health-related behaviours: a genealogical study', *Social Studies of Science*, 39:6 (2009), 909–26; R. Crawford, 'Healthism and the medicalization of everyday life', *International Journal of Health Services: Planning, Administration, Evaluation*, 10:3 (1980), 365–88.
11 N. Ayo, 'Understanding health promotion in a neoliberal climate and the making of health conscious citizens', *Critical Public Health*, 22:1 (2012), 99–105.
12 I. Kickbusch, 'The contribution of the World Health Organization to a new public health and health promotion', *American Journal of Public Health*, 93:3 (2003), 383–88.
13 M. Valverde, *Diseases of the Will: Alcohol and the Dilemmas of Freedom* (Cambridge: Cambridge University Press, 1998).
14 B. Harrison, *Drink and the Victorians: The Temperance Question in England 1815–1872*, 2nd edition (Keele: Keele University Press, 1994).
15 B. Thom, *Dealing with Drink: Alcohol and Social Policy in Contemporary England* (London: Free Association Books, 1999); B. Thom and V. Berridge, '"Special units for common problems": the birth of alcohol treatment units in England', *Social History of Medicine*, 8:1 (1995), 75–93.
16 B. Luckin, 'A kind of consensus on the roads? Drink driving policy in Britain 1945–1970', *Twentieth Century British History*, 21:3 (2010), 350–74; B. Luckin, 'Anti-drink driving reform in Britain, c.1920–80', *Addiction*, 105:9 (2010), 1538–44.
17 J. Nicholls, *The Politics of Alcohol* (Manchester: Manchester University Press, 2009), p. 204.
18 Royal College of Psychiatrists, *Alcohol: Our Favourite Drug* (London: Tavistock, 1986), p. 108.
19 Royal College of Physicians, *A Great and Growing Evil: The Medical Consequences of Alcohol Abuse* (London: Tavistock, 1987), p. 24.
20 Thom, *Dealing with Drink*, pp. 110–20.
21 J. Lewis, *What Price Community Medicine?: The Philosophy, Practice and Politics of Public Health Since 1919* (Brighton: Wheatsheaf Books, 1986); M. Gorsky, 'Local leadership in public health: the role of the medical officer of health in Britain, 1872–1974', *Journal of Epidemiology and Community Health*, 61:6 (2007), 468–72; J. Welshman, 'The Medical Officer of Health in England and Wales, 1900–1974: watchdog or lapdog?', *Journal of Public Health Medicine*, 19:4 (1997), 443–50.
22 M. Gorsky, K. Lock and S. Hogarth, 'Public health and English local government: historical perspectives on the impact of "returning home"', *Journal of Public Health*, 36:4 (2014), 546–51.
23 Berridge, *Marketing Health*.
24 Thom, *Dealing with Drink*, pp. 109–11.

25 Central Policy Review Staff, *Alcohol Policies in the UK: The Report of the Central Policy Review Staff* (Stockholm: Sociologiska Institutionen, 1982).
26 R. Baggott, *Alcohol, Politics and Social Policy* (Aldershot: Avebury, 1990), p. 74.
27 The National Archives, London (hereafter TNA) FP 1/1, Report by the Objectives Committee, 29 October 1973.
28 TNA FP 1/2, Pilot campaign on alcoholism, for consideration, 7 May 1974.
29 TNA FP 1/1, Services to local authorities: submission by the Director General for consideration on 8 May 1973.
30 J. Budd, P. Gray and R. McCron, *The Tyne Tees Alcohol Education Campaign: An Evaluation* (London: Health Education Council, 1983); A. Thorley, 'The role of mass communication in alcohol health education', in N. Heather, I. Robertson and P. Davies (eds), *The Misuse of Alcohol: Crucial Issues in Dependence Treatment and Prevention* (London: Croom Helm, 1985), pp. 255–75.
31 G. Cust, 'Health education about alcohol in the Tyne Tees area', in J. S. Madden, R. Walker and W. H. Kenyon (eds), *Aspects of Alcohol and Drug Dependence* (Kent: Pitman Medical, 1980), pp. 117–22.
32 TNA FP 1/2, Pilot campaign on alcoholism – provisional budget, 7 May 1974.
33 Berridge and Loughlin, 'Smoking and the new health education in Britain', pp. 956–64.
34 Cust, 'Health education about alcohol'.
35 Budd, Gray and McCron, p. 31.
36 Thorley, 'The role of mass communication in alcohol health education', p. 261.
37 Budd, Gray and McCron, p. 36.
38 TNA FP 1/2, Meeting of the HEC Council, 19 November 1974.
39 Budd, Gray and McCron; Thorley, 'The role of mass communication in alcohol health education'.
40 Cust, 'Health education about alcohol'.
41 Budd, Gray and McCron, p. 41.
42 Ibid., p. 32.
43 Thorley, 'The role of mass communication in alcohol health education', p. 262.
44 Ibid., p. 262.
45 Berridge, *Marketing Health*, pp. 187–94.
46 Budd, Gray and McCron, p. 35.
47 Thorley, 'The role of mass communication in alcohol health education', p. 263.

48 Budd, Gray and McCron, p. 36.
49 Ibid., p. 39.
50 Ibid., p. 67.
51 Thorley, 'The role of mass communication in alcohol health education', p. 266.
52 S. Shapin, 'How to eat like a gentleman: dietetics and ethics in early modern England', in C. E. Rosenberg (ed.), *Right Living: An Anglo-American Tradition of Self-Help Medicine and Hygiene* (Baltimore: Johns Hopkins University Press, 2003), pp. 21–58; P. Withington and others, *Intoxication and Society: Problematic Pleasures of Drugs and Alcohol* (Basingstoke: Palgrave Macmillan, 2012); see also Chapter 4.
53 Royal College of Psychiatrists, *Alcohol and Alcoholism* (London: Tavistock, 1979), pp. 139–40.
54 Budd, Gray and McCron, p. 41.
55 Nicholls, *The Politics of Alcohol*, p. 207.
56 Budd, Gray, and McCron, pp. 148–9.
57 Ibid., p. 154.
58 TNA JA 384/1, Points from the speech of the Secretary of State for Social Services at the Annual General Meeting of the National Council on Alcoholism on 21 July 1981.
59 TNA JA 384/1, HEC, Alcohol education programme: strategy and proposals for 1982–3.
60 G. Rose, 'Sick individuals and sick populations', *International Journal of Epidemiology*, 14:1 (1985), 32–8.
61 G. Rose, *The Strategy of Preventive Medicine* (Oxford: Oxford University Press, 1992).
62 Thom, *Dealing with Drink*, pp. 120–1.
63 Advisory Committee on Alcoholism, *Report on Prevention* (London: HMSO, 1977), p. 4.
64 TNA MH 154/692, Mrs P. A. Lee to Mr Woodlock: Prevention of Alcoholism. July 1975.
65 TNA MH 154/692, Alcoholism Advisory Committee: Sub-Group on Preventive Strategies, Minutes of the first meeting on 29 January 1976.
66 Advisory Committee on Alcoholism, *Report on Prevention*, p. 8.
67 Ibid., p. 11.
68 TNA MH 154/692, Alcoholism Advisory Committee Sub-Group on Prevention: Minutes of meeting on 26 May 1976.
69 TNA MH 154/692, Alcoholism Advisory Committee: Sub-Group on Preventive Strategies: Minutes of the meeting on 17 March 1976.
70 TNA MH 154/692, Letter from Mrs P Lee [DHSS] to ACL Mackie, HEC, 12 April 1976.

71 Advisory Committee on Alcoholism, *Report on Prevention*, p. 6.
72 TNA MH 154/693, ACA Sub-Group on Prevention: Note of a discussion on papers on fiscal policy and alcohol consumption and on the Ledermann model of alcohol consumption, February 1977.
73 Advisory Committee on Alcoholism, *Report on Prevention*, p. 11.
74 DHSS, *Prevention and Health: Everybody's Business*, p. 69. On ideas about prevention and health more broadly and how they manifested in this report, see P. Clark, '"Problems of today and tomorrow": prevention and the National Health Service in the 1970s', *Social History of Medicine*, online advance access, 21 February 2019.
75 C. Welch, 'No meddles for Ennals', *Daily Telegraph*, 27 June 1977.
76 Peter Simple, 'Warning', *Daily Telegraph*, 11 November 1977.
77 Anon., 'Alcoholism: problem drinkers, drinking problems', *The Economist*, 12 November 1977, p. 27.
78 TNA MH 154/1124, Press Release: Government to launch nationwide debate on alcohol abuse, 7 November 1977.
79 DHSS, *Prevention and Health*, Cmnd 7047 (London: HMSO, 1977), p. 45.
80 TNA MH 154/693, A. Yarrow to Mr Benham, 29 October 1976.
81 TNA MH 154/1139, Preventive [sic] and Health: Consultative Document on Alcohol (Draft February 1978).
82 TNA MH 154/1141, Letter from DJ Howard, HM Customs & Excise to Mrs Pearson, DHSS, 3 July 1979.
83 TNA MH 154/1141, Letter from AJ Gray, Department of Trade to Mr Budd, DHSS, 19 May 1979.
84 TNA MH 154/1528, Consultative document on alcohol misuse: meeting with MAFF on 6 February 1981.
85 TNA MH 154/1141, Letter from HM Griffiths, Treasury to Mrs MAJ Pearson, DHSS, 1 June 1979.
86 DHSS, *Drinking Sensibly* (London: DHSS, 1981), pp. 51–3.
87 Ibid., pp. 58–9.
88 Ibid., p. 6.
89 TNA MH 154/1137, KJ Moyes to Mrs Pearson, Prevention and Alcohol, 29 July 1977.
90 TNA MH 154/1531, Mrs MAJ Pearson to Mr Warren, printing and stationery, 2 November 1981.
91 Anon., 'Drive to halt big rise in heavy drinking', *Guardian*, 15 December 1981.
92 T. Bewley, 'Government reports: published and pirated', *British Medical Journal*, 285 (1981, 28 August – 4 September), 638–40.
93 TNA MH 154/1530, Michael Brown to Mrs Pearson, 20 August 1981.

94 TNA MH 154/1530, Consultative document on prevention of alcohol misuse: in the health department's prevention and health series, no date [December 1979].
95 DHSS, *Drinking Sensibly*, p. 7.
96 Ibid., p. 8.
97 Health Education Council, *That's the Limit* [alcohol information pamphlet] (London: Health Education Council, 1984).
98 Royal College of Physicians, *A Great and Growing Evil*; Royal College of General Practitioners, *Alcohol: A Balanced View* (London: Royal College of General Practitioners, 1987); Royal College of Psychiatrists, *Alcohol: Our Favourite Drug*.
99 S. Boseley, 'Experts call for warnings on alcohol as men refuse to believe risks', *Guardian*, 13 May 2016, available at www.theguardian.com/society/2016/may/13/warnings-alcohol-middle-age-men-refuse-believe-risks, accessed 3 June 2016.
100 J. Gornall, 'Under the influence: 1. False dawn for minimum unit pricing', *BMJ*, 348:f7435 (2014). At the time of writing (November 2017) minimum unit pricing had just been approved in Scotland.
101 P. Bennett, S. Murphy and C. Smith, 'Health promotion and alcohol: some sober reflections', *Health Education Journal*, 49:2 (1990), 80–4; P. Anderson, D. Chisholm and D. Fuhr, 'Effectiveness and cost-effectiveness of policies and programmes to reduce the harm caused by alcohol', *Lancet*, 373:9682 (2009), 2234–46.
102 C. Herrick, *Governing Health and Consumption: Sensible Citizens, Behaviour and the City* (Bristol: Policy Press, 2011).
103 Marquand, *Decline of the Public*; R. Sennett, *The Fall of Public Man* (London: Penguin, 2002); J. Newman and J. Clarke, *Publics, Politics and Power: Remaking the Public in Public Services* (London: Sage, 2009).
104 Habermas, *The Structural Transformation of the Public Sphere*; N. Fraser, 'Rethinking the public sphere: a contribution to the critique of actually existing democracy', *Social Text*, 25/26 (1990), 56–80; C. J. Calhoun (ed.), *Habermas and the Public Sphere* (Cambridge: MIT Press, 1992).

4

'Look After Yourself': visualising obesity as a public health concern in 1970s and 1980s Britain

Jane Hand

Introduction

In 1978 the Health Education Council (HEC), a centralised non-governmental body responsible for health education services, launched a campaign to increase public awareness of the health problems caused by overeating, inactivity and smoking. Their campaign used television, poster and newspaper advertisements to encourage people to 'Look After Yourself' by eating less, exercising more and quitting smoking. It was devised as a 'better health' campaign that could unite risk factors for coronary heart disease (CHD) as well as other chronic conditions such as hypertension and diabetes into one central generic message.[1] A principal promotional tool of the campaign was to use visual images to redraw the boundaries of what constituted a balanced diet and demonstrate how a healthy lifestyle could be visually inscribed on the body. In this context obesity became a key marker of the unhealthy body, and its centrality in health education messages showcased the significance of individual behaviour to the public health agenda. The campaign reached a large proportion of the population through its multi-media approach, and later evaluation studies suggested it was successful in securing more widespread awareness of the routes to 'better health'.[2]

The development of the 'Look After Yourself' campaign was the culmination of a major shift in public health that took place in the decades after the Second World War. The rise of risk factor epidemiology in

Western medical science and its importation into health policy-making from the 1960s instituted new styles of public health practice that focused on risk rather than direct causation.[3] This risk factor model focused on the role of lifestyle and behaviour across time, enabling a wide range of preventive programmes to identify individuals as important agents of change. This 'new public health' necessitated more effective and innovative methods for communicating with the public.[4] Virginia Berridge has emphasised the role consumerism played in health education programmes, with both the state and the self being important brokers in constructing individuals as self-regulated actors encouraged to modify their behaviour in ways that were sanctioned and supported by the state.[5] Population-level approaches to public health issues increasingly used the tenets of marketing and advertising to engage with at-risk individuals. In 1964, the Cohen report on health education published by the Central and Scottish Health Services Councils argued the need for health education to make more effective use of the mass media so that campaigns could productively influence individuals to act on the advice given and demonstrate 'self-discipline' in controlling their behaviours.[6] The centrality of mass media techniques to the construction of the new public health ensured that visual communication techniques became valued tools of persuasion.

Visual culture has much to offer historical examinations of public health. Historians of visual culture and medicine have examined depictions of disease in relation to the dichotomous relationship between the 'beautiful' and the 'ugly' body as an aesthetic norm.[7] Much of this research has focused on depictions of insanity during the eighteenth and nineteenth centuries and bodily representations of AIDS during the 1980s and early 1990s.[8] Yet, health education more broadly offers insights into how similar visual tropes for representing disease prevention utilised contemporary understandings of gender, beauty and the body to convey disease risk. The mid- to late twentieth century witnessed a distinct shift in the way the body was depicted for public health purposes with the adoption of a representational mode based on a new image of the body, itself enshrined in the concept of 'body image'.[9] Healthy behaviours were often gendered and coded in terms of bodily attractiveness, reinforcing the culturally contingent understanding that eating and the social body were inextricably linked.

Health education programmes also firmly established the idea that balancing individual diets and physical activity was essential to good health.

Such ideas of balance and selfhood permeated individualised notions of health education throughout the 1970s and 1980s. For heart disease prevention programmes, overweight and obesity were regularly constructed as an imbalance between caloric intake and energy expenditure, with the individual identified as the crucial agent in self-adjustment and self-improvement. Of course, this idea of dietary moderation for health preservation long pre-dated these post-war health education initiatives and had been evident since at least the early modern period in England, where dietetic culture was central to medical understandings of the self.[10] But personal body management techniques including the control of diet and exercise endured as an essential part of personal identity and social worth in post-war Britain, where the consumerist society contributed to the creation of new disease-focused diet cultures. The centrality of the self to risk factor epidemiology remained a salient aspect of post-war public health where the individual held new-found power in dictating health outcomes and contributing to chronic disease reduction.

This chapter examines the use of visual images to promote healthy eating as a tool of disease prevention in health education during the 1970s and 1980s across England, Scotland and Wales. It not only analyses the activities of the HEC, and especially its poster output, in reorienting nutrition as a major part of its activities, but also highlights the role of public information films and the work of the commercial television station ITV in providing ancillary educative content through the documentary format. These examples represent only a small proportion of the poster and filmic material produced during this time on the subject of nutrition, diet and chronic disease, but they reveal some of the ways in which scientific knowledge about dietetics and disease causation were entangled in a range of cultural and representational practices focused on tropes of gender, body image and the 'cult' of slimming. By coding disease risk in terms of particular visual attributes and specific practical preventive measures, these images functioned to express and articulate specific health ideologies. These ideologies promoted the idea that individualised health risks, often visualised by the obese body, could be overcome (at least in part) by complying with a myriad of health advice that together would construct individual balanced good health.

Health education and nutritional health policy

From the 1960s onwards body weights in Britain rose steadily, and so too did associated diseases such as heart disease, hypertension and diabetes.[11] In this respect Britain was not unique but rather part of the wider international proliferation of chronic disease in the post-war period.[12] Various scientific studies, especially the Framingham Heart Study in the United States and the Seven Countries study, suggested a strong correlation between diets high in saturated fat and the increased incidence of coronary heart disease (CHD).[13] This had particular implications for the understanding of heart disease and the development of disease prevention programmes in many countries.[14] For Britain, it was integrated into epidemiologically based health policy-making. The concurrent rise of technocracy and the establishment of expert committees, which united scientists, medical professionals and government in influencing policy, were central to introducing epidemiological findings into policy-making, public health priorities and health education strategies.[15]

The Committee on Medical and Nutritional Aspects of Food Policy (COMA) was a key organisation in creating new health policies to address the emergent scientific understanding of the role diet was playing in CHD causation. Established in 1957 and chaired by the Chief Medical Officer, the Committee advised the government on 'medical and scientific aspects of policy in relation to nutrition'.[16] In 1965 the Committee was reconstituted and the word 'nutritional' was dropped from its title. This change reflected the wider range of issues coming under the Committee's remit, including the bacterial, toxic and carcinogenic risks posed by food. In January 1969 the Committee discussed a Scandinavian research paper on the topic of unsaturated fats and agreed that COMA could not endorse it without examining the problem in greater depth.[17] The COMA panel on diet and heart disease was subsequently established in 1970 to advise on the 'significance of any relation between nutrition and cerebro-vascular and cardio-vascular disease, and on any indications for future action'.[18] Its report, *Diet and Coronary Heart Disease*, released in 1974, recommended that people should lower their consumption of fat, especially saturated fat; but the level of professional disagreement among panel members was such that John Yudkin, Professor of Nutrition and Dietetics at Queen Elizabeth University, included a caveat stating that the report 'exaggerated the possible role of dietary fat in causing I.H.D [ischaemic heart disease] and has minimised the role of sucrose'.[19] This debate severely limited the policy implications of the report. Its main impact related to advertising standards, giving COMA the power to reject any advertisement that made health claims unsupported by the conclusions of the report.[20]

Yet the environment in which this Committee was operating was dynamic and rapidly changing. The emergence of new lifestyle- and risk-focused community health coalesced with increased medical efforts to reduce rates of heart disease by emphasising prevention. In 1976 the Royal College of Physicians published a report on diet and cardiovascular disease recommending that saturated fat intake be lowered.[21] This coincided with the government's commissioning of various policy reports to better understand the health implications of diet. The Department of Health and Social Security (DHSS) published *Prevention and Health: Everybody's Business* in 1976, followed by *Prevention and Health: Eating for Health* in 1978. These documents emerged during a period of substantial challenges for the state in funding the welfare state.[22] In this context preventive medicine was viewed as a potentially cost-saving measure that might reduce pressures on financially stretched NHS services. Dietary recommendations were therefore conceptualised not only in a changing public health context, but also in a period of government retrenchment in health spending.[23] The National Advisory Committee on Nutrition Education (NACNE), established in 1979, similarly sought to determine pragmatic policy recommendations on diet and heart disease. It made more extensive recommendations for dietary change.[24] A second COMA panel updated their findings in 1984, which led to the development of the 'Look After Your Heart' campaign to replace the 'Look After Yourself' initiative, so that a more targeted message could be communicated to the public.[25] In this context, public health campaigning emerged as one platform for promoting overweight and obese body types as potential risk factors for coronary heart disease.

The move towards detailed advice campaigns reflected an effort to enlist consumers into adopting appropriate self-regulating health behaviours. By persuading consumers to engage in self-regulatory practices that aimed to prolong life, public health was contributing to new 'practices of the self' that convinced people to interiorise health advice and show self-restraint,[26] while at the same time consuming more (albeit different) products to secure the continued success of the consumer society. Health consumerism demonstrated respect for the development of new diet markets and consequently the marketisation of nutrition and health itself.[27] In this process images were key. They repeatedly constructed and coded notions of acceptable health behaviour within established modes of representation – notably those pertaining to gender, beauty norms and the role of the individual. Thus, government-sponsored health education campaigns took into account the varied and changing social environments in which they were operating. Health messages were linked to contemporary notions of health and beauty because – as so succinctly put by Professor James Halloran of the Centre for Mass Communication Research in 1975 – '[a] "message" is not dropped into a social vacuum. It enters into an existing social network, an established system of norms and values, an ongoing process of interactions and relationships'.[28] It was in this changing policy context that health education and community health more generally appropriated visual representations as important components of advertising healthy nutrition and diet behaviours.

'Look After Yourself' and visualising the healthy body

As international scientific findings linking diets high in saturated fat with raised risk of heart disease were securing political purchase, so too were the ways such information was disseminated to the public. Health education was repeatedly identified as an asset to prevention by encouraging the public to adopt healthy living habits.[29] From 1973 the HEC was particularly concerned with the proliferation of overweight body types and obesity in Britain and the potential connection to heart disease.[30] Committed to the development and launch of a positive health campaign 'Look After Yourself' in 1978 across England and Wales,[31] the HEC intended to address the health effects of diet, lack of exercise and cigarette smoking in a shared campaign that aimed to educate the public on the interconnectedness of many risk factors in chronic disease aetiology.[32]

Visualising obesity as a public health concern

The 'Look After Yourself' campaign was designed by the Saatchi & Saatchi advertising agency, which had been working with the HEC on a variety of campaigns since the early 1970s.[33] These campaigns were notable for their use of the persuasive tools of the mass media, and used a combination of humour, shock tactics and hard sell to import contemporary advertising approaches from the commercial world into public health.[34] The poster material for the campaign was particularly focused on clear interaction between image and text, as well as on using one central image to convey or associate the message effectively to the viewer. One poster showed a large pair of men's plimsolls alongside the tag line 'You'd enjoy more sex if you had a pair of running shoes', which stereotyped the unhealthy middle-aged man while cynically suggesting that sex rather than health would incentivise behaviour change. This approach was viewed as distasteful by some, with Conservative MP Michael Shersby asking the House of Commons, 'is it suitable to be read by young children or many women who would find such an advertisement embarrassing?', and asserting his hopes 'that the HEC will concentrate on providing information which is based on hard evidence and not merely on opinion'.[35]

Nevertheless, the 'Look After Yourself' campaign continued to use visual images to reinforce the primacy of the 'beautiful' over the 'ugly' body as an aesthetic norm and to link it with conceptions of health, fitness and personal attractiveness. Posters used images of male and female bodies to discuss weight loss, diet and exercise in a context that emphasised culturally contingent understandings of sex appeal.[36] The poster 'Is your body coming between you and the opposite sex?' (Figure 4.1) displays an overweight man, in swimming trunks, standing at the poolside looking at a group of women in the middle ground, swimming and playing with a ball. The inclusion of a solitary man in the background of the image, ready to catch the women's ball, visually suggests that it is his fitness, slimness and involvement in physical activity that ensures nothing is coming between him and the opposite sex. Contrastingly, the foregrounded figure is turned away from the viewer, his body in profile to emphasise his rotund form and to guide the viewer's eye past him to the pool scene in the middle ground of the image.

The man was presented as both within and without the scene, removing him visually and metaphorically from the 'action'. Consequently, the poster suggested the existence of a barrier between healthy and

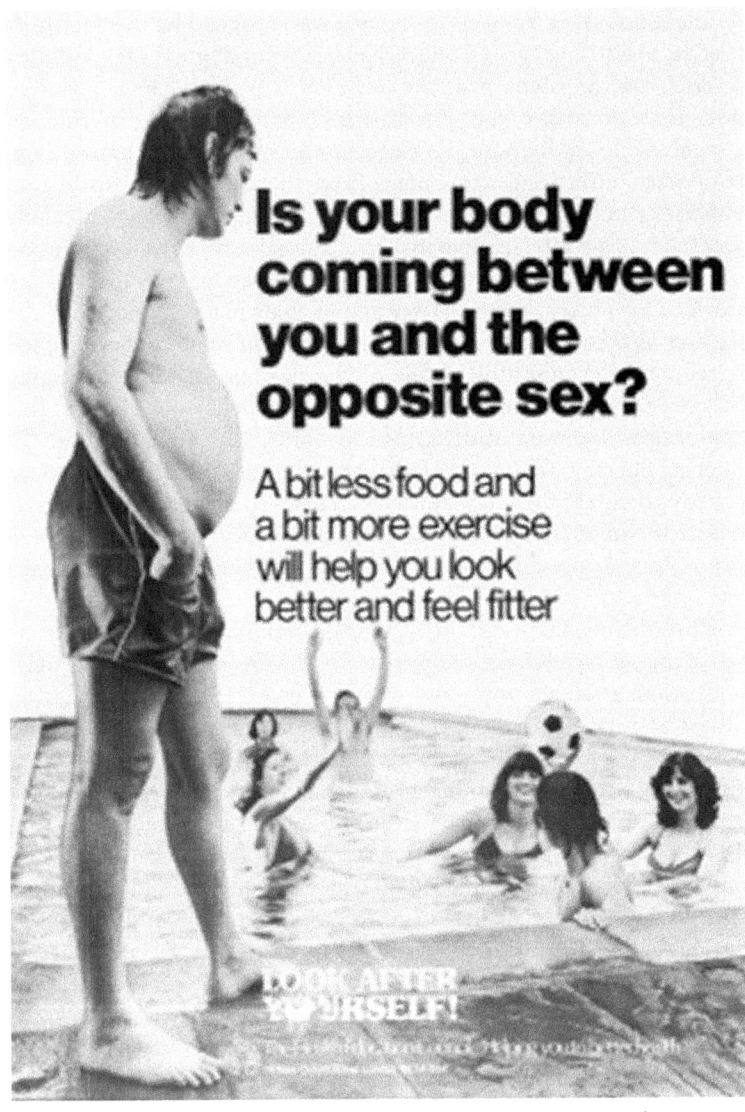

4.1 Is your body coming between you and the opposite sex? (Poster, Science & Society Picture Library, 10411400), 1978–80

unhealthy individuals in their ability to participate in a modern active life. This separation of the overweight male from other figures in the visual field underscores that overweight was not just a barrier between him and the opposite sex, but also from society more generally. The advice to eat a 'bit less food' and take a 'bit more exercise' suggests that a rebalance in diet and activity was needed to be attractive. This builds on nineteenth- and early twentieth-century understandings of physical energy expenditure that connected energy usage both at rest and at work with nutrient composition and caloric intake.[37] In this context balance was a scientific calculation that measured calories in relation to their expenditure. It also closely connected understandings of dietary balance with those of social 'modernity', where an individual's productive potential was linked to the ability of society to reduce social risks without restricting individual freedoms.[38] This poster is subconsciously connected to this longer heritage, similarly tying the post-war modern man with a particular understanding of dietary balance codified in terms of food intake versus energy expenditure as a social as well as a medical necessity. In juxtaposing the slim, swimsuited female bodies in the middle ground with the larger, overweight male figure in the foreground, as well as the depiction of a thinner man incorporated into the pool scene, the need to '*look* better and feel fitter' was framed as an aspiration for all and a reality for some.[39]

The poster visually and textually emphasised the centrality of the 'look' and 'looking' in society. Outward appearance was prioritised in visual terms over any genuine commitment to conveying specific instances of disease risk. The poster failed to reference any disease that would be affected by poor diet and lack of exercise. While HEC minutes reveal the campaign's commitment to reducing mortality rates from heart disease in particular, they expose a cautious approach to visualising disease risk openly.[40] The omission of any reference to specific health risks, especially in terms of mortality, was mirrored in other visual material produced for the 'Look After Yourself' campaign. The 'Do you hold your breath when a man looks at you?' poster (Figure 4.2) similarly avoided reference to disease types, instead fulfilling the campaign's aims to 'emphasis[e] ... the benefits of good health not the disadvantages of habits ... conducive to ill health'.[41] This absence of the diseased body from the visual components of the campaign, while still acknowledging the body 'at risk', marked a distinct break from previous cultural expressions of disease typified by eighteenth- and nineteenth-century representations of madness and syphilis. Earlier representations had asserted that the diseased body was visually marked as ugly, for 'ugly' and 'diseased' were identical categories.[42] In these 'Look After Yourself' posters, however, the relationship between the binaries of beautiful/ugly and healthy/diseased was reconceptualised in new, risk-centred ways. The 'ugly' – overweight – body was no longer the 'diseased' body, but the body at risk.

The use of photographs in these posters was an important aesthetic choice. Figure 4.2 used the photograph in a 'before and after' arrangement to visually 'show' the visible effects that a controlled balanced diet coupled with increased exercise could have on the body. While it may appear that this particular example of the 'after' showed nothing more than improved posture and stomach muscle tension (implying that these photographs were taken just minutes apart), the textual message implied a more meaningful change. The poster suggested that 'Tucking in your tummy isn't the answer', calling into question its own visual elements. This ambiguity suggested that while this tummy-tuck approach to achieving the beautiful/healthy body was not a long-term solution, the same body shape was attainable by 'eat[ing] more low calorie foods like wholemeal bread, fresh fruit and vegetables'.

Such dietary habits were constructed in positive terms and used to demonstrate the importance of having control over the body. In this campaign, food was classified into binary categories such as good or bad, masculine or feminine, healthy or unhealthy, self or other.[43] This duality in health advice enabled the HEC, and by extension the state, to 'shape food preferences and beliefs in everyday life, to support some food choices and militate against others, and to contribute to the construction of subjectivity and embodied experiences'.[44]

The role of the state in this process raises questions about the nature of citizenship in 1970s and 1980s Britain. The rise of social citizenship,[45] which provided rights of welfare, healthcare and housing, was part of a broader ethical focus on the relationship between the individual and society. Public health proved especially fertile ground for the reworking of citizenship not purely in terms of the provision of rights but also the fulfilment of responsibilities by both citizens and the state.[46] Preventive medicine in particular was an object of two balanced parties: the state and the individual.[47] In the context of the 'Look After Yourself'

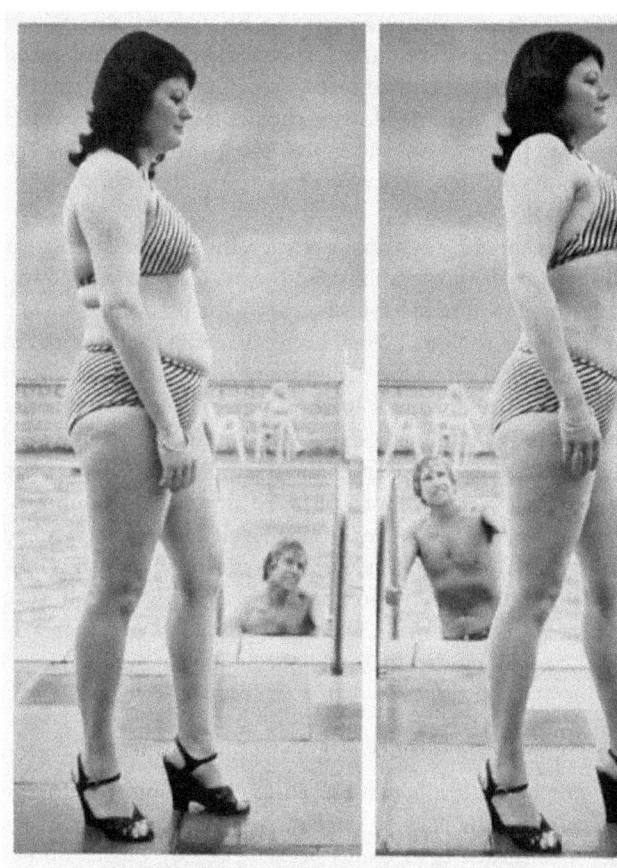

4.2 'Do you hold your breath when a man looks at you?' (Poster, Science & Society Picture Library, 10411688), 1980

campaign, the state was advocating a particular balance of duties, where the DHSS, through the HEC, assumed responsibility for informing and persuading the public to implement behaviour changes, and where the individual consented to institute lifestyle choices that promoted better health. In this way the state was an active agent in constructing the health citizen as a self-conscious consumer responding to scientific and state advice.

Rather than documenting behaviour change, the images comprising the 'Look After Yourself' posters imitated the 'real' as another educational tool that might inspire lifestyle change on the part of the viewer. By promoting the need to 'look better', both posters participated in the visual and psychological quest for bodily beauty. This contrasted with visual representations of madness in the eighteenth and nineteenth centuries and subsequent depictions of AIDS, which encouraged a sense of distance between the observer and the unhealthy subject of an image. This approach became more nuanced in the case of chronic disease.[48] In order to instigate behavioural change, public health relied on an internalisation of risk. The overweight or un-toned body was now used to bridge the distance between the healthy and the unhealthy, so that the majority of the population was framed as at risk and therefore targets for implementing individualised behavioural change.

Obesity on film

In the development of public health prevention programmes both film and television allowed the state to circulate a more nuanced message about obesity and health than could be achieved by poster output alone. The combination of moving image and voiceover created a different visual message from fixed images by firmly linking the specific health risks of obesity, alongside practices of prevention, with a clear narrative structure. The documentary film had long been an important mode of communication used by government to convey disease risk.[49] Despite the traditional narrative of a post-war 'collapse' in the British documentary film movement, the Central Office of Information (COI) continued to use public information films as a visual tool of health persuasion.[50] The COI in conjunction with the HEC, the Scottish Health Education Unit and the British Nutrition Foundation produced a short film entitled *A Way of Life* in 1976. Its production represented a moment of national cooperation across England, Scotland and Wales in using film to disseminate knowledge of the risk factors associated with coronary heart disease. A dramatised documentary, it narrativised the importance of healthy eating habits and regular exercise as forms of preventative medicine. Filmic techniques associated with fiction were linked with those related to documentary realism. This allowed the COI to focus on dramatisation to achieve the individual-as-representative and therefore universalise the experience of the protagonist.

A Way of Life depicts the medical and lifestyle implications of ill health for a taxi driver who becomes involved in a near-fatal collision. It takes place over the course of a single day. Following hospitalisation, he is diagnosed with hypertension and his body weight is identified as an important contributory factor. He is referred to an obesity clinic where the many health problems associated with being overweight, as well as the difficulties linked with surgical procedures for the obese, are discussed at length. At twenty-two minutes, this film contributes to the documentary film tradition of producing educational shorts based on a single theme. The choice of obesity is noteworthy. At a time when the link between diet and any specific disease, such as coronary heart disease, was still affected by policy inaction resulting from the divided COMA report of 1974, publicising possible risk factors became the central method for discussing health and disease more generally. Obesity was therefore used as a risk factor through which a myriad of health issues, including diet, could be visualised, discussed and debated. Its close link with overeating and lack of exercise constituted an important intersection for discussing associations between diet and exercise, on the one hand, and diseases such as coronary heart disease and diabetes, on the other.

The majority of the film is set in the present day of 1976. We follow a typical journey in the protagonist's cab, becoming increasingly aware that he is suffering from sight problems. Distorted focus is used to display the driver's difficulty in negotiating his journey safely. The camera shots alternate between subjective point-of-view shots, unassigned close-ups and medium shots of both driver and passenger. Sudden cuts to black fragment and temporally unhinge the scene, creating an uncertainty as to what occurs in the interim. As a visual tool this device expresses a sense of what the driver's physiological responses *feel* like. Similarly, the noise of traffic is halted during the visual blackouts.

This technique serves to visualise and make audible these somatic symptoms.

As the film continues the driver is diagnosed with hypertension, linked to his weight. A doctor warns him, 'If you don't lose weight now, you would end up a permanent invalid ... at best.' In contrast to the tactics of the later 'Look After Yourself' campaign, he laments that in contemporary culture 'too many people think the only reason to lose weight is to look more attractive'. Yet, he continues, the real stimuli – disease prevention and increased longevity – are repeatedly undermined or ignored: 'It's not just a matter of looks; being fat invites serious heart disease and heart disease can kill.' During these explanatory scenes, the doctor's interaction with the protagonist is visually interrupted by cuts to static images of the technology used by medical professionals to test for and treat coronary heart disease. After the protagonist's diagnosis he is referred to an obesity clinic for follow-up advice and further warnings.

The film's portrayal of an obesity clinic combines close-ups of overweight bodies separated into their distinct parts with a voiceover of real patients' opinions and thoughts on their respective body weights. These serve to situate the dramatised events concerning the taxi driver in a non-fiction, medical context, making the message of the film more pressing. Despite the focus on the taxi driver as a typical example of the proliferation of chronic disease in men, it is women that articulate these voiceovers. Therefore, the visual accompaniments (shown in Figure 4.3, Figure 4.4, Figure 4.5 and Figure 4.6) are implied to be female bodies. This gender dichotomy is particularly noteworthy considering that the death rates from diseases such as coronary heart disease and diabetes were rising more quickly for men than women during the 1970s.[51] However, in visual terms women were 50 per cent more likely to be overweight than men by age 30, and this only increased with age. Thus, the use of overweight female bodies to depict obesity visually was more striking, enabling a greater emphasis on 'fatness' as soft, white, wobbly and clearly comprehensible.

In a similar way to how the nexus between the beautiful/ugly and healthy/unhealthy was established in the posters discussed earlier, these sequences display the obese body as ugly and therefore unhealthy. The voiceover itself reinforces this position, with one interviewee highlighting how obesity makes her feel 'unattractive and nothing interests

Visualising obesity as a public health concern

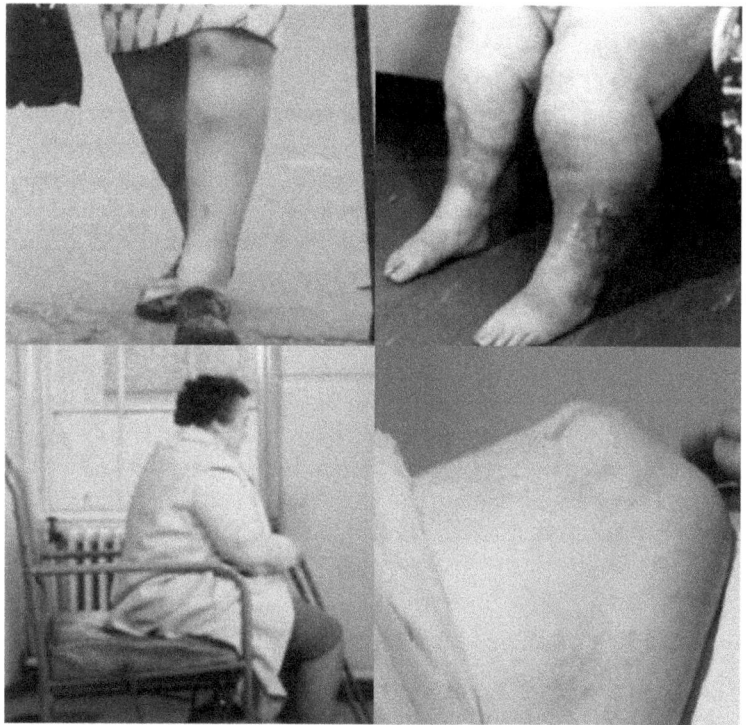

4.3, 4.4, 4.5, 4.6 (clockwise from top left): Stills from *A Way of Life* (S. Clarkhall, Central Office of Information, 1976)

you'. This visual and oral linkage emphasises how the long-term effects of obesity on the body could have tangible effects on personal quality of life.

The visual display of female bodies and body parts in this segment is an interesting representational choice. At no point in the dramatic narrative is the body of the named protagonist shown unclothed. Yet it was permissible to expose the unnamed female body, often separated visually into specific body parts, whether legs or stomach. The aural interplay contextualises and elevates the visual power of the images. As the doctor prefaces this sequence, 'the fat person's life can be extremely unpleasant and you may not discover that until it's too late'. These images are clearly linked, through the cinematic technique of the voiceover, to broader societal norms about personal attractiveness, body weight, self-control and self-esteem.[52] As seen in Figure 4.4, leg sores are depicted as one visually striking outcome of excess body weight. The camera zooms in to emphasise the sores themselves as they become the visual focus of the frame. This emphasis on an unsightly consequence of obesity is confirmed through a sense of inadequacy and personal failure that is revealed through the voiceover. It is autobiographical and used to authenticate the message of the dramatic format that underpins the film as a whole. By combining an aesthetic that emphasises the ugly and not the beautiful with the realist features of the docudrama, the film attempted to convey both information and alarm to encourage change in personal health behaviours. Despite using quite different visual techniques from the later 'Look After Yourself' campaign, and drawing very specific connections between diet, exercise, smoking and health outcomes, *A Way of Life* conformed to the same models of balance and selfhood that emphasised self-regulation, individual action and the role of lifestyle in disease prevention.

Investigative journalism and documenting nutritional health

Alongside documentary film, television was an important additional site for disseminating health information. In particular, current affairs programming provided the public with additional, non-government-sponsored advice about health, diet and disease. While televisual investigative journalism exposed different narrative foci for allocating responsibility for disease and health, the composition and visual arrangement of these documentaries revealed alternative notions regarding the role of individualism in the disease prevention process. They provided a counternarrative, emphasising how televisual media were engaging with broader health and social equality issues that impacted on health outcomes. Examining the structural and economic barriers to health was one part of this counternarrative, with poverty, environment, service delivery and healthcare access all contributing to the construction of another type of self – anyone unable to achieve balanced diets because of inherent health inequality. By examining a particular two-part edition of the current affairs programme, ITV's *This Week*, this section shows how community health and health education were developing a disease prevention agenda of their own that included direct discussion of inequalities in health.

This Week was first launched in 1956, was renamed *TV Eye* from 1978–86, and reverted to the title *This Week* from 1986–92. It was committed to investigative journalism with a 'social conscience'.[53] Operating in a shifting context of increased welfare state retrenchment, recurring NHS funding crises and the widespread existence of health inequalities, such current affairs programming constituted an important transmitter and translator of Conservative government policies aimed at 'roll[ing] back' social services to end the 'dependence culture'.[54] The airing of the two-part *Lessons from the Dead* and *Lessons for the Living* was instigated by the publication of a report carried out by the Heartbeat Wales initiative in 1987.[55] Heartbeat Wales was a pilot project conducted by the HEC from 1982 to 1987, when it was extended nationwide as the 'Look After Your Heart' campaign. The programme's opening dialogue clearly identified the imminent publication of this report into mortality statistics in Britain as the necessary impetus for carrying out its own independent inquiry into the health of the British population.

The programme focused on Sheffield as a case study to highlight the growing inequity in health that was evident in Britain at the time. The choice of Sheffield can be situated within a longer history of the city being identified as a region with poor health resources under the NHS.[56] This was one of the areas deemed in need of reform by the Resource Allocation Working Party (RAWP) system in the 1970s. RAWP struggled to bring about meaningful change in inequality, in part because it was a purely technical solution,[57] and because Conservative political priorities were focused on a 'two-nations' approach between North and South, which enabled the South East to benefit most from a Thatcherite emphasis on 'localism, self-help, entrepreneurship and marketisation'.[58] For investigative journalism, this continued inequality in health, especially in the North of England, enabled producers to showcase how inequality could be broken down to the individual and local level. The limited study carried out by the investigators of *This Week* used various visualisations of statistical information, first-person interviews and explanations of the structures of local health planning to illustrate similar health inequalities.[59] It used its ability to find the 'human face behind the news story' to imply that the same findings would apply to the rest of the country. The structure and content of the programme showed an awareness (at least in production terms) of the multi-faceted nature of disseminating information about individualised health behaviour at a national level, while at the same time appreciating the need for region-specific health practices that facilitated targeted services. To this end, the host Jonathan Dimbleby asserted that Sheffield was not unique and that 'as in other deprived areas of Britain, the poor are destined to grow up with an average life expectancy five, six or even seven years below that of the rich'.[60]

In the context of current affairs programming, *This Week: Lessons from the Dead* and *Lessons for the Living* framed disease in terms of a rich–poor divide. Recognition of such a divide gained national prominence with the publication of the Black Report (1980), which explored the social distribution of mortality and morbidity in the thirty years since the establishment of the National Health Service.[61] It documented widespread disparities between rich and poor in terms of health, which were not being adequately addressed by the NHS. Presented as it was to an incoming Conservative government intent on cutting public expenditure, the report was at first delayed, but later published with a short print run on a bank holiday weekend and with only limited same-day press coverage.[62] This resulted in a media furore with accusations of a cover-up, greatly increasing public awareness of the role that socio-economic status and poverty were playing in terms of mortality.[63]

In opposition, the Conservatives had bemoaned a focus on inequality, instead promoting the New Right perspective that inequality was not inherently structural but rather the outcome of personal choice, which could therefore be overcome by individual commitment, skill, energy and motivation.[64] This assessment maintained that poor conditions acted as a stimulus to encourage people to work harder, while the prospect of superior conditions was a further motivation. Thus, unsurprisingly, the Black Report prompted little in tangible policy terms, and by the mid-1980s the Director of the HEC, David Player, commissioned a follow-up research paper. The resultant *The Health Divide* (1987) was published directly by the HEC and further emphasised these health inequalities.[65] Together, the Black Report, *The Health Divide* and the Heartbeat Wales report received considerable press attention, thus provoking further televisual coverage.[66] Moreover, *Lessons from the Dead* suggested that heart disease could also be framed in terms of poverty and socio-economic status, complicating understandings regarding dietary excess and affluence.

Of the two-part *This Week* programme, *Lessons from the Dead* focused on the issue of health inequalities in 1980s Britain. It employed a number of visual tools aimed at exemplifying the health problems facing the nation in uncomplicated terms. In particular, the programme illustrated the widening gap in health issues and the probable effect on mortality by dividing a group of schoolchildren in a playground into two separate groups. Through narration, viewers are informed that those on one side represent the more affluent sections of Sheffield society, while the much greater number on the other side symbolise those from lower socio-economic backgrounds. In slow motion the children then fall to the ground. The glaring numerical difference emphasises that, as the voiceover states, 'these deaths are not evenly shared by the population of Sheffield'. As simply articulated by Dimbleby: 'If you live in a poorer part of the city then you are more than twice as likely to die before the age of retirement than if your home is on the richer side of town.'

These children are later used to illustrate how important good health in early life and childhood is in reducing premature mortality. The camera pans across their faces in close-up to make their youth more readily apparent to the viewer, underscoring issues of age and life expectancy in the context of health inequalities. The visualisation of these mortality statistics and their inherent inequity stress that just as 'healthy children make healthy adults' (as was stated in the lead-in interview to this section) the opposite is also true, that 'conversely, sick children make sick adults'. While the socio-economic background of the children involved in these visualisations of health inequity is unknown, it remains noteworthy that children served as an indicator of this disparity. Building on a visual lineage established during the Second World War and continued into the 1950s and 1960s of depicting children to emphasise health risk, by the 1970s and 1980s medical scientists were increasingly identifying childhood itself as a key period during which predisposition to disease is determined. A leading article in the *British Medical Journal* in April 1970 focused on obesity in childhood, addressing not only the dangers of obesity developmentally, but also its long-term effects on adult health.[67]

By focusing certain scenes on the child, *Lessons from the Dead* was not only coding premature mortality in terms of long-term risk but also identifying children as a central focus of disease prevention. The use of children as a metaphorical tool in this programme was particularly pertinent. As deaths from chronic diseases proliferated, possible causal links between childhood obesity and malnutrition motivated medical research.[68] These links in turn received press attention, particularly in the scientific and medical columns of local and national newspapers.[69] If predisposition to diseases was determined in infancy and/or childhood, then the onus of responsibility lay with the mother, who was still socially coded as the primary caregiver in society.

In exploring the many multi-faceted causes of health inequality in Britain, the programme identified numerous social, environmental and financial factors as contributing to the extension of a health divide between rich and poor. In contrast to the 'Look After Yourself' and 'Look After Your Heart' campaigns, which stressed individual action to redress imbalances between diet and exercise, *Lessons from the Dead* constructs the self as subject to external forces that inhibit the ability to act individually in improving health. As Martin Moore and Alex Mold suggest in Chapters 2 and 3, the role of the individual, as part of a broader collective, was central to public health approaches to disease prevention by encouraging the individual to demonstrate self-restraint in bodily management practices.[70] This contrasts with the message of *Lessons from the Dead*, which focused on limited employment opportunities, low pay and lack of education as additional contributory factors when investigating the widespread presence of chronic disease among lower socio-economic groupings.

To discuss and develop these topics further the programme used a range of instructive dissemination techniques including interviews, explanatory film shorts, footage of health planning and filmed examples of community health projects such as mobile cervical cancer screening units. In particular, Dimbleby conducted a number of short interviews with female factory workers from Sheffield in their workplace environment, thereby establishing the health of women as centrally important in improving mortality statistics in relation to socio-economic status.

In the course of these interviews the camera focused on cigarette smoking as a central concern. Two of the three women were smoking while being interviewed, and when this was addressed by the programme (through a cut-in to a close-up on an ashtray filled with cigarette ash rather than a direct interview question) one female interviewee explained her attitude: 'Gives me a bad health, smoking, but I need to smoke because I can't have any other pleasure out in life like going for a drink or anything else so I turn to cigarettes.' When asked how many she smoked a day, she responded 'forty, fifty a day. I should cut down really but it's one of the hazards of life. I have cigarettes instead of drink.' This personal approach to what constituted sufficient risk and how individuals assessed and balanced risky behaviours suggests that alcohol consumption could be traded for cigarette smoking as a justifiable vice. Prioritising one habit over the other allowed her to achieve a personal balance. From the 1960s, British public health policy conceptualised alcohol consumption within the epidemiological model of public health and measured it against concepts of lifestyle choice and behavioural risk.[71] As Alex Mold suggests, redefining alcohol in the same health policy rhetoric as smoking and unhealthy diets ensured that it was similarly constructed as personalised and individualised in the preventive approach of public health.[72] Therefore, during the 1970s and 1980s in Britain diet was being identified as just one among a number of factors considered to be contributing to high mortality rates from chronic disease. The government employed a multi-factorial approach that sought reduction in *all* personal behaviours considered detrimental to health.

The programme demonstrated that some health advice was being successfully communicated to the public, especially in the area of diet and food. When the interview discussed diet, the interviewee not only listed her daily dietary intake but also conceded that this 'junk food', which was the mainstay of her diet, is 'no good for you'.[73] Another female contributor agreed, but asserted that there were financial constraints on attaining a healthy diet and that on low incomes better quality food products were not an option.[74] In this context, dietary balance had been priced out of reach, and calls to engage the individual to self-regulate were not only impractical but also impossible. This counternarrative of inequality was shown to be structural, based on poverty, deprivation and environment. While the programme did not comment explicitly on the need for healthier, better diets for those on low incomes, it did imply that such improvements were necessary to break the fundamental link between poverty and poor health. The programme acted to provide information by highlighting and emphasising hazards to health and signalling ways to engage in healthier personal behaviours. Lived experiences therefore complicated prescriptive calls to the individual promoted by government campaigns and calls for dietary balance. While 'Look After Yourself' may have been successful in raising the profile of better health and communicating that message to the public,[75] the ability of individuals to act on this advice was more complex and multi-factorial.

This is particularly visible in *Lessons for the Living*, which spends much of its investigative content examining the health outcomes of North Karelia in Finland – a region where coronary heart disease prevention programmes had been particularly successful and mortality rates had dropped dramatically. This comparative element enabled the programme to demonstrate successful community interventions at work, emphasising the role that prevention could play in Britain alongside management and curative practices. By interviewing the Karelia Project's team leader, Pekka Purka, *Lessons for the Living* stressed that treatment did not really affect mortality statistics. Instead, it maintained that prevention was key. In line with the types of advice the programme espoused, Purka declared that the best advice was to stop smoking, change diets to reduce blood cholesterol, and reduce blood pressure.

Throughout the 1960s and 1970s, as quantitative methods of measuring disease risk became central to health policy creation, national public health strategies incorporated the use of the media to inculcate risk-avoidance behaviour in the population. From the late 1970s in particular, current affairs journalism had forged a role for itself in bringing issues of healthcare and health provision to a national audience. *This Week* alone had covered thirty-three different healthcare and medical topics in dedicated programmes between 1979 and 1987. Therefore, both *Lessons from the Dead* and *Lessons for the Living* contributed to a wider trend in current affairs programming, which enabled health promotion and the provision of specific and detailed health information to be provided to the public unrestricted by government policy or DHSS priorities. *This Week: Lessons from the Dead* and *Lessons for the Living* can be read as manifestations of health education shrouded in the mantle of current affairs programming. This emphasises the place that audio-visual forms of education can occupy in understanding how health behaviours are communicated to the public beyond the confines of government initiatives.

Conclusion

At the time that *This Week: Lessons from the Dead* and *Lessons for the Living* were broadcast, public knowledge about diet and chronic disease risk was firmly embedded in British social culture. A decade of public information campaigning had successfully transmitted the message that diet was a central risk factor and that individuals were responsible for reducing their own risk. Because risk was increasingly internalised and invisible, health educators used obesity as an externally visible risk factor for discussing a variety of chronic diseases, especially heart disease. These messages were framed in terms of an ugly/beautiful divide that emphasised gender and personal attractiveness. Balancing dietary intake and physical exertion not only for health, but also to secure bodily beauty, was an essential organising practice and metaphor through which the HEC sought corrective measures on the part of the public.

In this risk factor model, new conceptions of balance and the self were formulated by a variety of actors including government, scientists and the mass media. While different models of balance were promoted, they all relied on some form of self-regulation – some reworking of how selfhood was related to healthiness and disease prevention. The individualisation of risk in this period enabled the state to reframe individuals as a new type of health citizen incorporated into a balanced conception of rights and responsibilities. This meant persuading the individual to act as a self-conscious and self-regulated consumer engaged in healthful behaviours, thereby establishing a new social contract with the state.

The centrality of persuasion to the 'new public health' agenda ensured an important role for health education in public health, especially in its ability to incorporate and utilise mass media techniques to speak to the public. Visual forms of communication were fundamental in the way health education constructed the individual-at-risk as the key arbiter of change. The 'Look After Yourself' campaign alongside the public information film *A Way of Life* emphasised how visual representations were central to health education on chronic disease in the 1970s and 1980s. Eating less and exercising more were presented as straightforward and easy methods to rebalance personal risk. Perhaps unsurprisingly at a time of government retrenchment, both 'Look After Yourself' and *A Way of Life* reinforced the primacy of the individual over and above any potential need for increased service provision in the NHS. They emphasised simple prescriptive changes and placed responsibility firmly with the citizen-consumer.

While it is clear that government-sponsored public health messages were penetrating and remaking perspectives on health, individuals still acted independently to reinterpret these messages for themselves in highly personalised contexts. They produced their own balance of risk that challenged the view that behaviour change was easy. Especially in socially deprived communities, access to healthy foods could be compromised by a number of inherent health inequalities. *This Week: Lessons from the Dead* and *Lessons for the Living* were able to show a counternarrative about chronic disease risk and the place of the individual. Its production by commercial television allowed *This Week* to discuss the wider determinants of ill health and examine their impact on chronic disease causation. By focusing on health inequalities, it served to undermine the efficacy of the government's focus on individual responsibility and suggested that wider social and structural changes would be needed alongside education to make any great inroads into disease prevention.

An emphasis on balance, especially in terms of diet and exercise, provides important traction on understanding the disparate and personalised ways health advice was consumed and practised during the 1970s and 1980s. *This Week* presented different perspectives on balance, selfhood and regulation. While contributors to the programme were well aware of the health risks posed by smoking, drinking and eating nutritionally poor food, they were involved in a trading of risks to achieve a personal balance that took account of their financial and social situations. This form of balance was less explicitly focused on adjusting dietary intake in relation to energy expenditure, evident in the 'Look After Yourself' campaign and *A Way of Life*. Instead, balance in this context involved offsetting risk factors against one another in very personal ways. This complicates our understanding of the place of the self in post-war public health and exposes the importance of recognising how health messages were internalised, reworked and adopted in specific social and cultural contexts.

Notes

1 The National Archives, London (hereafter TNA) FP 1/5, FP 1/6, FP 1/7, Health Education Council papers: Health Education Meetings 1977, 1978, 1979.
2 J. Thomas, 'Look after yourself: monitoring the effects of a campaign', *Journal of Human Nutrition*, 33:5 (1979), 376–82.
3 L. Berlivet, 'Association or causation? The debate on the scientific status of risk factor epidemiology, 1947–c.1965', in V. Berridge (ed.), *Making Health Policy: Networks in Research and Policy after 1945* (Amsterdam: Rodopi, 2005), pp. 39–74; G. M. Oppenheimer, 'Becoming the Framingham Study 1947–1950', *American Journal of Public Health*, 95:4 (2005), 602–10; R. A. Aronowitz, *Making Sense of Illness: Science, Society, and Disease* (Cambridge: Cambridge University Press, 1998), pp. 111–44.
4 V. Berridge and K. Loughlin, 'Smoking and the new health education in Britain 1950s–1970s', *American Journal of Public Health*, 95:6 (2005), 956–64.
5 V. Berridge, 'Medicine and the public: the 1962 report of the Royal College of Physicians and the new public health', *Bulletin of the History of Medicine*, 81:1 (2007), 286–311.
6 Central Health Services Council and Scottish Health Services Council, *Health Education* (London: HMSO, 1964).
7 S. Gilman, *Picturing Health and Illness: Images of Identity and Difference* (Baltimore: Johns Hopkins University Press, 1995); P. Burke, *Eyewitnessing: The Uses of Images as Historical Evidence* (London: Reaktion Books, 2001), pp. 9–20.
8 S. Gilman, *Seeing the Insane* (Lincoln and London: University of Nebraska Press, 1995); Gilman, *Picturing Health*, pp. 51–66 and 115–72; A. Ingram and M. Faubert, *Cultural Constructions of Madness in Eighteenth-Century Writing: Representing the Insane* (Basingstoke: Palgrave Macmillan, 2005), pp. 170–201; R. Cooter and C. Stein, 'Coming into focus: posters, power, and visual culture in the history of medicine', *Medizinhistorisches*, 42:2 (2007), 180–209.
9 Gilman, *Picturing Health*, pp. 33–50 and 115–72; J. J. Brumberg, *The Body Project: An Intimate History of American Girls* (New York: Vintage, 1988), pp. 97–137.
10 S. Shapin, 'How to eat like a gentleman: dietetics and ethics in early modern England', in C. E. Rosenberg (ed.), *Right Living: An Anglo-American*

Tradition of Self-Help Medicine and Hygiene (Baltimore: Johns Hopkins University Press, 2003), pp. 47–8.

11 T. Khosla and C. R. Lowe, 'Height and weight of British men', *Lancet*, 1:7545 (1968), 742–5; J. N. Morris, J. A. Heady, P. A. B. Raffle, C. G. Roberts and J. W. Parks, 'Coronary heart disease and physical activity of work', *Lancet*, 48:8 (1953), 1485–96; J. Morris, 'Coronary thrombosis: a modern epidemic', *The Listener*, 8 December 1955, pp. 995–6.

12 E. Giroux, 'The Framingham Study and the constitution of a restrictive concept of risk factor', *Social History of Medicine*, 26:1 (2012), 94–112; G. Weisz, *Chronic Disease in the Twentieth Century: A History* (Baltimore: Johns Hopkins University Press, 2014), pp. 171–232; J. Madarász-Lebenhagen, 'Perceptions of health after World War II: heart disease and risk factors in East and West Germany, 1945–75', in M. Fulbrook and A. I. Port (eds), *Becoming East German: Socialist Structures and Sensibilities after Hitler* (New York: Berghahn, 2013), pp. 121–40; C. Timmermann, 'Appropriating risk factors: the perception of an American approach to chronic disease in the two German states, c.1950–1990', *Social History of Medicine*, 25:1 (2012), 157–74.

13 A. Keys, *Seven Countries: A Multivariate Analysis of Death and Coronary Heart Disease* (Cambridge, MA: Harvard University Press, 1980); W. G. Rothstein, *Public Health and the Risk Factor: A History of an Uneven Medical Revolution* (Rochester: University of Rochester Press, 2003).

14 J. M. Parr, 'Obesity and the emergence of mutual aid groups for weight loss in the post-war United States', *Social History of Medicine*, 27:4 (2014), 768–88; D. Lupton, *Fat* (London: Routledge, 2012); A. Offer, 'Body weight and self-control in the United States and Britain since the 1950s', *Social History of Medicine*, 14:1 (2001), 79–106.

15 V. Berridge, *Marketing Health: Smoking and the Discourse of Public Health in Britain, 1945–2000* (Oxford: Oxford University Press, 2007), pp. 132–60.

16 TNA MH 56/442, Correspondence – 'Mr Sinson', 1961.

17 M. W. Bufton and V. Berridge, 'Post-war nutrition science and policy making in Britain', 1945–1994: the case of diet and heart disease', in D. F. Smith and J. Phillips (eds), *Food, Science, Policy and. Regulation in the Twentieth Century: International and Comparative Perspectives* (London: Routledge, 2001), p. 211.

18 DHSS, *Annual Report of the Chief Medical Officer for 1970* (London: HMSO, 1971), p. 115.

19 DHSS, *Diet and Coronary Heart Disease: Report of the Advisory Panel on the Committee on Medical Aspects of Food Policy (Nutrition) on Diet in Relation to Cardiovascular and Cerebrovascular Disease* (London: HMSO, 1974).

20 Bufton and Berridge, 'Post-war nutrition science', p. 212.

21 Ibid., p. 211.
22 R. Klein, 'The crises of welfare states', in R. Cooter and J. Pickstone (eds), *Companion to Medicine in the Twentieth Century* (Routledge: London and New York, 2003), pp. 159–62.
23 Public expenditure suffered real terms cuts in both 1976/77 and 1977/78: R. Lowe, *The Welfare State in Britain since 1945* (London: Palgrave Macmillan, 2005), pp. 333–4.
24 For more on the recommendations of NACNE and the hostile government reaction, see Bufton and Berridge, 'Post-war nutrition science', pp. 213–17.
25 The COMA panel was deemed more acceptable to the DHSS than NACNE because the evidence against saturated fat fell short of proof and guidelines could therefore remain tentative. See: Bufton and Berridge, 'Post-war nutrition science', p. 215; DHSS, *Annual Report of the Chief Medical Officer of Health for 1988* (London: HMSO, 1989), pp. 49–53.
26 E. Hofman, 'How to do the history of the self', *History of the Human Sciences*, 29:3 (2016), 8–24.
27 J. Hand, 'Marketing health education: advertising margarine and visualising health in Britain from 1964–c.2000', *Contemporary British History*, 31:4 (2017), 477–500.
28 I. Sutherland: *Health Education – Half a Policy, 1968–1986: Rise and Fall of the Health Education Council* (London: Health Education Authority, 1987), p. 11.
29 DHSS, *Prevention and Health: Everybody's Business* (London: HMSO, 1976).
30 TNA FP 1/1, 'Health Education Council meetings', 1973.
31 TNA FP 1/10/1, 'Health Education Council discussion paper', 1981.
32 TNA FP 1/5, FP 1/6, FP 1/7, 'Health Education Meetings', 1977, 1978, 1979.
33 Berridge and Loughlin, 'Smoking and the new health education', pp. 960–2; A. Mold, 'Everybody likes a drink. Nobody likes a drunk': alcohol, health education and the public in 1970s Britain', *Social History of Medicine*, 30:3 (2017), 622.
34 A. Fendley, *Saatchi & Saatchi: The Inside Story* (New York: Arcade Publishing, 1995), pp. 35–7.
35 M. Shersby MP, 'Debate: preventive medicine', House of Commons, 12 June 1978, col. 766.
36 'Debate: "Look After Yourself" (Health Campaign)', House of Commons, 11 July 1978, col. 477.
37 A. Rabinbach, *The Human Motor: Energy, Fatigue and the Origins of Modernity* (Berkeley: University of California Press, 1992), pp. 130–3.

38 Rabinbach, *The Human Motor*, pp. 292–5.
39 Italics added by this author.
40 TNA FP 5/1, 'Health Education Council discussion paper', 1977.
41 TNA FP 5/1, 'Health Education Council discussion paper', 1977.
42 Gilman, *Picturing Health*, pp. 33–66.
43 D. Lupton, *Food, the Body and the Self* (London: Sage, 1996), pp. 1–2.
44 Lupton, *Food, the Body and the Self*, p. 2.
45 T. H. Marshall, *Citizenship and Social Class and Other Essays* (Cambridge: Cambridge University Press, 1950).
46 D. Porter, *Health Citizenship: Essays in Social Medicine and Biomedical Politics* (Berkley: University of California Press, 2011), pp. 204–20; J. K. Seymour, 'Not rights but reciprocal responsibility: the rhetoric of state health provision in early twentieth-century Britain', in A. Mold and D. Reubi (eds), *Assembling Health Rights in Global Context: Genealogies and Anthropologies* (Oxford and New York: Routledge, 2013), pp. 24–5.
47 Seymour, 'Not rights but reciprocal responsibility', p. 34.
48 Gilman, *Picturing Health*, pp. 51–66 and 115–72.
49 T. Boon, *Films of Fact: A History of Science in Documentary Films and Television* (London: Wallflower, 2007); T. Boon, 'Health education films in Britain, 1919–1939: production, genres and audience', in G. Harper and A. Moor (eds), *Signs of Life: Cinema and Medicine* (London: Wallflower Press, 2005), pp. 45–57; S. Anthony and J. G. Mansell, *The Projection of Britain: A History of the GPO Film Unit* (Basingstoke and New York: Palgrave Macmillan, 2011).
50 This 'collapse' consensus has come under revision. See: P. Russell and J. P. Taylor, *Shadows of Progress: Documentary Film in Post-War Britain* (London: BFI, 2010); B. Winston, *The Documentary Film Book* (London: British Film Institute, 2013).
51 DHSS, *Diet and Coronary Heart Disease* (London: HMSO, 1976), p. 26.
52 Various contributors, *A Way of Life*, 11.58–12.40 minutes.
53 P. Holland, *The Angry Buzz: This Week and Current Affairs Television* (London: I. B. Tauris, 2006), pp. xiv–xv.
54 Lowe, *The Welfare State in Britain since 1945*, pp. 332–3.
55 Heartbeat Wales operated concurrently with the last phase of the 'Look After Yourself' campaign. TNA FP 1/14, 'Health Education papers', 1982/3; TNA FP 1/15, 'Health Education Council papers', 1983.
56 J. Welshman, 'Inequalities, regions and hospitals: the Resource Allocation Working Party', in Martin Gorsky and Sally Sheard (eds), *Financing Medicine: The British Experience since 1750* (London: Routledge, 2006), pp. 221–41.
57 Welshman, 'Inequalities, regions and hospitals', p. 238.

58 J. Mohan, 'Uneven development, territorial politics and the British health care reforms', *Political Studies*, 46:2 (1998), 326.
59 *This Week: Lessons from the Dead* (ITV, 1987).
60 Ibid.
61 W. D. Dressler, 'Explaining health inequalities', in C. Panter-Brick and A. Fuentes (eds), *Health, Risk and Adversity* (Oxford and New York: Berghahn Books, 2009), p. 175.
62 V. Berridge, 'Introduction: inequalities and health', in V. Berridge and S. Blume (eds), *Poor Health: Social Inequality Before and After the Black Report* (London: Frank Cass, 2003), pp. 1–12.
63 V. Berridge, 'The Black Report: interpreting history', in A. Oliver and M. Exworthy (eds), *Health Inequalities: Evidence, Policy and Implementation Proceedings from a Meeting of the Health Equity Network* (London: The Nuffield Trust, 2003), available at www.nuffieldtrust.org.uk/sites/files/ nuffield/publication/health-inequalities-mar03.pdf, accessed 4 May 2014.
64 M. Thatcher, 'Speech to the Institute of SocioEconomic Studies: Let our children grow tall', 15 September 1975, available at www.margaretthatcher.org/ document/102769, accessed 28 November 2017.
65 M. Blythe, *David Player in Interview with Max Blythe*, MSVA 032.
66 P. James, 'Their life in their hands', *Guardian*, 16 October 1980, p. 14; P. Chorlton, 'Closing the class health gap', *Guardian*, 9 September 1981, p. 4; A. Veitch and N. Hart, 'How the government buried its dead reckoning', *Guardian*, 30 July 1986; J. Sherman, 'Report confirms strong link between deprived areas and poor health', *The Times*, 18 September 1986, p. 3; A. Veitch, 'Health chief put under pressure over report ban', *Guardian*, 26 March 1987, p. 4; Anon., 'Health report "not suppressed"', *Guardian*, 27 March 1987, p. 9; R. Wilkinson, 'Does poverty equal poor health?', *The Times*, 2 April 1987, p. 14; S. Hughes and A. Kirkwood, 'Ill-times for improving the nation's health', *Guardian*, 3 April 1987, p. 10.
67 Anon., 'The overweight child', *British Medical Journal*, 2:5701 (1970), 64–5.
68 Ibid.; J. J. Nora, 'Identifying the child at risk for coronary heart disease as an adult: a strategy for prevention', *Journal of Paediatrics*, 97:5 (1980), 706–14; D. J. P. Barker and C. Osmond, 'Infant mortality, childhood nutrition and ischaemic heart disease in England and Wales', *Lancet*, 327:8489 (1986), 1080.
69 For example: Anon., 'Children face heart risk', *The Times*, 18 April 1972.
70 Mold, 'Everybody likes a drink', pp. 612–36. J. Hand, 'Visualising food as a modern medicine: gender, the body and health education in Britain, 1940–1992' (PhD dissertation, University of Warwick, 2015). George Weisz provides a useful counter to this, suggesting that individualism fitted

less comfortably in British models of public health: Weisz, *Chronic Disease in the Twentieth Century*, pp. 196–7.
71 V. Berridge, R. Herring and B. Thom, 'Binge drinking: a confused concept and its contemporary history', *Social History of Medicine*, 22:3 (2009), 597–607; B. Thom, *Dealing with Drink, Alcohol and Social Policy: From Treatment to Management* (London: Free Association Books, 1999); Mold, 'Everybody likes a drink', pp. 612–36.
72 See Chapter 3.
73 *This Week: Lessons from the Dead* (ITV, 1987).
74 Ibid.
75 Thomas, 'Look after yourself', pp. 376–82.

Part II
Regulating imbalance

5

Self-help and self-promotion: dietary advice and agency in North America and Britain
Nicos Kefalas

Introduction

'PEOPLE CAN CHANGE: YOU HAVE IN YOUR HANDS a tool for changing your life'.[1] The title and first sentence of Dr Andrew Weil's bestseller *8 Weeks to Optimum Health*, first published in 1997, encapsulates the style and language used in self-help and health advice literature on both sides of the Atlantic across the second half of the twentieth century. Analysis of this literature reveals cultural preoccupations with notions of balance and efforts to reframe the self under medical direction, as well as concerns about the detrimental effects of modern living on diet and health. More particularly, a key feature of the self-help genre, in relation to diet at least, was a commitment to providing readers with the knowledge and agency necessary to achieve ideal selfhood, health and well-being themselves through what the authors thought to be balanced diets or lifestyles.

Drawing on self-help books that were in the *Publishers' Digest* top ten, *The New York Times'* bestsellers and books with multiple reprints, this chapter considers the self-help genre as one of the key sources and promoters of thinness, youthfulness, vitality, longevity and health as necessary pillars of twentieth- and twenty-first-century selfhood, but also of the concept of balance as a means of achieving health. More specifically, this chapter draws on the work of popular authors, such as Gayelord Hauser, Robert and Violet Plimmer, Linus Pauling and Robert Atkins, in order to understand the development of preoccupations with healthy eating and diet in both the US and Britain. The self-help books analysed in this chapter were often similar in their promotion of balance as the way to health, but each of the authors used their own expertise and had differing interpretations of balance. The first section explores the historical contexts that enabled self-help and dietary advice to become increasingly popular during the second half of the twentieth century, as well as reflecting on the authors, readers and popularity of self-help books. The second section analyses the manner in which self-help authors promoted themselves, their ideas and their products to the public, and the ways in which they legitimised self-help as a respectable practice in the Anglo-American public sphere. The final main section of the chapter explores the multiple ways in which self-help authors argued that responsibility for health lay with the individual, the language and terms used to empower readers to lose weight and be healthy, and the methods and techniques that self-help authors used to encourage readers to take care of their own health.

Self-help and dietary advice in context

The 1950s marked the beginning of what Eric Hobsbawm refers to as the quarter-century 'Golden Age' of the Anglo-Americans, marked by the spirit of post-war reconstruction and a monopoly in production and the growth of consumerism in the Western world.[2] Advances in home and store refrigeration techniques and the growth of expendable income introduced new ways of purchasing, storing and consuming food.[3] As Harvey Levenstein, Warren Belasco and Derek Oddy have argued, in the post-war years there were considerable changes in food processing and manufacturing, with an increasing number of pre-packaged and convenience foods.[4] More importantly, as Claude Fischler argues, during the twentieth century many regions of the developed world underwent a 'McDonaldization of culture', in which the major change was 'a shift toward more individualised, less structured patterns of eating'.[5] Social factors also shaped food consumption. As Derek Oddy has suggested, in Britain 'single-person households gradually increased', partly as a product of rising levels of divorce.[6] In addition, shifting food preparation and consumption practices were driven by 'patterns of daily life … profoundly altered by urbanisation, industrialisation, the entry of women in the workforce, the rise in standard of living, the ubiquity of the automobile, and expanded access to leisure activities, vacations and travel'.[7] Such changes created an increased need for self-sustenance as the number of occasions on which individuals ate outside the home – at school or the workplace, for example – became more frequent.

On both sides of the Atlantic during the middle decades of the twentieth century, there was increased medical, political and popular interest in, and concerns about, balanced diets and lifestyles, degenerative diseases, graceful ageing and optimal nutrition. Driven largely by the conditions generated by interwar economic recession and the ravages of the Second World War, providing better nutrition, fighting cancer and heart disease, reducing obesity and promoting healthy ageing became key targets of state health systems.[8] Often drawing directly on ancient medical formulations of health in Hippocratic and Galenic traditions, as well as on nineteenth-century studies of calories and optimal standards of nutrition by Nicolas Clément and Justus Leibig, early and mid-twentieth-century self-help authors in these areas regularly mobilised notions of balance. Preoccupations with balance in the area of dietary advice reflected a more widespread scientific and clinical interest in the physiology and psychology of balance in the interwar years: as Mark Jackson has argued in his study of stress, 'the physiology of self-regulating bodies emerged most decisively during the middle decades of the twentieth century'.[9] The significance of balance for health, for example, figured particularly strikingly in the work of Walter Cannon and Hans Selye. Indeed, Cannon's concept of homeostasis, which captured the ability of organisms to maintain stability or equilibrium in the face of changing external conditions, dominated many biomedical accounts of physiological and psychological health as well as popular advice literature.[10]

During the post-war years, society – like individuals – was also often construed as 'unbalanced' or at risk. As Ulrich Beck argued in his seminal book *Risk Society*, 'in advanced modernity the social production of wealth is accompanied by a social production of risks'.[11] Although technology and science offered the potential for new forms of medicine and healthcare, they also brought death and destruction.[12] Many self-help accounts of health and disease emphasised how balance could be achieved by adhering to natural diets. Diseases in the developed Western world, it was argued, were a direct result of 'unbalanced diets', such as eating too much and consuming large amounts of fat, sugar or processed foods. Stories of the wisdom of the noble savage, the lifestyle of the Mediterranean grandparent and the longevity of the Japanese elder thus gained new cultural currency in the West in the context of rising rates of chronic degenerative disease and new accounts of risk.

The concept of the self also played a key role in the lives of people in the Western world, as the idea of 'being', 'becoming' or 'realising' yourself through education, leisure and new patterns of consumption became more prominent during the middle decades of the twentieth century. In Chapter 4, Jane Hand argues that in the post-war period diet and exercise were accepted as components of British identity and social worth, as vehicles for self-realisation. At the same time, as Giddens has argued, the process of 'detraditionalisation' associated with modernity meant that people increasingly came to rely on forms of expert knowledge and guidance in the construction of new selves through consumption practices.[13] Other factors instilled notions and practices of self-preservation, self-care and self-help, particularly the growing critiques of medical elitism and the power of the food industry. According to Warren Belasco, during the 1960s a counterculture against fast food, processed food and unnatural food spread rapidly: 'young cultural rebels began to emerge against mainstream foodways ... their rebellion deserves careful reconsideration, for it raised important questions about our food system and also suggested serious alternatives, a countercuisine'.[14] Those rejecting mainstream foodways or criticising the power of orthodox medicine often targeted individual moral choice: eating organic and natural products or turning to alternative medicine was necessary to improve health and preserve the natural environment.

The readership of self-help books on diet and nutrition expanded as a result of increasing preoccupations with slim, young bodies and the rise of what Levenstein refers to as 'Negative Nutrition', which shifted foods from being regarded in positive terms to becoming dangerous.[15] As Belasco argues, historically salvation of the soul has been more important than the maintenance of healthy and slim bodies. But during the twentieth century it was the body, and not the soul, that became the central focus of efforts to maintain health and promote a positive self-image. The advertisements examined by Jane Hand in Chapter 4 demonstrate how obesity was viewed by the late 1970s. The ugly/beautiful divide and the emphasis on gender and attractiveness made obese bodies not only more visible, but culturally unattractive. As magazines such as *Playboy* began to sell pleasure and consumption,[16] preoccupations with bodily fitness accelerated the quest, perhaps particularly among the middle-aged and elderly, for optimal diets, supplements and exercise routines that would promote health and longevity.[17] Self-help authors also often directed their advice at women, especially wives and mothers, who bought these books as guides to feeding their families correctly.

The self-help authors explored in this chapter – notably Gayelord Hauser, Robert and Violet Plimmer, Linus Pauling and Robert Atkins – all advocated different diets and possessed different qualifications, but they also had elements in common. They were all scientists or had some connection with medicine or the biomedical sciences, and most of them had reputations and long careers in health-related disciplines.[18] As Matthew Smith has emphasised in his study of the popular allergist, Ben Feingold, many self-help authors in the mid-twentieth century were middle-aged men – at least in their forties and often older – who exploited their status as mature and established scientists to promote their work.[19] For example, Atkins was 41 when *Diet Revolution* was printed, Hauser was 55 when he published *Look Younger, Live Longer*, and Robert Plimmer was 62 when *Food Values* was first seen in bookshops.

As Matthew Smith and Mark Jackson have pointed out in their reflections on the work of authors such as Ben Feingold and Richard Mackarness, many self-help authors were dissatisfied with, and critiquing, the contemporary authority of science.[20] Both Feingold and Mackarness wrote popular books to promote their ideas, often drawing on neo-romantic aspirations to disseminate advice on how readers could restore natural equilibrium to their lives without recourse to conventional medicine. While Plimmer was dissatisfied with inadequate education on nutrition that caused imbalances and deficiencies, Hauser criticised artificial foods that disrupted normal bodily function, Pauling promoted vitamin C supplements to combat deficiency, and Atkins argued that obesity was the result of carbohydrate poisoning which was the product of an imbalance when humans shifted away from 'natural' diets.

Most self-help authors were men; if women were involved they were often authors' wives. Some books in this genre were written by women, such as *Let's Eat Right to Keep Fit* (1954) by Adelle Davis and the *Beverly Hills Diet* (1981) by Judy Mazel, but the genre was dominated by men. Readers of these books, by contrast, were more often women, or at least male authors deliberately targeted women as those responsible for family diet and health.[21] Rima Apple has argued that in the early to mid-twentieth century women were encouraged to adopt and apply scientific knowledge correctly to household duties, or to perform what Apple refers to as 'scientific motherhood'.[22] However, it is also possible to identify shifts in this pattern. If women – notably wives – were responsible for the health of the household including their husbands, women joining the workforce and rising levels of divorce forced men both to learn more about food, cooking and health and to take care of their own health. Combined with the increasing visibility of professional athletes, performing artists, actors and singers, which brought nutrition, dieting and slimness to the forefront of debates about appearance and performance, these transitions gradually made the self-help genre more inclusive of men.

Many of the self-help books analysed here were bestsellers and their authors often made public appearances in the media, attracting readers from all socio-economic and religious groups. Contemporary debates about an obesity epidemic, concerns about food additives and chemicals, and preoccupations with vitamins promoted public interest in healthy eating and encouraged the sale of self-help books.[23] Post-war Britons and Americans demonstrated the reach of governmentality as they wanted to maintain their health, energy and productivity in line with normative body standards. A fetishism for goods also attracted readers to this genre. Discussing the popularity of dietary advice during the Renaissance, the early-modernist historian of food Ken Albala has argued that a 'literate audience with enough leisure and money to be choosy about diet appears to have been a prerequisite for the genre to flourish'.[24] Anglo-Americans in the post-war era had an increasing amount of leisure time and disposable income to begin experimenting with advice to eat balanced diets. Healthy eating became more fashionable and readers wanted to display their knowledge of contemporary health foods. Mel Calman, cartoonist for *The Times*, argued that 'dieting almost feels like being a member of a club that revolves around calories, effective diets and foreign health foods'.[25] The success of the 'health food' industry, Fabio Parasecoli suggests, was the effective imposition on society of the idea that a better body and better health, highlighted by notions such as the 'Adonis complex', could both be purchased.[26] According to Jill Dubisch the manner in which 'health' food became almost a religion, with its own system of symbols and meanings, reinforced the commodification of healthy and balanced eating.[27] By reading these books and following their advice, readers chose to be part of a wider belief system. As John Coveney has argued, eating well and dieting replaced Christian asceticism in modern Western societies.[28]

Some dietary self-help books were targeted at informed audiences, but also at sceptical readers. According to Marion Nestle, the US government actively informed the public about healthy food choices: from home economics being taught in schools, to the promotion of food pyramids and reports from the Surgeon General. This led to what Gyorgy Scrinis has referred to as 'nutritionism', a preoccupation with eating correct amounts of micro- and macro-nutrients, which encouraged more people to buy self-help books.[29] Self-help authors eager to promote their diets not only wrote books, but also began to lecture, instruct and debate in public the benefits of a 'balanced' diet. Partly through self-promotion to an audience already sensitised to the importance of natural living in an artificial world, writers such as Hauser, the Plimmers and Atkins popularised the promotion of health through self-regulation and agency.

Self-promotion and self-help

The authors analysed in this chapter used their views of what constituted 'balanced' diets and lifestyles – but also idealised notions of selfhood revolving around slimness, youthfulness, energy, vitality and longevity – to achieve higher status and notoriety, earn money from book sales, and to promote self-care and self-help as the most important concepts in maintaining health. They thought of themselves as agents of change and education, locating agency at the individual level. Gaylord Hauser was a German immigrant to the US who had suffered from bovine tuberculosis as a teenager, and was cured while in Europe.[30] He claimed that he learned about the healing properties of food in Dresden and Vienna in 1923, which were prominent centres for fringe medicine at the time.[31] Hauser probably undertook his formal education, however, in the Chicago College of Naturopathy and the American School of Chiropractic.[32] Hauser was among the first advocates of whole grains, vitamin supplements and what he called 'wonder foods', such as yogurt, brewer's yeast, powdered skimmed milk and blackstrap molasses, which had all the necessary nutrients for an optimal, balanced diet.[33]

Hauser styled himself as an 'Internationally Famous Young Viennese Scientist'.[34] He sparked discontent from the American Medical Association (AMA), because he dismissed one of the most significant scientific initiatives of the time, fortified white bread, as devitalised. In turn the AMA seized copies of Hauser's *Look Younger, Live Longer* on the grounds that it promoted only one brand of blackstrap molasses.[35] The AMA's investigation of Hauser did not stop his health crusade, however, as he went on to write more than twelve books on food, diet, health and beauty.[36] Hauser referred to himself as a doctor, not of medicine but of natural science,[37] a strategy designed to increase his credibility. In *Look Younger, Live Longer*, he wrote in a quasi-scientific way, trying to maintain a level of readability appropriate for the general reader, but nevertheless resorting to scientific terminology and methodology.[38] He also argued that he was qualified to advise because of his 'great relish for living', his 'great relish for people' and 'great relish for longevity'.[39] He proudly informed his readers that he had met 'society leaders, stage and screen stars, statesmen, business executives, sportsmen, writers, philosophers, doctors, artists, scientists, teachers, preachers and – yes – a Civil War veteran'[40] – an approach that helped to legitimise his methods and promote trust in his advice.

Hauser became a popular public figure, often making appearances in the media and giving lectures; AMA opposition might even have given him greater notoriety. He was one of the bestselling authors in the *New York Times* for more than a year in 1950 and one of the leading commentators on diet, health and beauty in Europe and the United States in the 1950s and 1960s.[41] *Look Younger, Live Longer* was popular when it was first published, and it was reprinted multiple times until the 1970s and translated into at least twelve languages.[42] In the UK, the book was published by Faber and Faber, an independent publishing house with a reputation for supporting bold new authors and ideas.

Hauser's diets are considered to be among the first 'celebrity' diets, as one of his early followers was Swedish actress and international film star of the 1920s and 1930s, Greta Garbo.[43] Simon Doonan, Creative Ambassador for Barneys, a chain of US department stores famous for its wide range of luxury brands, has commented on Hauser's popularity: 'His influence was far-reaching … in the 1950s my mother and my blind Aunt Phyllis both joined his cult, albeit trans-Atlantically ... they rejected white sugar and white flour and began ladling Brewer's Yeast and molasses down their throats, and mine. They also favoured a rock-hard Hauser-approved breakfast cereal called Fru-Grains, which resembled lumps of charred bark and played havoc with their dentures.'[44] Carstairs attributes Hauser's popularity to his target audience, which was usually white, healthy and mostly middle-aged women.[45] This segment of the self-help market, Carstairs argues, was eager for knowledge on beautiful ageing and the preservation of femininity in old age: 'Hauser was ... drawing on a significant tradition of men teaching women, especially older women, on how to perform femininity.'[46] Additionally, Hauser's sexuality may have helped enhance his status as a diet and health authority. Carstairs argues that the ambiguity of Hauser's sexuality intrigued his audience, since 'gay men, like women, were expected to take a special interest in style and performance'.[47]

The authors of *Food Values at a Glance* were dissimilar to Hauser in many respects. Robert Plimmer and his wife Violet had a more solid claim to scientific credibility: Robert was a biochemist and Violet a biologist, both fields embedded in mainstream biomedical science.[48] Robert's career as a prominent biochemist can be seen in the fact that at the age of 34 he was one of the founding members of the Biochemical Society.[49] His interest in nutrition was stimulated while in the Directorate of Hygiene War Office during the First World War,[50] where his main duty was to analyse common foodstuffs; he published the results in 1921 as *Analyses and Energy Values of Foods*.[51] Using results from the Army report, Plimmer and his wife published a number of books in the genre of food, diet and health. Like Hauser, Robert Plimmer gave public lectures and made appearances in the popular media, but with far less controversy than Hauser. The credibility of the Plimmers' *Food Values at a Glance*, which was reprinted many times between 1935 and 1959,[52] was perhaps enhanced by the fact that it was published by Longman Press, which had a reputation for publishing educational books written by scientific authorities. Violet's frequent appearance in the media as a commentator on food and health was of equal importance to the public image of their books.[53] In the first instance, it demonstrated that science was no longer an exclusively male realm. Secondly, the fact that the primary audience for their books, namely middle- and upper-class women who could afford to buy advice literature in a period of austerity, was being offered advice by both a man and a woman arguably added an element of trust in the nutritional information provided.

Vitamin C and the Common Cold was not strictly a diet book, but its cultural influence was (and still is) great. Its author, Linus Pauling, was one of the most distinguished scientists of the twentieth century. Pauling is the only person to have been awarded two unshared Nobel prizes: the Nobel Prize in Chemistry for 'his research into the nature of the chemical bond and its application to the elucidation of the structure of complex substances'(1954); and the Nobel Peace Prize (1962) for his efforts to ban nuclear bomb testing.[54] Pauling was thus a respectable scientist but also a pacifist with frequent media exposure, making his claims about vitamin C more credible to the general public. In the UK, as in the US, the government had played an important role in popularising vitamins and nutrition facts since the interwar period. Like their US counterparts, the UK public had already been initiated into the principles of 'vitamania' and supplementation through the *Food Facts* campaign, the *National Milk Scheme* and the *National Loaf*. By providing cod liver oil, orange juice and rosehip oil to lactating mothers, infants and young children, the state had prepared the ground for Pauling's success.[55] Equally, in the UK by the 1960s health food stores had begun opening their doors in many cities. Pauling was thus presenting his work to a receptive audience.

Pauling's interest in the health-restoring and health-promoting benefits of vitamin C stemmed from a letter he received from Dr Irwin Stone. Following Stone's advice, Pauling and his wife found that the number of colds they suffered decreased. In 1969, Pauling presented his findings in a lecture at Mt Sinai Medical School.[56] This incident attracted a reporter from the magazine *Mademoiselle* to ask him whether she could write an article on the information he presented, and Pauling accepted. Pauling's promotion of vitamin C prompted debate. The nutritional expert Dr Frederick Stare responded in another *Mademoiselle* article by insisting that a thorough study conducted by the University of Minnesota had concluded that vitamin C did not prevent colds.[57] He also declared that Pauling, even though he was a great American man of peace and chemistry, was not an authority on nutrition. However, as Rima Apple has argued, the tendency for Pauling's critics to articulate '*ad hominem* invective weakened their own claims to be objective, dispassionate observers of medical research and undoubtedly attracted even more attention to Pauling and his cause'.[58]

Controversy surrounded Pauling for most of his life. His decision to publish his findings in a popular format, for example, was condemned by his academic peers.[59] Even before the publication of *Vitamin C and the Common Cold*, however, he had experienced professional friction from conservative administrators and trustees because of his circulation of a petition to stop nuclear testing and because he wrote a popular book called *No More War!* (1958).[60] This forced him to leave the California Institute of Technology (Caltech), where he had worked for nearly forty-two years, to become a research professor at the Center for the Study of Democratic Institutions in Santa Barbara, California.[61] Pauling also faced hostility from within the American Chemical Society due to his choice to use the status he had achieved from earning the Nobel prize to promote pacifism and prevent nuclear testing, leading to his resignation.[62] The rejection Pauling faced, both publicly and privately, institutionally and professionally, made him more passionate than ever about vitamin C and he coordinated his own health crusade, giving interviews, making appearances on television and radio, and researching the role of vitamins in a range of conditions. However, the credibility of his message was compromised by his tendency to exaggerate the effects of vitamin C, which was linked to a grandiose aspiration to eradicate the common cold from human existence,[63] and to advocate the consumption of the vitamin for a wide range of other conditions, including back pain, cancer and the promotion of intelligence.[64]

Pauling presented the available data, but also offered his own interpretations and evaluations of research studies. For example, in response to Stare's criticisms, Pauling insisted that:

> The study to which Dr. Stare was referring had been carried out by Cowan, Diehl, and Baker ... in 1942. When I read this article I found that the study involved only about four hundred students, rather than five thousand, that it was continued for half a year, not two years, and that it involved use of only 200 milligrams of vitamin C per day, which is not a large dose. Moreover, the investigators reported that the students receiving the vitamin C had 15% fewer colds than those receiving a placebo.[65]

The restoration of balance in the human body was a central theme in Pauling's work. Pauling argued that human ancestors had traditionally consumed a diet much higher in vitamin C, generating the optimal balanced state for the human immune system. His recommended dosages, though, were much greater than those suggested as optimal by scientific and medical orthodoxy. The solution to the common cold, according to Pauling, was not a gradual increase in the uptake of vitamin C, but the stabilisation of vitamin C levels through the consumption of megadoses of the vitamin, an approach that echoed Galenic treatment of excess humours with bloodletting, purgatives, emetics and diuretics.[66]

Pauling's argument about vitamin C penetrated popular culture via television, radio, magazines and later the internet. Recommendations of vitamin C in other self-help books,[67] as well as celebrity endorsements, attracted further attention to vitamin C as a supplement to remedy colds and flu. For example, Sofia Loren told the *Daily Mail*: 'The only pill I take is vitamin C – I'm afraid of getting the flu.'[68] Further support for Pauling came from the food and supplement industries, which used the opportunity to market their products to health-conscious consumers.[69] Some products such as Ribena had been exploiting public beliefs in vitamin C as a 'protective' against the cold prior to the publication of Pauling's book, but Pauling's work helped to strengthen their advertising claims.[70] The benefits of vitamin C were incorporated into debates about other health issues, to the point that it was often hailed as a panacea.[71]

The final author considered here, Robert Atkins, was perhaps the most controversial of the self-help authors in the field of diet and health. He was a descendant of Russian-Jewish immigrants to the US, and undertook his pre-medical degree from University of Michigan and gained an MD from Cornell's Medical School in 1955. After completing medical training, Atkins chose to specialise in cardiology, serving cardiologist residencies at the University of Rochester's Strong Memorial Hospital and Columbia University's St Luke's Hospital in New York City.[72] According to his biography, written by journalist and author Lisa Rogak, Atkins always wanted to work with patients rather than becoming a researcher. According to Rogak, he also despised hospital politics. Wanting to establish his own medical practice, he worked initially as a freelance cardiologist, acting as an on-call emergency physician. Atkins had an entrepreneurial instinct, opening his first office close to Cornell (and was thus somehow perceived as a Cornell cardiologist) and choosing to cover night shifts as more celebrities and members of the elite from the nearby New York's Theatre district had emergencies in the evening. This allowed Atkins to make connections with people in show business: in 1962, for example, he assisted in an electrocardiogram for the actor Edward G. Robinson.

According to the introduction to *Dr Atkins' Diet Revolution* (1972), Atkins's road to fame began when he was battling his own obesity. Atkins tried various diet plans available at the time, but felt that none of them helped him lose weight and that they all promoted unacceptable levels of hunger. On the basis of his own research, Atkins lost twenty-eight pounds in just six weeks. In 1964, in his capacity as a corporate physician, he tested his diet on sixty-five executives working for the American telecommunications company AT&T. Rogak argues that sixty-four of the executives lost weight, and from that moment Atkins's practice began to boom and his diet appeared on live television. This weight loss experiment received a high level of notoriety, encouraging celebrities like Buddy Hackett to consult Atkins for weight loss concerns. Hackett answered the question put by the audience of *The Tonight Show* with Johnny Carson: 'You know how I lost this weight? Dr Atkins used to call me every hour and say "Are you eating?"'[73] By 1970, the popular magazine *Vogue* had dubbed the Atkins diet 'the *Vogue Diet*', and Atkins became an international diet icon.[74]

Atkins's own narrative account of how he discovered his diet drew on a tradition of the scientist as detective. He had researched past medical journals, where he found a number of studies suggesting that *ketosis* was an effective weight loss mechanism.[75] In ketosis, the body switches its main source of fuel from carbohydrates to fat. Burning ketones instead of glucose means that the body burns stored fat. Atkins was not the first author to recommend a low-carbohydrate diet – in *Dr Atkins' Diet Revolution* he recognised the first documented promoter of such a diet, William Banting,[76] a nineteenth-century funeral director in London, who had successfully adopted a high-protein diet to lose weight.[77] Atkins was also not the first to condemn carbohydrates in the twentieth century, as Gaylord Hauser, Adelle Davis and others had forbidden the use of white sugar, white flour and 'devitalised' industrial food.[78] Other books recommended similar restraints on the consumption of carbohydrates, such as Vilhjalmur Stefansson's *Not By Bread Alone: Eating Meat and Fat for Stay Lean and Healthy* (1946), Richard Mackarness's *Eat Fat and Grow Slim* (1958), Herman Taller's *Calories Don't Count* (1961), and Robert Cameron's *The Drinking Man's Diet* (1964).[79]

Atkins's popularity can be explained in a number of ways. He was an ambitious Cornell-educated cardiologist, who wanted to spend time with patients rather than deal with hospital administrators. Determination and focus were qualities that Atkins showed from the beginning of his career; he chose the path less travelled by his peers, working as a freelance physician, covering night shifts, opening his own practice and becoming a physician and diet advisor to celebrities. Celebrity endorsement played a fundamental role in popularising his diet, as stars such as Jennifer Aniston, Renée Zellweger and Catherine Zeta Jones began to follow and publicise his diet. Although he did not conduct clinical studies himself, he used the success stories of the AT&T executives to bolster his claims. Lisa Rogak argues that another reason for Atkins's popularity was that he had a reputation for being 'a ladies' man', allegedly having relationships with female patients and nurses working at his practice.[80] Rogak suggests that many women began to visit his practice just to meet Atkins, who was well dressed, handsome and spoke with confidence and authority.[81] Men also became interested in the Atkins diet because it spoke to dominant cultural tropes of masculinity: 'The best part was that these men who so prided themselves on their masculinity – some were veterans of World War II – could eat beef and still lose weight without being hungry.'[82] Atkins's diet presented men with the opportunity to display and perform their masculinity and achieve weight loss. With an Ivy League medical education, Atkins's authority was not questioned by AT&T personnel at the beginning of his career or by dieters later on. Atkins's authoritative voice and strict mannerisms – in person and through his books – led to him being regarded by dieters as a father figure, a role that Atkins often exploited by bullying them when they cheated on their diets.[83]

Atkins wrote in an exaggerated and sometimes aggressive manner. In his attempt to demonise carbohydrates, he often resorted to unbalanced and extreme positions. Indeed, hyperbole was a pivotal element of Atkins's style, evident in an episode recounted by Rogak: Atkins once told a boy that the sugar in his sweets was dangerous, and the boy then asked: 'What's wrong with sugar?'; Atkins replied: 'Nothing, as long as you don't swallow it.'[84] Like an evangelist, he used vivid language and imagery, referring to 'carbohydrate poisoning' or 'no carbohydrates also means no hunger!'[85] Atkins was radical in his views as he believed that modern diets were imbalanced due to their high carbohydrate and sugar content. He opposed previous dieting rules – as he stated that eating more resulted in losing weight – and subsequently opposed orthodox Western medicine by opening the Atkins Center for Complementary Medicine.[86]

Another feature of Atkins's success was the controversy he attracted from mainstream medicine. Like Gayelord Hauser, Atkins's ideas were opposed by the AMA and the Medical Society of the County of New York. Atkins countered such opposition to his work by pointing out that, although the AMA had supposedly rejected his claims, one of his studies had in fact been published in the *Journal of the American Medical Association*. He also had feuds with other diet authors such as Nathan Pritikin, which generated further publicity and media exposure.[87] A keen opportunist and entrepreneurial maverick, Atkins accepted Oscar Dystel's book offer from the Bantam publishing house, with a signing bonus of $30,000.[88]

Luck was on Atkins's side. Dystel was struggling to make Bantam Books profitable again and was willing to take big risks; *Dr Atkins' Diet Revolution* was one of them.[89] Bantam Books hired a ghost writer, Ruth West, to help Atkins write the book plainly and without footnotes or a bibliography.[90] Although Atkins was sceptical initially, the publisher convinced him that the book was intended for a lay audience rather than the scientific community.[91] His books proved immensely successful; together, they sold more than 45 million copies worldwide, and 1,054,196 copies in the UK.[92] According to the British Broadcasting Corporation (BBC), in 2003 there were 3 million people in the UK following the diet. To this day, *Dr Atkins' Diet Revolution* is the fifty-seventh bestselling book of all time in the UK, and until 2004 it was the bestselling book in the category Fitness & Diet, later replaced by Gillian McKeith's *You Are What You Eat: The Plan That Will Change Your Life*.[93]

Through self-promotion, their perceived status and their 'anti-establishment' rhetoric, all of these self-help authors promoted individual agency in the pursuit of health and slimness. Readers, they all agreed, should take responsibility for their own health and for ensuring that they followed balanced, health-promoting diet and exercise regimes. By empowering citizens to make healthier choices to enable them to live more balanced lives, maintaining or restoring health became a responsibility – but also a possibility – for individuals as well as a benefit to the state in terms of reducing the healthcare burden and increasing industrial productivity.

Human agency and technologies of the self

Drawing on Anthony Giddens's assertions on the nature of the self in modernity, David Bell and Joanne Hollows argue that 'self-help books offer advice on how to construct the self, but also contribute to changing ideas about the self'.[94] For example, self-help books on food and diet emphasise that readers possess not only the power to manage their own health, but also a moral obligation to do so.[95] This rhetoric stemmed from different cultural and societal ideals that emerged during the twentieth century. Notions of agency, for example, can be seen in the context of deepening commitments to neo-liberal theories of political economy, which as David Harvey has suggested propose that 'human well-being can be best advanced by liberating individual entrepreneurial freedoms and skills within an institutional framework characterized by strong property rights, free markets, and free trade'.[96] The neo-liberal state distanced itself from many responsibilities by placing the onus for maintaining health on individuals and the market. John Coveney has explored certain aspects of governmentality and its impact on food consumption, in particular in relation to Foucault's discussion of what he referred to as technologies of the self: 'the way in which individuals internalise modes and rules of behaviour, emotion and thought in their everyday lives'.[97] Food and eating constitute one category in which individuals make sense of their surroundings, emotions and selves, and these diet books gave advice that resonated with contemporary technologies of the self.

By offering readers a way of preventing or treating modern illnesses, self-help authors promised readers hope. Many of the authors had themselves struggled with weight problems in the past, such as Robert Atkins, who lost twenty-eight pounds on his diet, and Dr Berger, who claimed that he had once weighed 420 pounds.[98] Testimonials from patients were also mobilised to emphasise the value of restoring agency. Atkins used them extensively in his book to complement his own success story. One patient history, for example, recounted how he had 'lost that 90 pound without hunger and without cravings', by eating one and a half pounds of meat and salads.[99] At the turn of the twenty-first

Self-help, dietary advice and agency 143

century, Dr Andrew Weil responded to letters that he received, reminding correspondents that they had the power to change:

> And this from Shelley Griffith of Massena, New York: I was on a program of my own due to the tragic (suicide) death of my twenty-year-old son, which took my health down the tubes. Then I ran across your book when I was searching for advice to bring my physical body back to good alignment ... Your consciousness-raising methods are so ahead of Western, sterile, nonspiritual methodology, anyone with any sense of the greater picture will take heed. ... I brought flowers indoors, did away with all vegetable oils, brought in extra-virgin olive oil, worked with garlic ... And I went to the health food store for organic flours, grains, and beans. I decreased animal protein and bought green tea. I take echinacea and practice 'news fasts.' My personal development has been super, with renewed energy. The deep breathing has almost eliminated the grief, pain, and anxiety. Depression has lessened considerably, my weight has dropped, my chest pain has disappeared, and my circulatory system is back in balance. I also take some of the tonics you recommend, especially ginger and dong quai. I'm learning all I can.[100]

Weil's message was clear: by taking simple steps such as changing elements of the diet, practising deep breathing or buying health foods, it was possible to achieve good health. By providing stories of 'everyday' and 'ordinary' individuals, the authors implied that their advice could be followed by anyone, a strategy that was reinforced by numerical evidence of success. For example, Stuart Berger used figures from 3,000 patients who had consulted him and lost a total of thirty-seven tons of fat between them.[101]

Cultural reverence for rational truth, revealed by experts, was exploited by self-help authors, who demystified the process of losing fat at the same time as reinforcing belief in science. Distaste towards body fat, or lipophobia, was increasingly evident through the twentieth century, leading to moral panics triggered by the perceived threat of obesity to societal values and interests.[102] Controlled, healthy eating offered a route to social, as well as personal, change: dieting could bring secular salvation in the form of health, fitness and youthfulness. Dietary advice literature offered a rational means of conforming to body ideals through individual agency. Evidence for this comes from *Dr Berger's Immune Power Diet*, which was a bestseller in the 1980s. Berger took a direct approach to invoke a sense of responsibility in his readers.

Berger's first section in the first chapter, 'The immune power diet commitment', urged readers to take their fate into their own hands, to move away from passivity towards actively pursuing better health.[103]

Self-help books also promoted the 'best' diets and lifestyles for what each author considered the most balanced or 'optimum' health, energy and productivity. For example, Dr Berger wrote: 'CONGRATULATIONS! Why? Because you have decided to become a healthier, happier more vital person.'[104] Similarly, Gayelord Hauser's first page states: 'A new theory on the treatment and prevention of a wide variety of ailments – the common cold, hay-fever, arthritis, high blood-pressure, chronic fatigue, overweight and many others – and holds out a promise of zestful good health for young and old.'[105] This reflects a wider cultural phenomenon, the preoccupation of the Western world with efficiency, with generating healthy producers and consumers who actively pursued and achieved their own health, productivity, longevity, energy and happiness. John Coveney has referred to this as 'the formation of a self-reflective, self-governing individual or collective subject'.[106] Adverts for various food brands also stressed agency, urging consumers to take care of their own health. As Alex Mold and Jane Hand show in Chapters 3 and 4, British advertisers and the Ministry of Food both reinforced this notion of agency through the middle decades of the century.

The moral responsibility and obligation that citizens had for maintaining their own health were often expressed in militaristic terms and linked explicitly to collective social interests. For example, Robert and Violet Plimmer argued that food was 'the first line of defence against disease and in wartime against the enemy'.[107] A woman's obligation to provide 'good nutrition' for her husband and children was addressed often in *Food Values*. By discussing the effects of malnutrition on men, especially their physical unsuitability for joining the army, and the impact of improper nutrition on schoolchildren, the Plimmers stressed that women could serve their country by providing proper nutrition at home. A prime example of the influence of biopolitics at that time was that the Plimmers emphasised the impact of improper nutrition on productivity by including facts provided by insurance companies: 30,000,000 weeks of productivity were lost in 1933 due to illnesses lasting from one to four days, costing approximately £300,000,000 per year.[108] Pauling, too, framed individual obligations to consume adequate amounts of vitamin C in economic terms: 'the damage done by the common cold to the people of the United States each year can be described roughly as corresponding to a monetary loss of fifteen billion dollars per year and in the United Kingdom to a loss of seven hundred million pounds per year'.[109] In addition, according to Pauling parents were obliged to give vitamin C to their children, because the vitamin had been shown to produce higher IQ scores.[110] Other self-help authors similarly discussed the benefits of their diets in terms of productivity, memory, concentration, feeling positive about oneself and leading long, healthy, active and productive lives. The line between self-help and societal help was blurred in these writings: healthier, more productive and longer-living individuals made society more productive and efficient.

Some readers expressed concerns about the hunger that attended dieting. Deborah Lupton has argued that in modern societies hunger is not just a physiological response to the absence of food.[111] Cravings and hunger were thought to be irrational and burdensome, especially to people with extra weight; in particular, they represented a lack of will that readers could overcome through rational self-control. Self-help authors assured readers that they would not experience 'negative' emotions such as hunger if they followed their eating programmes. Robert Haas, for example, tackled the issue of hunger by recommending that his readers could eat unlimited raw or steamed vegetables with their meals, and if they were active individuals that they should eat six times per day.[112] To fight cravings Haas instructed his readers: 'There is no point in worrying about cheating occasionally. Enjoying a variety of foods is one of the luxuries of eating to win, as long as you stick to the Peak Performance Programme in the long run.'[113]

Berger also addressed the issue of deprivation by stating that his diet restored people to a 'state of *homeostasis*, which eliminates nutritional spikes and drops, removes cravings and stops binges'.[114] Self-help authors thus mobilised dominant notions of balance and constancy evident also in popular and scientific accounts of stress that 'emerged from the traditional matrix of modernity and its preoccupation with stability',[115] which, as Jackson argues, constituted 'the apotheosis of the modern urge to impose order and control on natural, social, and cultural systems'.[116] Balance also figured in other ways. According to the Plimmers, the 'satisfactory supply of vitamins is a question of the proper balance of the whole diet ... How much vitamin A is required daily? ...

A diet that is well balanced and contains a proper supply of the other vitamins will provide from 4.000 to 6.000 units.[117] Berger similarly used concepts of balance and imbalance:

> THE FIRST STEP – CORRECTING IMMUNE IMBALANCE ... Sometimes an immune imbalance makes our immune cells attack healthy parts of our bodies in what is called an *autoimmune response* ... Zinc is perhaps the most vital immune mineral. Without enough zinc in our bodies, many of the lymph system tissues actually shrink, including the thymus where crucial T cells develop.[118]

Notions of balance were routinely accepted, but each author drew different conclusions as to what constituted a balanced state. Robert Haas, for example, rejected what mainstream science and medicine referred to as a balanced diet:

> Forget the 'Balanced Diet'. For years, nutritionists have recommended a balanced diet built from the four food groups for people concerned with physical fitness. Yet this kind of diet is actually very unbalanced. It contains too much protein and fat and too little carbohydrate. The only way to reach your level of peak performance, is by radically changing the amounts of protein, fat and carbohydrate in your meals and snacks.[119]

Self-help authors had to find ways to cope with what Belasco has referred to as a cultural 'antipathy towards "healthy" foods', which in itself was another obstacle to individual agency.[120] The palate's aversion to 'healthy foods' could be catastrophic to diets; broccoli and Brussel sprouts did not look as appetising as burgers, pizza and ice cream, at least for most people. Self-help books had to portray eating healthily as an easy process that involved appetising and filling food in order to provide a viable alternative to the variety and superior taste offered by unhealthy foods. For instance, Atkins's diet offered people a way to lose weight on: 'bacon and eggs for breakfast, on heavy cream in their coffee, on mayonnaise on their salads, butter sauce on their lobster; on spareribs, roast duck, on pastrami; on my special cheesecake for dessert'.[121]

Self-help books exemplify how health was increasingly marketed as a commodity. Readers' control over their own bodies depended on following advice given by self-help authors, but also on purchasing specific foods, drinks and supplements. The promotion of such goods included reference to the fact that they were inexpensive, easy to obtain and painless to ingest, as well as healthy in so many ways. According to

Plimmer, 'headache, constipation, anaemia, dyspepsia, nervous debility, wasting, obesity, lung weakness and kidney trouble ... were all signs of malnutrition', implying that purchasing and eating 'healthy' foods enabled readers to nourish their bodies to a state of perfect health.[122] The message here was clear: readers were no longer helpless, but lived in an age of affordable wonders in which they could combat not only malnutrition, but almost every condition imaginable, through buying 'health' foods and products. This is evident in the way Linus Pauling urged his readers to have a life without colds by buying vitamin C supplements. He firstly argued that the common cold caused unnecessary suffering and resulted in a loss of productivity and income.[123] Having offered advice on how to prevent and ameliorate a cold, Pauling then compared vitamin C with other over-the-counter medicines and antibiotics. Vitamin C, he argued, offered the easiest, cheapest and most efficient choice with fewer side effects, making health foods and supplements desirable commodities that readers could purchase and ingest for their own health's sake. 'By the proper intakes of vitamins and other nutrients', Pauling argued, 'and by following other healthful practices from youth or middle age on, you can, I believe, extend your life and years of well-being by twenty-five or even thirty-five years.'[124]

Although they shared some characteristics, self-help authors each possessed their own notions of balance, distinct dietary and lifestyle philosophies and writing styles. Each of these authors exploited their language, tone and expressions and used metaphors and similes to explain and encourage dietary change. Gaylord Hauser, for example, stated: 'You are holding a passport to a new way of living ... You are beginning a new adventure, a journey of discovery.'[125] His advice offered a reinterpretation of the cosmos, or what the anthropologist Anthony Wallace referred to as a 'mazeway resynthesis'.[126] Salvation was promised through adherence to new worldviews: youth and longevity lay purely in the hands of the individual. In addition to balanced diets, Hauser also recommended that readers manage or regulate their emotions and thoughts, and emphasised the need for balanced reciprocity in marriage; in later years, he argued, marriage should revolve around 'mutual interests, mutual accomplishments, as well as mutual affection'. Atkins adopted an alternative approach to Hauser's, capitalising sentences in order to urge readers to join his 'revolution': 'A REVOLUTION IN OUR DIET THINKING IS LONG OVERDUE'; and 'WE

ARE THE VICTIMS OF CARBOHYDRATE POISONING'.[127] These books were motivational, inspiring and easy to read; their conversational style made them appear more accessible and their goals more achievable.

Personal agency was also reinforced by stressing the fact that readers themselves could improve their own health without doctors, expensive and invasive treatments, or pills. In *Folk Medicine*, for example, D. C. Jarvis promoted the different uses of apple cider, honey and kelp for the prevention or treatment of a plethora of health conditions such as chronic fatigue, headaches, high blood pressure, sleep disorders and infertility.[128] Pauling's belief in the efficacy of self-care can be seen in his advice that, by not seeing 'the "doctor as God", you can avoid serious errors in your own care'.[129] Pauling also challenged the medical establishment and pharmaceutical industry as he compared vitamin C supplements favourably to commercial remedies such as aspirin and phenylpropopanolamine hydrochloride.[130] In *Life Extension*, Durk Pearson and Sandy Shaw promoted consumer choice as a route to better health and questioned the guidelines set by the Food and Drug Agency's (FDA) recommended daily allowances (RDA) of vitamins and minerals.[131]

Self-help authors echoed the views of clinicians – discussed by Martin Moore in Chapter 2 – that the health of diabetics depended to an extent on their own intelligence and reliability. Knowledge, agency and 'intelligence' had to be taught to diabetic patients and similarly to self-help readers. For example, being healthy was not a difficult endeavour, as Plimmer stressed that 'the ordinary person can plan his or her daily food without elaborate calculations'.[132] More flatteringly, Hauser's readers were reminded that simply by choosing to read his book they had taken a smart decision to live longer and feel younger. Hauser offered his readers a way to eat 'intelligently'; his books would enable people to expand their knowledge of foods, vitamins and minerals, as well as learning other holistic methods to maintain their youth.[133] A similar message was conveyed by Pauling and by Pearson and Shaw, who presented all the available information about vitamin C and antioxidants respectively, allowing readers to evaluate and criticise the recommendations of orthodox medicine and the FDA. Atkins went further, offering his readers a way to monitor their weight loss through the self-application of scientific methods. He urged his readers to purchase a home urine chemistry kit, Ketostix, which they could use to track whether or not, or to what extent, they were in ketosis.[134] 'Happiness is a purple stick' Atkins used to say, referring to the Ketostix, which constituted a physical manifestation of successful self-care. Pearson and Shaw also wanted readers to perceive themselves as scientists, as they dedicated a whole chapter to life-extending experiments in the home such as the cooking oil shelf-life test and vitamin C urine test using C-stix.[135] Robert Haas taught readers about high-density and low-density lipoproteins, blood glucose levels, triglycerides and uric acid.[136] The significance of these scientific endeavours lay in the fact that readers actively sought ways to measure, quantify and evaluate their own health, which reinforced a sense of control and mastery over their own bodies and allowed them to achieve a healthy state of physiological and psychological balance.

Conclusion

This chapter has considered some of the most popular self-help books in the genre of diet and health in order to understand more clearly how self-promotion, self-help, individual agency and personal responsibility for health came to dominate advice literature in the second half of the twentieth century. The authors of self-help books promoted self-care firstly through reference to their scientific expertise and scientific evidence. Self-help authors, who were almost exclusively men, published routinely on popular platforms instead of scientific, peer-reviewed journals, which made them appear to their readers as pioneers and revolutionaries.

All of the books explored in this chapter emphasised that readers could and should take care of their own bodies and safeguard their own health. The narratives were replete with notions of balance and neo-romanticism, and reflected interest in constructing new forms of selfhood through consumption and healthy lifestyles. The inclusion of insurance-related statistical figures by Plimmer and Pauling suggests that Western societies embraced and internalised a form of self-reflective, self-governing individualism, as well as the notion of efficiency, which most authors dealt with, if sometimes remotely. While Plimmer emphasised the impact of malnutrition on productivity and the strength of armies, Hauser promoted a graceful, youthful and productive old age, and Atkins offered people an escape from the carbohydrate poisoning, hunger pangs and mood swings that caused illness and loss of productivity.

The cultural capital of rationality and knowledge, a legacy of Enlightenment ideology, is also evident in these books as authors portrayed themselves as visionaries in the field of dietetics, supplementation and health. They emphasised how rationality, education and intelligence could lead to better health; facilitated the use of charts and graphs; recommended exact quantities and foods; and encouraged readers to undergo specific tests and to purchase supplements. Health, according to these authors, was observable, quantifiable and measurable, and they wrote in a way that made clear to their readers that good health was the product of the victory of mind over body, of rationality over primitivism. As Parasecoli has argued, through the promotion of specific foods, drinks, supplements, stores, products, tests and practices, these authors contributed to the commodification of health.[137] Readers could relatively affordably – but with sufficient willpower – improve their own health. According to self-help authors, rejection of the cultural authority of orthodox medicine and the adoption of more carefully balanced pathways to health constituted the most intelligent and rational form of self-care.

Notes

1 A. Weil, *8 Weeks to Optimum Health*, 2nd edition, 4th reprint (London: Time Warner Press, 2002), p. 1.
2 E. Hobsbawm, *Age of Extremes: The Short Twentieth Century 1914–1991* (London: Abacus, 1998), pp. 258–60.
3 D. Oddy, *From Plain Faire to Fusion Food: British Diet from the 1890s to the 1990s* (London: Boydell, 2003), p. 173.
4 Ibid.; W. Belasco, *Appetite for Change: How the Counterculture Took on the Food Industry*, 2nd edition (New York: Cornell University Press, 2007), pp. 15–16; H. Levenstein, *Fear of Food: A History of Why We Worry About What We Eat* (Chicago: University of Chicago Press, 2012), p. 2.
5 C. Fischler, 'The McDonaldization of culture', in J. L. Flandrin and M. Montanari (eds), *Food: A Culinary History from Antiquity to the Present*, 2nd edition (New York: Penguin Books, 2000), pp. 530–48.
6 Oddy, *Plain Faire to Fusion Food*, p. 188. For a discussion of changing rates of divorce, see Chapter 8.
7 Fischler, 'The McDonaldization of culture', pp. 533–4.
8 A. Bentley, 'Introduction', in A. Bentley (ed.), *A Cultural History of Food in the Modern Age* (New York: Berg, 2014), p. 12.

9 M. Jackson, *The Age of Stress: Science and the Search for Stability* (Oxford: Oxford University Press, 2013), p. 11.
10 W. B. Cannon, 'Organization for physiological homeostasis', *Physiological Reviews*, 9:3 (July 1929), 400.
11 U. Beck, *Risk Society: Towards a New Modernity*, trans. M. Ritter (London: Sage, 1992), p. 19.
12 C. E. Rosenberg, 'Pathologies of progress: the idea of civilization as risk', *Bulletin of the History of Medicine*, 72:4 (1998), 714–30.
13 A. Giddens, *Modernity and Self-Identity: Self and Society in the Late Modern Age* (Cambridge: Polity Press, 1991), p. 8.
14 Belasco, *Appetite for Change*, p. 4.
15 H. Levenstein, *Paradox of Plenty: A Social History of Eating in Modern America* (Oxford: Oxford University Press, 1993), p. 195.
16 M. Jancovich, 'The politics of *Playboy*: lifestyle, sexuality and non-conformity in American Cold War culture', in D. Bell and J. Hollows (eds), *Historicizing Lifestyle: Mediating Taste, Consumption and Identity from the 1900s to 1970s* (Hampshire: Ashgate, 2006), pp. 70–87.
17 For more work on anti-ageing, see: J. Stark, 'The age of youth', *Lancet*, 388:10059 (2016), 2470–1; and K. Heath, *Aging by the Book: The Emergence of Midlife in Victorian Britain* (New York: State University of New York Press, 2009), p. 16. See also Chapter 9.
18 Gayelord Hauser was a doctor of natural science (homeopathy and naturopathy); R. H. A. Plimmer was a biochemist and a nutrition expert; Dr Atkins was a medical doctor; Linus Pauling was a Nobel laureate in biochemistry and peace; and Pearson and Shaw are researchers.
19 M. Smith, *Hyperactive: The Controversial History of ADHD* (London: Reaktion Books, 2012), p. 136.
20 Feingold, an allergist from San Francisco, argued that ingestion of food additives caused hyperactivity and that the disorder could be alleviated with an additive-free diet. Mackarness was a clinical ecologist who argued that mental conditions could be attributed to food allergies – Jackson, *The Age of Stress*, pp. 172, 209.
21 G. Hauser targeted middle-aged, upper-class white women and Plimmer targeted literate housewives.
22 R. Apple, *Vitamania: Vitamins in American Culture* (New Jersey: Rutgers University Press, 1996), pp. 19–20.
23 C. Carstairs, '"Look younger, live longer": ageing beautifully with Gayelord Hauser in America, 1920–1975', *Gender and History*, 26:2 (2014), 334; Belasco, *Appetite for Change*, p. 68.
24 K. Albala, *Eating Right in the Renaissance* (Berkeley: University of California Press, 2002), p. 15.

25 M. Calman, 'Affairs of the heart: the day I got my just desserts', *The Times*, 4 July 1984, p. 13.
26 F. Parasecoli, 'Gluttonous crimes: chew, comic books, and the ingestion of masculinity', *Women's Studies International Forum*, 44 (May–June 2014), 236–46; and F. Parasecoli, *Bite Me: Food in Popular Culture* (New York: Berg, 2008), pp. 85–102.
27 J. Dubisch, 'You are what you eat: religious aspects of the health food movement', in C. Delaney and D. Kaspin (eds), *Investigating Culture: An Experiential Introduction to Anthropology*, 2nd edition (Chichester: Wiley, 2011), pp. 284–5. John Coveney has also discussed new dieting concerns as a modern iteration of Christian asceticism in Western societies, in J. Coveney, *Food, Morals, and Meaning: The Pleasure and Anxiety of Eating* (London: Routledge, 2000), p. 10. Sander Gilman argues that obesity generated a moral panic in the twentieth century and that dieting adopted both 'the lexicon and characteristics of a religious movement', in S. Gilman, *Obesity: The Biography* (Oxford: Oxford University Press, 2010), p. 77. The adoption of various lifestyle practices to achieve better health, whether mental, spiritual or physical, could be seen in the philosophy and activities of Esalen, including massages, naked baths and organic free-range food, which promoted a religion of no religion – see J. J. Kripal, *Esalen: America and the Religion of No Religion* (Chicago: Chicago University Press, 2007), p. 8.
28 Coveney, *Food, Morals, and Meaning*, p. 156.
29 G. Scrinis, 'On the ideology of nutritionism', *Gastronomica*, 8:1 (Winter 2008), 39.
30 Carstairs, '"Look younger, live longer"', p. 336.
31 Ibid.; and P. Kerr, 'Gayelord Hauser, 89, Author: proponent of natural foods', *New York Times Online* (originally published 29 December 1984), available at www.nytimes.com/1984/12/29/obituaries/gayelord-hauser-89-author-proponent-of-natural-foods.html, accessed 15 January 2016.
32 Carstairs, '"Look younger, live longer"', p. 336.
33 G. Hauser, *Look Younger, Live Longer* (New York: Farrar Straus, 1950), p. 32.
34 Carstairs, '"Look younger, live longer"', p. 336.
35 Ibid., p. 342.
36 Bureau of Investigation, 'Bengamin Gayelord Hauser: fruits, vegetables – and nuts', *Journal of the American Medical Association*, 108:16 (1937), 1360.
37 Hauser, *Look Younger, Live Longer*, p. 4.

38 Hauser's chapter on 'Bodily resistance' refers to how many grams of protein and how much vitamin C should be ingested: Hauser, *Look Younger, Live Longer*, pp. 54–5.
39 Ibid., pp. 4–5.
40 Ibid., p. 5.
41 Ibid., p. 332. *Look Younger, Live Longer* was in the top three bestsellers in non-fiction two years in a row: Berkeley's The Books of the Century initiative, which gives comprehensive lists of *Publishers' Weekly* bestselling books, *The Books of the Century: 1950–1959*, available at www.ocf.berkeley.edu/~immer/books1950s, accessed 1 November 2015.
42 Carstairs, '"Look younger, live longer"', p. 332.
43 S. Doonan, 'Eating gruel and loving it: strange celebrity diets, explained', *The Slate Online* (March 2012), available at www.slate.com/articles/life/doonan/2012/03/gayelord_hauser_the_man_who_invented_the_celebrity_diet_.html, accessed 11 January 2016.
44 Ibid. Hauser's legacy continued into the twenty-first century. In 2013, Rebecca Harrington from *New York Magazine* tried his nutritional plan for ten days. Some of the responses to Harrington's article refer to Hauser as a 'quack', while others refer to him as the father of the 'real' or 'wholefoods' movement.
45 Carstairs, '"Look younger, live longer"', pp. 332–3.
46 Ibid., pp. 335–6.
47 Ibid., p. 342. *Look Younger, Live Longer* also resonates with auto-suggestion as a self-help genre: N. V. Peale, *Power of Positive Thinking* (New York: Prentice-Hall, 1952).
48 J. Lowndes, '[R. H. A. Plimmer] Obituary notice', *Journal of Biochemistry*, 62:3 (March 1956), 353–7.
49 Ibid.
50 Ibid.
51 R. H. A. Plimmer, *Analyses and Energy Values of Foods* (London: HM Stationery Office, 1921).
52 R. H. A. Plimmer, *Practical Organic and Bio-Chemistry* (London: Longmans, 1918).
53 See, for example, V. Plimmer, 'Diet fallacies in the quest for slimness', *Daily Mail Atlantic Edition*, 31 March 1928, p. 10.
54 B. Marinacci, *Linus Pauling Biography*, Oregon State University, Linus Pauling Institute website, available at lpi.oregonstate.edu/linus-pauling-biography, accessed 1 November 2015.
55 Oddy, *From Plain Faire to Fusion Food*, p. 163.

56 A. Serafini, *Linus Pauling: A Man and his Science* (San Diego: ToExcel, 2000), pp. 240–9.
57 Apple, *Vitamania*, pp. 54–5.
58 Ibid.
59 Serafini, *Linus Pauling*, p. 249.
60 C. Mead and T. Hager, *Linus Pauling: Scientist and Peacemaker* (Corvallis: Oregon State University, 2001), p. 94; Marinacci, *Linus Pauling Biography*.
61 R. Paradowski, 'Linus Pauling: American scientist', *Encyclopaedia Britannica Online*, available at www.britannica.com/biography/Linus-Pauling, accessed 20 November 2015.
62 Mead and Hager, *Linus Pauling*, pp. 94–5.
63 L. Pauling, *Vitamin C and the Common Cold* (London: Ballantine, 1972), p. 7.
64 Ibid., pp. 35–8.
65 Ibid., p. 3.
66 Albala, *Eating Right in the Renaissance*, p. 49.
67 Around one thousand milligrams of vitamin C per day. R. Atkins, *Dr Atkins' Diet Revolution: The High Calorie Way to Stay Thin Forever: The Famous Vogue Superdiet Explained in Full* (New York: Bantam, 1972), p. 126.
68 L. Avedon, 'Look younger – longer', *Daily Mail*, 31 May 1971, pp. 14–15.
69 For example, 'Big value Yeoman potatoes enriched with vitamin C', *Daily Mail*, 26 April 1976, p. 4.
70 'Ribena', *The Times* (London), 9 September 1960, p. 14; 'Ribena', *Daily Mail*, 12 November 1979, p. 14 – 'nothing like … Ribena for keeping out the winter cold and chill'.
71 'Contraception: pill may cause vitamin deficiency', *The Times*, 7 August 1972, p. 9.
72 L. Rogak, *Dr Robert Atkins: The True Story of the Man behind the War on Carbohydrates* (London: Robson, 2005), p. 72.
73 Ibid.
74 Atkins, *Dr Atkins' Diet Revolution*.
75 Using Rogak's list of names, the studies Atkins probably consulted were: W. L. Bloom and G. Azar, 'Similarities of carbohydrate deficiency and fasting', *Archives of Internal Medicine*, 112:3 (1963), 333–7, and a series of studies between the 1950s and 1960s by A. Kekwick and G. L. S Pawan, such as 'Calorie intake in relation to body weight changes in the obese', *Lancet*, 268:6935 (1956), 155–61. In *Dr Atkins' Diet Revolution* it is evident that Atkins was aware of Dr John Yudkin's work, such as *Pure, White and Deadly* (1972) and other studies such as J. Yudkin and J. M.

Carey, 'The treatment of obesity by the "high-fat" diet. The inevitability of calories', *Lancet*, 276:7157 (1960), 939–41.
76 W. Banting, *Letter on Corpulence: Addressed to the Public* (London: Harrison, 1863).
77 R. Harrison, rev. V. Smith, 'Banting, William (1796/7–1878)', *Oxford Dictionary of National Biography Online*, available at www.oxforddnb.com/view/article/1320?docPos=1, accessed 4 April 2016.
78 Hauser, *Look Younger, Live Longer*, p. 63; A. Davis, *Let's Cook it Right* (San Diego: Harcourt, Brace and World, 1947), p. 22; H. Taller, *Calories Don't Count* (New York: Simon & Schuster, 1961); and R. Cameron self-published his book under the noms de plume Elliott Williams and Gardner Jameson, *The Drinking Man's Diet* (San Francisco: Cameron & Company, 1964).
79 V. Stefansson, *Not by Bread Alone: Eating Meat and Fat for Stay Lean and Healthy* (New York: Macmillan, 1946); R. Mackarness, *Eat Fat and Grow Slim* (London: Harvil Press, 1958); Taller, *Calories Don't Count*; Williams and Jameson [Cameron], *The Drinking Man's Diet*.
80 Rogak, *Dr Robert Atkins*, pp. 68–9.
81 Ibid., pp. 32, 37.
82 Ibid., p. 57.
83 Ibid., p. 59.
84 Ibid., pp. 5–9.
85 Atkins, *Diet Revolution*, p. 23.
86 Now the Center for Balanced Health, run by Dr Keith Berkowitz MD.
87 Rogak, *Dr Robert Atkins*, p. 89.
88 This equates roughly to $192,120 in 2017.
89 D. Martin, 'Oscar Dystel, who saved Bantam Books, dies at 101', *New York Times Online*, 29 May 2014, available at www.nytimes.com/2014/05/29/business/media/oscar-dystel-who-saved-bantam-books-dies-at-101.html?_r=0, accessed 20 February 2016.
90 Rogak, *Dr Robert Atkins*, p. 75.
91 Ibid.
92 Nielsen Book Scan, 'Top UK book sales of all time', available at https://docs.google.com/spreadsheets/d/1dhxblR1Vl7PbVP_mNhwEa3_lfUWiF__xSODLq1W83CA/edit#gid=0, accessed 20 February 2016.
93 Ibid.
94 D. Bell and J. Hollows, 'Towards a history of lifestyle', in Bell and Hollows (eds), *Historicizing Lifestyle*, p. 4; Giddens, *Modernity and Self-Identity*, p. 3.
95 J. Kirby, 'Working too hard: experiences of worry and stress in post-war Britain', in M. Jackson (ed.), *Stress in Post-War Britain, 1945–1985* (London: Pickering & Chatto, 2015), pp. 59–74.

96 D. Harvey, *A Brief History of Neoliberalism* (Oxford: Oxford University Press, 2007), p. 2. For a more in-depth historical analysis: D. Stedman Jones, *Masters of the Universe: Hayek, Friedman, and the Birth of Neoliberal Politics* (Princeton: Princeton University Press, 2014). See also: M. D. Moore, *Managing Diabetes, Managing Medicine: Chronic Disease and Clinical Bureaucracy in Post-War Britain* (Manchester: Manchester University Press, 2019).
97 D. Lupton, *Food, the Body and the Self* (London: Sage, 1996), p. 3; M. Foucault, 'Technologies of the Self', in L. H. Martin, H. Gutman and P. H. Hutton (eds), *Technologies of the Self: A Seminar with Michel Foucault* (London: Tavistock Press, 1988), pp. 16–49.
98 Atkins, *Diet Revolution*, p. 27.
99 Ibid., p. 19.
100 Weil, *8 Weeks to Optimum Health*, pp. 11–12.
101 S. Berger, *Dr Berger's Immune Power Diet* (New York: New American Library, 1985), p. 26.
102 S. L. Gilman, *Fat: A Cultural History of Obesity* (Cambridge: Polity Press, 2009), p. 7.
103 Berger, *Immune Power Diet*.
104 Ibid., p. 3.
105 D. C. Jarvis, *Folk Medicine* (London: Pan Books, 1968), title page.
106 J. Coveney, *Food, Morals and Meaning: The Pleasure and Anxiety of Eating*, 2nd edition (New York: Routledge, 2006), p. 23.
107 V. Plimmer and R. H. A. Plimmer, *Food Values at a Glance*, 9th edition (London: Longmans, 1959), p. 7.
108 Ibid., p. 17.
109 Pauling, *Vitamin C and the Common Cold*, p. 13.
110 Ibid., p. 37.
111 Lupton, *Food, the Body and the Self*, p. 33.
112 R. Haas, *Dr Robert Haas: Eat To Win, The High-Energy Diet for Peak Performance and Physical Fitness*, British reprint 2nd edition (Harmondsworth, Middlesex: Penguin Books, [1983] 1986), pp. 39, 90.
113 Ibid., p. 75.
114 Berger, *Immune Power Diet*, p. 25.
115 Jackson, *The Age of Stress*, p. 267.
116 Ibid.
117 Plimmer and Plimmer, *Food Values*, pp. 56–8.
118 Berger, *Dr Berger's Immune Power Diet*, p. 6.
119 Haas, *Eat To Win*, p. 7.
120 W. Belasco, *Food: The Key Concepts* (New York: Berg, 2008), p. 29.
121 Atkins, *Diet Revolution*, p. 3.

122 Plimmer and Plimmer, *Food Values*, p. 14.
123 Pauling, *Vitamin C and the Common Cold*, pp. 11–13.
124 L. Pauling, *How to Live Longer and Feel Better* (New York: Freeman & Company, 1986), p. 4.
125 Hauser, *Look Younger, Live Longer*, p. 4.
126 A. Wallace, *Religion: An Anthropological View* (New York: Random House, 1966), p. 237.
127 Atkins, *Diet Revolution*, pp. 3–5.
128 Jarvis, *Folk Medicine*, pp. 72–9.
129 Pauling, *Vitamin C and the Common Cold*, p. 5.
130 Ibid., pp. 91–3.
131 D. Pearson and S. Shaw, *Life Extension: A Practical Scientific Approach* (New York: Warner Books, 1982), p. 398.
132 Plimmer and Plimmer, *Food Values*, p. 11.
133 Hauser, *Look Younger, Live Longer*, p. 36.
134 Atkins, *Diet Revolution*, p. 14.
135 Pearson and Shaw, *Life Extension*, pp. 390–1.
136 Haas, *Eat To Win*, pp. 28–9.
137 See the discussions in Parasecoli, 'Gluttonous crimes', and Parasecoli, *Bite Me: Food in Popular Culture*.

6

Your life in your hands: teaching 'relaxed living' in post-war Britain

Ayesha Nathoo

Introduction

In 1968, a short Disney film, *Understanding Stresses and Strains*, narrated by actor, writer and director Lawrence Dobkin, opened with the following statement:

> A modern concept of well-balanced health may be visualised as an equilateral triangle composed of a physical side, a mental side and a social side, each of equal importance. This is a soundly based concept and those who live within it, keeping all sides in balance, enjoy good health.[1]

Accompanying a visual representation of a spinning and rapidly shrinking equilateral triangle, the narrator continued: 'But how does one maintain this balance when driven by pressures of our modern world?' The animators of this film, part of the Upjohn Company's 'Triangle of Health' series, included Eric Larson, one of Disney's original core artists, whose famous animations included Peter Pan's magical flight over London to Neverland. In contrast, *Understanding Stresses and Strains* included no fantastical scenarios or solutions, instead remaining firmly grounded in the contemporary reality of a Western metropolis. It posed the serious question of how to maintain 'well-balanced health' in a perpetually stress-inducing environment.

One regular set of audience members who were shown this film were relaxation class students. With the aid of the film, relaxation teachers would explain how chronic states of tension were responsible for a wide array of modern maladies. To counter and reverse this effect, students were told that duly practising neuromuscular relaxation would provide an effective means of developing and maintaining a healthy, balanced life – physically, mentally and socially.

Owing to the work of early pioneers, most notably that of the Chicago physician Edmund Jacobson, a particular understanding of 'relaxation' as neuromuscular 'tension control' was forged in the twentieth century, distinct from its vernacular usage implying recreation or 'being languid'.[2] Instead, relaxation was recharacterised as a technical, scientifically validated skill that required precise teaching and long-term cultivation. Once learned, relaxation methods could be applied as both prophylactic and therapy for a whole spectrum of physical and mental health conditions, and used to improve states of well-being.[3] As Jacobson had argued in his seminal texts, *Progressive Relaxation* (1929) written for a medical readership, and *You Must Relax* (1934) for a popular audience, it was impossible to be tense and relaxed at the same time. He claimed that even thought manifested in muscular tension, and hence it followed that systematically recognising and releasing bodily tension would both relax the body and quieten the mind. In line with the principles of psychosomatic medicine that garnered widespread support from the 1940s, relaxation advocates considered physical and mental states to be interconnected, indeed inseparable.

A range of relaxation methods were developed during the twentieth century that spanned diverse Western socio-political contexts. Yet a common explanatory framework made them therapeutically appealing to successive populations beset by 'neurasthenia', 'exhaustion', 'nerves' and 'stress'.[4] Notions of balance featured predominantly in relaxation and stress discourse: therapeutic strategies were framed as a means to restore and retain bodily equilibrium, and provide a counterbalance to the mental and physical stresses of modern life. A relaxed individual would supposedly not only cope better with his or her environment – balancing personal needs and social demands – but would also positively impact on their wider environment by fostering healthier dispositions and better social relations.

To support the remedial claims of relaxation, advocates drew heavily on the developing scientific literature on stress, spearheaded by the physiologist Walter Cannon (1871–1945) and the endocrinologist Hans Selye (1907–82). For example, Cannon's notions of 'homeostasis', the body's 'fight or flight' response to biological, psychological and social 'stressors', and the supposed destabilising effects of chronic stress on the endocrine, digestive and circulatory systems were routinely incorporated into relaxation teachings.[5] From the late 1960s, the Disney film *Understanding Stresses and Strains* was one entertaining yet serious way of engaging relaxation class attendees with these concepts.

Although recent historical studies have highlighted that relaxation practice, primarily used as an antidote to 'stress', proliferated in the post-war period, we so far know very little about how these therapeutic ideologies were promulgated.[6] What were the cultural platforms and processes by which relaxation discourse reached different populations? Who were the practitioners and what were the sites, modes and methods of teaching and learning relaxation? Moreover, what did relaxation teaching entail, why and to whom did it appeal, and how did it impact on modern formations of selfhood? Through a focus on Britain from the 1950s to the late 1970s, this chapter analyses the processes by which neuromuscular relaxation functioned and proliferated as a taught practice. It is a study of health communication, education and management, which pays attention to material and audio-visual cultures and uncovers the mechanisms, expectations and consequences of teaching and learning relaxation. Whereas state-sponsored public health campaigns relating to smoking, alcohol, diet and exercise have been well documented by historians, the processes by which stress-management strategies were contemporaneously popularised and consumed have received little scholarly attention. This chapter therefore extends growing historical interest in stress, well-being, chronic-disease prevention, health education and medical communication in the post-war period.[7] It is informed by sociological and historical analyses of how 'psy' therapeutics gain traction, utilise expertise, operate and (self-) govern individuals in advanced liberal democracies.[8] But while sympathetic to such perspectives, it takes a detailed, localised, cultural-historical approach that complements more recent cultural sociological scholarship – in particular the work of Eva Illouz. Using sociologist Philippe Corcuff's designation of 'bulldozer' concepts, Illouz criticises notions of 'governmentality', 'surveillance' and 'biopower' for a tendency to produce overly homogenising interpretations. Instead, through 'a thick and contextual analysis' her work aims to uncover the 'mechanism of culture: how meanings are produced ... how they are used in daily life to shape relationships and cope with an uncertain social world, and why they come to organise our interpretation of self and others'.[9] This chapter shares a similar orientation, and contributes a medical historical grounding to such sociological studies on the 'therapeutic turn'.

Piecing together a diverse array of rich archival material, the following sections uncover the varied particularities of relaxation advice and experience, the range of sources and the multiple processes by which relaxation discourse and practice was created, circulated and appropriated. In line with the work of historian Jim Secord, this analytical stance lays bare how 'knowledge-making itself' is a form of communication, exchange and interaction.[10] Although relaxation practices proliferated across Europe and the United States, the geographical focus of this chapter on Britain permits a focused analysis across myriad sources, and brings to the fore a largely undocumented narrative of how and why post-war relaxation ideology and practice paved the way for an expansive stress-management industry in later decades.

The first section details the pedagogy of neuromuscular relaxation, surveying the spectrum of teachers and the competing sites, modes and channels of teaching that facilitated debate, popular awareness and uptake. The second section examines notions of professionalism and expertise and the relationship between relaxation and biomedical practitioners, models and therapeutics. It investigates how relaxation practices were framed as a viable alternative to common pharmaceuticals, especially through tapping into and co-creating the market established by minor tranquillisers. The last section documents what relaxation teachings comprised over and above physical exercises, uncovering the diffuse meanings and requirements that constituted a healthy, relaxed way of life. It places relaxation in the wider contexts of self-care and health education, and allows for an assessment of the consequences of teaching individuals to cultivate relaxed, balanced selves.

Mediating relaxation

Although therapeutic relaxation strategies were taken up in a number of clinical settings in the post-war decades, this section concentrates on the methods by which relaxation instruction circulated in popular culture, including self-help books, radio and television programmes, group classes and teaching aids such as cassette tapes and biofeedback equipment. These various modes of communication were differentially accessed, promoted and evaluated, and reinforced one another as part of a larger communication circuit that co-established a specific health discourse and a growing market for relaxation teachings.

'Modern man lives at a speed and under a strain unknown to his forefathers', opened a popular book, *Relaxation: Nature's Way with Tension* in 1968: 'Constant tension must inevitably take its toll on health and efficiency: strained faces, unsightly posture, irritable behaviour ... heart trouble, high blood pressure, stomach ulcers and other results of the speed and stress of the times are on the increase.'[11] The reader is subsequently advised: 'if the health-destroying tension is to be banished or kept away you need to learn the techniques of relaxation.'[12] Alongside numerous other twentieth-century relaxation teaching resources, this text signalled to readers: a) that they were living in an age of unprecedented stress and strain; b) that this was having a detrimental impact on their minds, bodies, social relations and well-being; and c) that relaxation was a solution available to those prepared to learn and practise regularly. But how and where could one learn to relax, and through what means was this discourse created, diffused and reaffirmed among British publics?

Relaxation ideology was most widely communicated via the mass media. Newspapers and magazine articles, radio and television programmes were key channels through which thousands of people gained awareness of neuromuscular relaxation, conceptualised as a therapeutic skill. Health items traditionally featured heavily across different media sources, targeting and attracting large numbers of media consumers, especially women. Items on 'nerves' and advice on managing 'nervous tension' held considerable traction, as media channels and medical and psychological frameworks opened up new discursive spaces for articulating both the challenges of and potential solutions to emotional, domestic and everyday experiences.[13] As the Health Editor of *Woman* magazine wrote in 1960, she received over 6,000 letters, mainly from 'young wives and mothers', in response to one of her magazine articles on nervous tension. Conditions such as 'chronic tiredness and indigestion, persistent backache, recurring headache, and difficulty in breathing or swallowing' were frequently referenced. To help these women 'sort themselves out', she encouraged 'essentials' such as 'wise eating habits, the regular practice of muscular relaxation and deep breathing, plus the instigation of a more satisfactory way of life.'[14] Relaxation, therefore, readily sat alongside dietary and other 'lifestyle' advice that increasingly characterised post-war public health education.[15]

Health matters were an integral part of BBC radio broadcasting from its inception in the interwar years.[16] Unlike printed sources, radio could utilise vocal qualities, and relaxation proponents featured regularly on programmes such as *Woman's Hour* – a 'daily programme of music, advice, and entertainment for the home', which started in 1946 on what was then BBC Light (the precursor to BBC Radio 2). Antenatal care was one of the first and most central forums for incorporating relaxation teachings in Britain, and a number of radio relaxation programmes from the 1950s focused on preparation for childbirth.[17] Other programmes appealed to wider audiences, such as 'New Year Resolution: Let's Remember to Relax in 1952' on *Woman's Hour*, which was followed by three weeks of daily guided relaxation exercises for stiff necks, backaches, strained faces and breathing.[18] Audience reach increased as other radio programmes and airwaves were established, such as the medical magazine *In Practice*, which started in 1968, and the lunchtime *You and Yours* programme in 1970, mainly directed at housewives.

By the late 1960s, the medium with the potential to reach the largest audience was television, which by that time was broadcasting in colour with a choice of three channels and an ever-increasing variety of programme formats. Relaxation teachers were keen to take advantage of this audio-visual medium, but their material had to make good television – entertaining as well as informative – and they faced stiff competition. As Dr Claire Weekes, who featured regularly on British radio, bemoaned at a study day for relaxation teachers in 1977: 'I can't get on television – not even for 10 minutes. Been on *Nationwide* – they gave me 3 minutes. I can say a lot in 3 minutes but not enough.'[19] Given the overall intentional lack of activity involved in a relaxation exercise, practical teachings tended to feature as part of programmes that included more eye-catching content, for example alongside demonstrations of hypnosis or within yoga programmes – both of which incorporated more visually striking material than relaxation practices alone.[20] Less constrained by time pressures and the need for visual entertainment, it was radio, rather than television, that proved more conducive to broadcasting detailed neuromuscular relaxation advice and instruction.

Physiotherapist Jane Madders' six-part radio series, 'Relax – and Enjoy it', broadcast on *You and Yours* in 1972, for example, proved extremely popular with listeners, who were systematically taught neuromuscular methods. Madders was a leading proponent of relaxation, who made regular radio appearances and provided training to National Childbirth Trust (NCT) antenatal teachers and instructors from the charity Relaxation for Living which had recently formed around the time that 'Relax – and Enjoy it' was broadcast.[21] The widespread popularity of this series led the BBC to publish a book, *Relax: The Relief of Tension Through Muscle Control* (1973), and an accompanying cassette tape.[22] The foreword to the book, written by the producer of the *You and Yours* radio series, explained that she had hoped listeners to the series would find lasting help from relaxation. 'However', she continued, 'it's not always possible to be near your radio when you want to be – or to remember every word you hear.' She noted that one listener had complained that someone came in while she was listening to the programme, and so she 'missed the arms and legs'. Another wrote: 'As my husband is at work during the day it is impossible for him to hear your programme on relaxation and I feel he is missing out on something that could change his life in a very positive way.' Other listeners requested that the ideas be written down, 'so they could refer to them whenever they wanted'.[23] Radio, therefore, had the advantage of reaching wide audiences simultaneously, and making the most of the vocal instructions, but was by no means a replacement for written resources, which had the major advantage that they could be referenced repeatedly, whenever and wherever suitable.

Self-help books such as *Relax* were key sites of detailed relaxation teachings. Although not at first categorised as a specific genre, the number and sales of such publications burgeoned over the course of the twentieth century, particularly in the United States, but also in Britain.[24] Increased literacy rates and access to education, and the development of paperback printing in the 1960s, significantly helped to boost demand and supply in the post-war period, reinforcing this popular yet private channel by which health advice and information could be obtained outside of and alongside formal medical encounters. Therapeutic relaxation practices were promoted especially in books on: combating 'stress' or 'nerves'; preparation for childbirth; and, as it gained popularity from the 1960s, secularised modern yoga.[25]

Following earlier traditions of self-help that encouraged self-reliance, some books signalled the wider benefits of relaxation, over and above combating ill health, reflected in titles such as *Relax and Be Successful* (1951) and its sequel *The Art of Relaxed Living: A Guide to Health, Happiness and Success in an Age of Stress* (1955) by journalist and health writer James Hewitt. Many relaxation books underwent successive reprints and new editions, and relaxation advice was included in widely popular series such as Tandem publishing house's 'Do Something' series, and Hodder and Stoughton's 'Teach Yourself' series in the 1960s and 1970s.

As with Madders's book *Relax*, audio recordings often accompanied relaxation books as supplementary teaching aids. Following the development and commercial availability of long-playing records in the 1950s and cassette tapes in the early 1960s, these objects circulated widely among consumers and practitioners, and were available for loan through libraries. The Graves Medical Audiovisual Library, initially housed by the College of General Practitioners, for example, stocked a range of relaxation cassettes, allowing the medium and method to become more widely accessible to medical practitioners and their patients.[26] The organisation Relaxation for Living also housed its own audio and printed-source library for relaxation teachers and their students. Relaxation recordings brought to life the written information, providing a 'vicarious presence' of the author, which could make listeners feel as though they were 'sitting beside' the teacher. Commenting positively on the value of cassettes over written instruction, the author of *The Art and Practice of Relaxation*, psychiatrist Ian Martin, remarked: 'Every attempt is made in vocal technique to capitalise on the recording medium by inducing a soothing and reassuring atmosphere.'[27] Martin also commended the use of cassette tapes as a means of improving the availability of the technique while reducing the therapist's routine involvement.[28]

Not all practitioners, however, favoured the use of cassette tapes and other teaching tools. Notably, Jacobson argued that the foundational therapeutic skill to be learned was subtle self-recognition and self-control of muscular tension without reliance on any external aid. For this reason, Jacobson supported neither the use of cassette tapes nor another key teaching aid developed in the 1960s – biofeedback devices.[29] These machines were designed to provide usually auditory or visual feedback in order to 'make conscious what is happening inside [the] body as it responds to various subjective or behavioural states.'[30] Measurable functions included heart rate, blood pressure, electrical resistance of the skin via sweat gland activity and electrical activity across muscles, skin temperature and brainwave patterns shown via an EEG (neurofeedback). Biofeedback instruments measured and displayed physiological changes that users were not normally aware of, to help develop conscious control over these bodily processes.

The term 'biofeedback' was coined at a conference in 1969 in Santa Monica, building on and bringing together research into cybernetics and feedback, operant conditioning and physiological investigations into homeostasis and self-regulation.[31] Measuring and displaying the functions of the autonomic nervous system was not new – for example, equipment had been developed in the nineteenth century to determine heart rate and skin resistance – but biofeedback devices helped demonstrate that these physiological functions could not only be measured and displayed but also voluntarily controlled. Jacobson himself had devised a neurovoltmeter in the 1920s, capable of detecting tiny changes in muscular electrical activity; indeed, making tension measurable was central to his formulation of relaxation therapy as a demonstrable, verifiable, scientific enterprise.[32] But despite his support for accurate measuring equipment, Jacobson considered biofeedback training to be 'self-defeating'.[33] Requiring an external aid to learn how to relax, he believed, took away from the process of tuning into the body's own feedback and the ability to recognise and eliminate subtle residual tension.

Other practitioners, such as Madders, found biofeedback devices to be an important and successful teaching aid, and the field attracted widespread attention. Devices were often introduced during group and individual teaching sessions to demonstrate how tension states could be altered through relaxation exercises. By the 1970s, biofeedback equipment was put to a diverse range of therapeutic uses in British hospitals – including the Royal Free and Bartholomew's in London, and the Queen Elizabeth Hospital in Birmingham – to help to treat stammering, tension headaches, anxiety and phobias.[34] The Cambridge company Aleph One Ltd, established in 1972, was a key distributor of this equipment, and helped raise awareness of biofeedback and relaxation research and training via a monthly newsletter. As well as supplying equipment for clinics, for home training Aleph One offered for sale the mini 'relaxometer'. Users placed two fingers on the device's small metal plates and the relaxometer provided auditory feedback on fingertip sweat levels, producing a corresponding tone that lowered in pitch as arousal decreased. The uptake of this small, affordable technology in domestic environments coincided with the development and circulation of a wide range of home medical monitoring and diagnostic devices that granted patients a greater sense of agency, autonomy and responsibility.[35]

Self-care practices such as relaxation therapy reoriented relationships between health-seeking populations and practitioners, but by no means did away with the need for professional support and oversight. Books, magazine articles, radio and television programmes were forums for introducing large audiences to the principles and merits of relaxation practice, but most practitioners advocated lessons with a teacher as the most effective means to learn properly. Jacobson's original progressive relaxation technique required months of 'live training' with a teacher for at least two hours per week, as well as up to two hours' daily home practice.[36] Although less intensive, shorter styles and formats of muscular relaxation teachings were subsequently developed, the role of the teacher remained primary. As Madders explained in a radio interview: 'It is important to have interaction with a caring person. If one can extrapolate from other psychological treatments, the teacher is crucial.'[37] In support of group classes, one relaxation advocate reflected that 'people find it easier to relax when other people are doing it'.[38] But not all practitioners agreed. Favouring individual tuition over group training, one practitioner at a relaxation teacher study day argued: 'I think groups are dangerous. If they start to exchange symptoms … you can get an exhibitionist … people get upset by others in a group.' She also had concerns that 'you get people who have been ill for a long time and have no intention of getting better because they like being a member of the group'.[39] Nonetheless, by the mid-1970s demand for group relaxation classes was outstripping supply. Through widespread promotional practices and a rich material culture, the market for relaxation had been firmly established.

Individual practitioners and small organisations such as the Relaxation Society, Relaxation for Living, Stress Watch and the Institute of Applied Meditation helped to both create and meet the demand for relaxation classes in Britain. Some classes were drop-in, and others were offered as a course. The set of six lessons offered through the charity Relaxation for Living, for example, was modelled on relaxation classes for migraine sufferers and NCT antenatal courses.[40] Given the strong association forged between relaxation and childbirth, practitioners had to work harder to make the techniques appealing and relevant to men.

In *Relaxation: A Key to Better Living* (1965), health educator Joe Macdonald Wallace reflected on the difficulties of introducing a weekly neuromuscular relaxation class for men in an English college: 'it was obvious that to some students this kind of learning is associated rather exclusively with having a baby. Frequently, I have found this opinion to be held by many others, and some of my men pupils have been somewhat hesitant to begin lessons because of this connection.'[41] Through increasing research and publicity surrounding chronic stress, hypertension and heart disease, and a developing public health discourse around 'risk' and 'lifestyles', relaxation practice became more appealing and accessible to men. Specific classes and literature were developed for male 'executives', drawing on contemporary epidemiological, psychological and clinical research and terminology, often targeting supposed 'Type A', 'coronary-prone', middle-aged men. In tandem with the rising marketing and prescription of pharmaceuticals for chronic-disease prevention, relaxation practitioners promoted their practices as safe, effective means of lowering the risk of having or repeating a heart attack.[42] Modelling relaxation as a path to increased physical and mental efficiency, and hence productivity, was also central to encouraging uptake among men and in the workplace.[43]

Antenatal teacher and physiotherapist Laura Mitchell was one leading relaxation teacher in post-war Britain who catered for both men and women. In the 1970s, she started to offer lunchtime relaxation classes to 'overtired city workers' at St Mary Woolnoth Church in Lambeth, London. Mitchell had developed her own relaxation method, devised while recovering from a serious neck injury. A billboard outside the church advertised the relaxation classes: 'STRESS. Learn to recognise it. Learn to cope with it.' An image depicted two hands clutching either end of a stick, bending it to breaking point. These classes were arranged by the church Vicar, Reverend Geoffrey Harding, a member of the Churches' Council of Health and Healing and the Institute of Religion and Medicine, and founder of the Relaxation Society. Through the society he produced and distributed booklets on the benefits of relaxation as an antidote to the ill-effects of tension derived from Western urban living – physically, mentally, socially and spiritually. Harding himself offered weekly classes in the church on relaxation and meditation, which, although grounded in a Christian perspective, were open 'to anyone who needed help, without theological strings attached'.[44] The church relaxation classes attracted considerable media attention, featuring on ITN's *News at Ten*, and in newspaper articles, which steadily increased the flow of attendees.[45]

For those who wanted close interaction with a teacher but could not attend a class in person, private correspondence courses were also available. Relaxation for Living started a correspondence course in 1972, but there had been a number of precursors. Desmond Dunne, author of numerous popular yoga-relaxation books, offered correspondence courses from the 1940s when he established Britain's first yoga school.[46] Relaxation featured heavily in yoga teachings, which were made more widely available from the 1960s through nationwide adult education classes. Yoga-relaxation teachers in London, Birmingham and Liverpool established notable local followings.[47]

During the post-war decades, then, relaxation material was widely distributed via multiple modalities. Authors of relaxation self-help books frequently featured on radio and television programmes, gave talks, produced cassette tapes and vinyls and taught classes. Different media sources reinforced one another – with books often recommending 'further readings' and other resources, and classes promoted through media interviews, magazine articles and newsletters, and recommended through word of mouth. The variety of teaching modes, including biofeedback equipment and educational films, prompted lively debates over the respective merits and drawbacks of different media and ways of teaching. As the next sections will discuss, relaxation teachers were also concerned with the legitimacy and status of who was imparting relaxation instruction, and offered multiple perspectives on what relaxation training could and should entail.

Biomedicine, education and expertise

Relaxation teachers came from a variety of professional backgrounds. They shared a common aim of promoting the field of relaxation therapy, but in a competitive and diverse marketplace they also sought to differentiate themselves from one another. Although relaxation was widely advocated as a 'simple' and essential means of self-care, practitioners also warned of the need for professional guidance and regulation. This section analyses how relaxation practitioners negotiated claims to professional expertise, related their discipline to medical science and health education, and presented relaxation therapy as a safe, effective alternative to pharmaceuticals.

In the preface to the first edition of *You Must Relax* (1934), Jacobson opened with the drawbacks of writing such a book: 'a popular book on fatigue and nervous ills might prompt many to try to use it for self-healing, when what they really need is instruction in the method by a physician or else some other form of medical attention.'[48] Nonetheless, he believed that better informed laymen might aid and stimulate physicians in dealing with the common maladies of the nervous, digestive and circulatory systems that resulted from 'high nerve tension'. He also hoped that the book would meet the demands for a 'popularly written volume' by instructors in the performing arts, and in physical education (PE), who noticed that 'proficiency in their pupils depends upon the attainment of a certain relaxation during execution.'[49] By the 1960s, Jacobson considered PE teachers, rather than physicians, the most suitable professional group to teach neuromuscular relaxation, but the foundational authority still lay with medical science. Jacobson consistently and adamantly differentiated his 'scientific relaxation' method from any esoteric practices or traditions that were not firmly grounded in the biomedical model – in particular practices stemming from the mesmeric tradition.[50]

Debates concerning the need and place for professional, medical and scientific expertise ensued as relaxation practitioners grew in number. Writing in 1965, Joe Macdonald Wallace, health educator and lecturer in anatomy and physiology, argued that teaching relaxation required no 'medical halo'.[51] Relaxation, according to him, was best left in the hands of health and PE teachers, who had sufficient knowledge of physiology and anatomy and had the potential to influence young people at a critical point in their lives. Relaxation for Living teachers also primarily positioned themselves as health educators: 'We make no claim whatsoever to be medically qualified', stated the founder in a magazine interview.[52] Many of the organisation's original instructors were antenatal teachers who were not medically trained, and later teachers included former students from a range of professional spheres, whose understanding of relaxation therapy derived primarily from their own prior experience as class attendees.

Nonetheless, relaxation teachers still had claims to expertise that warranted their status and fees as professionals. One of Relaxation for Living's core teachers, Penny Wade, was asked to justify this position during an interview on the Radio London programme *Woman in Town* in 1974: 'What qualifications do you need to be a relaxation teacher?', the presenter asked. Wade responded: 'You need a knowledge of anatomy, physiology of course, and you need to know how to teach.'[53] She explained to listeners, in advance of broadcasting a lesson, that relaxation was in fact a very simple undertaking. The interviewer proceeded to press her on why then, if it was so simple, people needed to be taught how to relax. For some teachers, framing relaxation training as simple was pedagogically intended, presupposing the needs and capacities of potential learners. As one teacher, who trained under Madders, recalled: 'Jane Madders' watchword was "keep it simple", as a group of women could have varied levels of understanding and could be intimidated by wordy physical explanations.'[54]

Physiotherapist Laura Mitchell also stressed simplicity, evidenced from her bestselling book *Simple Relaxation*. The jacket advertised 'a simple and effective antidote to stress that anyone can learn and apply in a matter of hours'. It was a tension-relieving system with 'no complicated exercises or complex psychological regimens' and 'simple in the extreme'.[55] Simplicity could also act as a deterrent, however. Writing in 1968, when technically ground-breaking undertakings such as heart-transplant surgery and space travel dominated medical and scientific news, psychiatrist and relaxation practitioner Ainslie Meares, lamented:

> I have found that one of the greatest difficulties in helping people by this approach has been getting them to accept its simplicity. People always want the newest form of medical treatment. The modern trend in medicine is continually toward greater and greater complexity ... We have come to associate complexity of therapy as an advance over more simple treatment.[56]

Leading practitioners such as Meares and Madders tended to encourage combining elements from a number of available techniques, without privileging one method over another. Concerns abounded, however, over the status and qualifications of the increasing number of self-fashioned relaxation teachers, impacting on the reputation of the field as a whole. As Madders told attendees of a conference on 'Stress in Everyday Life' in 1974:

> During the past ten years there has been an unprecedented interest in somatic enterprises which claim to affect the mind through bodily processes ... Almost the only common component is muscle relaxation. Some of these systems are soundly based, taught by highly qualified teachers ... others may well be dangerous in the hands of unqualified enthusiasts ... It is hardly surprising therefore that the medical profession as a whole is sceptical and cautious about the claims of these self-help methods.[57]

Madders supported teachers who based their teachings on 'evidence and research' rather than 'conjecture', and was wary of the commercial aspect of teaching relaxation, where sessions could become 'an expensive trap for those who are especially vulnerable and gullible when they are under stress'. Relaxation for Living teachers were told to stick on their wall the following note from Madders, who was the organisation's lead trainer and technical advisor:

> I stress objective teaching based on research because it is too easy for the passionately fringe, pseudo-psychology eccentrics to blossom in this powerful role of teacher to those under stress.[58]

Historian Elizabeth Siegel Watkins has noted that 'medicalization of stress allowed for an expansion of therapeutic options available to practitioners and recipients of mainstream medicine by opening up space for the legitimation of alternative healing practices'.[59] Relaxation therapy was certainly a part of this expanded, pluralistic terrain of what historian Roberta Bivins usefully describes as 'medical heterodoxies',[60] but relaxation therapists rarely identified themselves as 'alternative' practitioners. Instead, teachers who were not medically qualified tended to adopt the terminology and cultural authority of biomedicine and psychology, generally allying themselves to the medical profession in a complementary, rather than alternative fashion. One practitioner, for example, declared at a teacher study day: 'I refuse to see people without the knowledge of their doctor.' Many practitioners who were not medically qualified made close ties with local GPs, who in turn referred patients to their classes; doctors who were sympathetic to the aims of relaxation organisations were often appointed as trustees, invited to speak at study days and review advice literature.[61] Relaxation teachers generally positioned themselves as aiding rather than challenging medical models and practice, often framing their work as helping to ease the burden on the already overstretched NHS.

Although some medical professionals were sceptical about relaxation training, doubting the vague concept and long-term health consequences of 'stress', there were also many supporters. Relaxation teachings were increasingly incorporated into healthcare practices in the post-war decades, especially in physiotherapy and osteopathy for pain management, physical and cardiac rehabilitation, and also in psychiatry and psychotherapy for anxiety treatment. Interest among London medical practitioners was high enough by 1973 for a 'Relaxation Therapy Study Group' to form and meet weekly to discuss therapeutic applications of relaxation.[62] Indeed, some of the most widely circulated relaxation books were written by doctors or physiotherapists, advising readers on how to identify, prevent or remedy specific medical conditions. Contrasting the brief consultation times available in general practice, the 'Do Something' series advertised on the cover sleeves: 'It is as though by some miracle, your own doctor had an hour to spare ... with you.'[63]

Scientific research into the efficacy of relaxation training also greatly contributed to increasing popular and professional acceptance. In the United States, cardiologist Herbert Benson's investigations into the physiological effects of meditative practices and his bestselling publication *The Relaxation Response* (1975) were no doubt seminal, but there were also influential British investigators. In the 1970s, GP and researcher Chandra Patel, in particular, furthered relaxation therapy's scientific credibility and perceived utility. Her longitudinal studies on the efficacy of yoga, biofeedback and relaxation therapy demonstrated encouraging results for reducing hypertension. Through medical journals and conferences, popular books, cassettes, television and radio programmes, Patel advocated relaxation as therapy and prevention for a range of chronic conditions including heart disease. GPs, she thought, should be at the forefront of teaching and promoting relaxation therapies that had the potential to reduce, or even provide a substitute for, pharmaceutical drugs. In 1976, a *British Medical Journal* editorial, 'Meditation or methyldopa', identified Patel's studies, and commented that although 'there is no immediate suggestion that physicians' efforts to lower blood pressure with drugs will be replaced wholesale by relaxation techniques ... in a few years, who knows?'[64] In 1981, Patel and other prominent researchers, including renowned epidemiologist Michael Marmot, suggested from their studies thus far that 'relaxation-based behavioural methods might be offered as a first-line treatment to patients with mild hypertension' and reduce coronary risk.[65]

In relation to pharmaceuticals, relaxation therapy could, therefore, offer an 'alternative' to standard biomedical treatment. For many conditions, including asthma, diabetes, hypertension, insomnia and anxiety, relaxation practices were promoted as a means to either reduce or eliminate the consumption of long-term medication. In the 1970s, populations looked towards pharmaceuticals with ambivalence. The high-profile thalidomide tragedy – when the morning sickness drug resulted in thousands of birth defects – was still playing out in the pages of the press. Nonetheless, demand and supply of pharmaceuticals were high: in 1965, British general practitioners wrote 39.7 million prescriptions for psychotropic drugs – comprising tranquillisers, antidepressants and sedatives – increasing to 47.2 million in 1970.[66]

The extensive popular uptake of minor tranquillisers had altered the threshold of what was considered to be tolerable and acceptable emotional and behavioural responses to the trials and tribulations of everyday living. Tranquillisers promised to restore a sense of physical and emotional equilibrium, by chemically rectifying supposed neurological imbalances. Marketed from the 1950s, particularly (though not exclusively) to women, anxious housewives and mothers made up a significant proportion of tranquilliser users. In Britain, women were twice as likely as men to be prescribed psychotropic drugs by general practitioners. Following Miltown and Equanil in the 1950s, Valium (introduced in 1963) became the single most successful drug in pharmaceutical history until Prozac entered the market in the 1990s. As various scholars have argued, minor tranquillisers such as Miltown and Valium performed a potent social as well as chemical function, encouraging and enabling women to cope with and better perform their social duties, without necessarily addressing or changing environments, expectations or patriarchal frameworks.[67] For certain demographics such as white, middle-class women and men, the uptake of relaxation therapies and minor tranquillisers share a combined history of intersecting populations and goals, which helped to co-create their markets.

A Ciba-sponsored medical conference in 1971, 'Relaxation therapy for psychosomatic disorders', for example, centred on tranquillisers and the new Ciba anti-anxiety drug Tacitin, which claimed to 'reduce muscle tension in man'.[68] Indeed, pharmaceutical companies used the pre-existing discourse of neuromuscular relaxation to promote their own drug therapies when tranquillisers first entered the market. In 1957, pharmaceutical company Pfizer released *The Relaxed Wife*, a short film showing a highly flustered man, neither coping with his working days nor enjoying time with his family, contrasted with his smiling, composed, efficient wife. She modelled the perfect middle-class housewife, looking after her happy children in her clean, orderly house. In the film, the husband tries and fails to follow relaxation self-help books and exercises. Only at the end of the film do viewers learn of an alternative way to achieve these demonstrably beneficial relaxation effects: through Pfizer's new drug Atarax – 'the Greek word for relaxation'. The film concludes: 'today, medical science recognizes that some folks aren't helped by relaxing exercises … in cases of difficult tension, and nervous apprehension, doctors are now prescribing an ataraxic medicine', leading to 'fewer breakdowns and insomniacs, when more of us have learned to be relaxed. We'll be free to relish the joys of life, no longer tense over daily worries and strife.'[69]

In later decades, relaxation proponents built on the popular markets for tranquillisers, sleeping tablets and anti-hypertensive drugs, highlighting the advantages of attaining the desired outcomes without suffering the side effects of drugs.[70] Self-help books often promoted relaxation therapy as a 'natural' way to improve physical and mental well-being, following in the fashion of the interwar naturopathy movement, which carried the slogan 'drugless healing'.[71] Prominent relaxation and antenatal teacher Betty Parsons proclaimed: 'dropping shoulders is as good as taking a Valium. It is much better … You carry it within you, it works instantly and has no nasty side-effects.'[72] Practitioners also claimed that neuromuscular relaxation was cheaper to administer than drugs, and far less time-consuming than psychotherapy. Without challenging and in fact through co-creating understandings of what physical and emotional experiences drugs such as tranquillisers could help with, relaxation was presented as a safe, simple, non-pharmaceutical alternative, that appealed to a common market of nervous middle-class men and women seeking more balanced lives.

The path to well-balanced living

Relaxation teachings incorporated far more than bodily exercises for releasing muscular tension. As the 1968 Disney film *Understanding Stresses and Strains* suggested, good health comprised a physical, mental and social side, all of which had to be kept in balance. Technical instructions therefore formed only one part of a larger package of health education circulated by professionals, which also included advice on managing 'lifestyles', poise and posture, encouraging self-discipline and self-reliance, and understanding physiological models and environmental inducers of 'stress'. Equipped with this wider understanding, students of relaxation would seemingly then be in a better position to 'help themselves'.

Drawing on Selye's formulation of 'biological stress', according to health educator and relaxation practitioner Joe Macdonald Wallace, the very 'function of the health educator is to help the individual to learn how to avoid excessive stress reaction'.[73] Macdonald Wallace, who had been teaching health education in Britain since the 1950s, wrote with disappointment in 1976 that health educational classes were still not offered in adult education programmes, even though demand was clearly there. Although noting that there had been state health education campaigns on 'alcoholism, cigarette smoking, cancer, VD, contraception, etc.', he regretted that there had been 'nothing about overcoming stress'. The responsibility for teacher provision and the development of health education classes on the topic of overcoming stress, he thought, should have been with the 'Health Education Council, the Royal Society for the Promotion of Health, the Society for Health Education ... in co-operation with the Department of Health and Social Security, and the Department of Education and Science'.[74] Relaxation teachings, however, were not high on the agenda for these institutions.

In the post-war decades, in response to new epidemiological findings, state-sponsored health education campaigns started to focus on managing 'risk factors' linked to the rising incidence of chronic diseases. From the 1960s, public health campaigns raised awareness of how individual 'lifestyles' impacted on health and chronic diseases:

healthy diets, quitting smoking and undertaking regular exercise were key state-promoted preventative strategies, designed to encourage health-seeking behaviours among informed, responsible citizens.[75] 'Stress-management', including relaxation training did not, however, feature in state-supported public health campaigns. Despite the promotion and proliferation of research into the topic, 'stress' was not unanimously accepted as a 'risk factor' for chronic diseases, on a par with smoking, diet or exercise. On the whole, doctors and public health officials were more concerned to promote active, productive lifestyles than to encourage slowing down.[76] Yet as Porter has noted: 'state organized health education did not have a monopoly'.[77] Utilising a plethora of communication channels, the growing network of relaxation teachers was one significant group that helped to shape and expand the concept of self-managed healthy living.

Learning relaxation involved first recognising states of tension. As one woman told listeners to BBC radio programme *Under Pressure*, she was surprised when her doctor suggested relaxation classes 'because I thought I was relaxed'. Jane Madders reaffirmed: 'many people don't know they are suffering from stress until they are educated'.[78] In order to uncover and demonstrate 'hidden tension', some teachers found biofeedback machines particularly helpful. One practitioner professed: biofeedback technology was especially useful for 'showing men (the sceptics) that they are NOT relaxed when they think they are'.[79]

Relaxation students were taught how to identify visible indicators of tension such as clenched teeth, frowns and hunched shoulders, and how to release this tension through various means such as massage, 'loosening exercises' and progressive muscle relaxation. An important distinction was made and taught between lengthy, restorative 'deep relaxation' methods, best done lying down, and what Jacobson had termed 'differential relaxation', which could be practised while carrying out everyday activities. Differential relaxation involved using minimal energy and reducing muscle tension to only what was required for the task at hand. If daily tasks such as speaking on the telephone, washing up, driving and reading were carried out with significantly reduced tension, teachers claimed, this would lead to healthier, happier, more efficient lives. Linking relaxation to efficiency helped to decouple it from notions of laziness and recreation, and relate it to working lives already bound by markers of productivity.[80] Middle-class lifestyles tended to be more amenable to learning and incorporating relaxation practice, and this was often reflected in the teachings. As a reviewer of Madders' *Relax* book and cassette noted: 'One limitation is that the material, especially the cassette, aims mainly at an upper middle-class audience. Thus the listener, presumably an executive, is advised to relax during committee meetings, or after an exciting business deal. The steelworker and the shopkeeper would be justified in feeling a little left out.'[81]

Relaxation, as a way of living, was also intimately linked to posture, poise and movement, not just stillness and rest. Many aspects of relaxation teachings encouraged a change of conduct, rather than a lessening of activity, in both domestic and working lives. Charles Neil, one of F. M. Alexander's first students who founded the 'Re-Education Centre' in London in the 1950s, reminded those learning to relax: 'Graceful effective movement in a calm, well-poised, alert person is good relaxation in practice ... Remember, you can't be completely relaxed until you are dead!'[82] Neil had developed his own training system, based on Alexander's method, but with an emphasis on relaxation. He featured on radio, taught classes, made a relaxation record, and in the mid-1950s authored a 'Family Doctor booklet', *Poise and Relaxation*, published by the British Medical Association. Among detailed discussions on posture – for when walking, standing, knitting, driving, lifting and gardening, for the young child, the adolescent, the housewife, the 'man of the family', the middle-aged and the elderly – lay the section 'learn to relax'. This included not only instructions in breathing and muscular relaxation techniques, but also recommendations on time management. Picturing a woman in her dressing gown at the breakfast table, Neil advised:

> First, start the morning well ... That extra ten or fifteen minutes makes all the difference to your poise. You can then enjoy your morning toilet and your breakfast. Discipline yourself to go over in your mind quietly as you sip your tea or coffee, the plan of activities for the day ... A well-ordered day makes the work of even a very busy person very much easier and pleasanter.[83]

In relaxation classes, group discussions provided a central forum for health and lifestyle advice to be shared, debated and circulated. Relaxation for Living founder, Amber Lloyd, described how discussions peppered throughout the classes allowed teachers to share 'philosophical tit-bits' such as 'a problem that you run away from becomes a dragon with two heads. The problem you face up to becomes a mouse.'[84] Although Lloyd lightly referred to such teachings as being popular among students, 'amusing, perhaps, and not to be taken too seriously', such material often derived from major global religious ethical frameworks and cultural traditions. Echoing elements from Christian doctrines and the 'Serenity Prayer', which was appropriated and popularised by Alcoholics Anonymous and other 'twelve-step programmes' from the 1940s, one relaxation teacher provided her class members with a 'Formula to Maintain Calm':

> Cultivate a positive attitude, combining: Acceptance of what you can't change, gratitude for the many blessings you have, compassion for those who annoy you, pride in yourself, an excited optimism for the future.
> The reverse of these: frustration, envy, anger, shame and pessimism are all destructive emotions and can cause mental and physical decay.[85]

'Acceptance of what you can't change' was not supposed to be interpreted as resignation to the status quo. There was a lot that an individual could do with a difficult situation. Practitioners stressed that relaxation was 'not a panacea' but, characterised by the newly formulated psychological frameworks of the time, a means of 'coping' better with personal and social situations. Lloyd stated in a magazine interview that clearly Relaxation for Living 'is not designed to help achieve the ambitions of those who are deeply unhappy with their jobs or general way of living and seek radical change'.[86] Although relaxation teachings did not overtly address underlying causes and could not fundamentally transform stressful environments, they encouraged a change in the individual's emotional and physical response to those environments. Relaxation proponents encouraged an acceptance that social and psychological 'stressors' were impossible to fully eradicate, but that the individual's stress reaction could be more easily modified. This attitude was reflected in teaching methods: Madders, for example, explained, 'I do not "spoil" the class. They bring a rug, I have a small pillow for each and that's all. It's part of the training to ignore discomfort and noise.'[87]

It should be noted, however, that changing stress-inducing environments and responses to such environments were not mutually exclusive. Indeed, symptoms of tension, once identified, often unveiled and implicated underlying causative factors. Relaxation practitioners did not encourage people to passively accept their fate. Rather, they framed relaxation methods as a means of taking greater control of one's life, demanding an active intervention in all aspects of everyday living: practically, emotionally and socially. 'We have to accept that there is a factor which some people might like to call "Fate", but there is an immense amount we can do to help ourselves', declared one practitioner.[88]

The overriding aim of relaxation teaching was to 'help people help themselves'. As teacher Penny Wade explained to BBC Radio London listeners: 'People like to be independent. They don't want to be dependent on another person or on a drug. This is something they can do themselves.'[89] Supporters of biofeedback characterised this form of training as one of the most successful means of empowering individuals: 'it places the power for change and control in the hands of the individual, not with an external authority. Of all the techniques for adjusting behaviour, this is the first to rely on the individual's ability to guide his own destiny', proclaimed early advocates.[90] Paraphrasing the World Health Organization's Expert Committee on Health Education, Macdonald Wallace told readers of the *Health Education Journal* that the central aim of health education was 'to equip individuals with knowledge and skills … and to influence their attitudes in such a way as to help them to solve their own health problems'.[91]

But to reap the benefits of relaxation training, it had to be consistently and diligently practised. Jacobson had noted in *You Must Relax* that a central function of the relaxation teacher-physician was 'police duty' – seeing to it that the patient practises regularly, and providing frequent reminders 'until differential relaxation becomes habitual'.[92] Unlike taking a drug, relaxation was in fact labour-intensive, and for many relaxation students 'dropping shoulders' was not 'as good as taking a Valium'. Relaxation, unlike taking a tablet, required a constant, active, multi-dimensional reworking of the self. Placing the onus onto the learner, Wade asserted '[relaxation] does need self-discipline. I think that this is the main problem – people not prepared to do it.' She postulated that this might be the case because 'it is so simple that people feel it can't really help'.[93]

Yet, as this section has demonstrated, relaxation constituted far more than 'simple' exercises. Relaxed living manifested in how individuals walked, talked and breathed; how they ate their breakfast and drove their cars; how they managed their time and relationships with others. Through this practical and ideological assemblage, proponents argued that relaxation could not only prevent disease – or 'dis-ease' – but was also the 'key to a longer, healthier life'.[94] Achieving these therapeutic outcomes required the adoption of a normative set of behaviours and attributes, including self-discipline, organisation, motivation and assertiveness. Teachers provided essential guidance as health educators, but ultimately, as one practitioner signalled in his book *The Western Way of Death*, it was a case of 'your life in your hands'.[95]

Conclusion

In *The Wellness Syndrome* (2015), Cedeström and Spicer reflect on contemporary 'prevailing attitudes towards those who fail to look after their bodies. These people are demonised as lazy, feeble or weak-willed.'[96] Relaxation, as a popular, secularised, Western self-care approach, could be seen to fall within the set of health and well-being methods that their book addresses, and is therefore open to similar critiques. Advice and teaching literature that valorised relaxed individuals as productive, efficient, healthy, responsible, proactive and self-reliant people implicitly characterised tense individuals as lacking these qualities. Such sentiments have been reinforced by a developing public health framework that emphasises the virtues of personal effort and healthy lifestyle choices, situated in an increasingly individualistic, consumerist society. However, as philosopher Hanna Pickard has indicated through her 'Responsibility without Blame' framework, it is possible to hold patients 'responsible and accountable for their behaviour, but not [blame] them, in order to facilitate learning and change'.[97] The development of organised patient consumerism, pressure groups and activism from the 1960s certainly signalled a desire among patients for greater autonomy and agency in healthcare.[98] In this context, positioning relaxation as a self-empowering tool has held wide appeal.

By encouraging and challenging responsible individuals to achieve, regulate and maintain healthy, well-balanced lives, to an extent relaxation therapies functioned under the Foucauldian rubric of 'technologies of the self'. Nevertheless, these practices are not inherently characterised by or limited to individualistic ends. Studies of comparable teachings in other geographical and temporal contexts usefully demonstrate the potential for a diversity of meanings and applications of such strategies, and their effects on formulations of selfhood. For example, as

Salmenniemi and Vorona (2014) discuss in their sociological work on self-help literature in Russia: 'in Soviet society the work on the self was to be performed for the common good – self-improvement was to support the building of communism.'[99]

Relaxation strategies appealed to a wide spectrum of people who held multiple identities as students, patients, citizens and consumers. Relaxation education therefore impacted on lifestyles and therapeutic outcomes in myriad ways as heterogeneous populations differentially and selectively appropriated the teachings. Middle-class women and men in particular were drawn to relaxation practice as a pharmaceutical alternative and a means of directing control over personal health and attaining greater emotional stability. As this chapter has demonstrated, the generation and circulation of relaxation ideology, and the growing popular demand and uptake of these practices were mutually reinforcing. Post-war health-seeking populations were clearly responsive to the therapeutic promise of stress-management techniques, which continue to proliferate today.[100]

Through a close contextual analysis of how relaxation ideologies have been formulated, communicated, debated and promulgated, this chapter has brought into focus the processes by which these teachings became woven into the social fabric of late twentieth-century Britain. As a therapeutic method, a cultural resource and a way of life, proponents positioned relaxation training within a growing assemblage of modern health and well-being strategies as a compelling means to cultivate more balanced, healthy lives.

Acknowledgements

The research on which this chapter is based was generously supported by the Wellcome Trust, through a postdoctoral Research Fellowship, 'Cultivating Relaxation in Twentieth-Century Britain', Grant No. 104411/Z/14/Z.

Notes

1 Walt Disney Productions and Upjohn Company, *Understanding Stresses and Strains* (Coronet/MTI, 1968), available to view at Wellcome Moving Image and Sound Collection, London.

2 Alongside neuromuscular relaxation techniques, which are the focus of this chapter, other 'mental relaxation' methods influenced by mesmeric and Eastern meditative traditions were developed. See A. Nathoo, 'Relaxation and meditation', in D. Brazier, M. Farias and M. Lalljee (eds), *The Oxford Handbook of Meditation* (Oxford: Oxford University Press, 2019), doi: 10.1093/oxfordhb/9780198808640.013.22. For a detailed historical analysis of the development and contextualisation of Edmund Jacobson's early work, see K. Kroker, 'The progress of introspection in America, 1896–1938', *Studies in History and Philosophy of Biological and Biomedical Sciences*, 34:1 (2003), 77–108.
3 A. Nathoo, 'Initiating therapeutic relaxation in Britain: A twentieth-century strategy for health and wellbeing', *Palgrave Communications*, 2 (2016), article 16043, doi: 10.1057/palcomms.2016.43.
4 Much of Jacobson's early work was directed at populations suffering from 'neurasthenia' – a diagnostic category that was fading by the 1930s. For historical studies on neurasthenia and exhaustion, see: M. Gijswijt-Hofstra and R. Porter (eds), *Cultures of Neurasthenia from Beard to the First World War* (Amsterdam: Rodopi, 2001); and A. K. Schaffner, *Exhaustion: A History* (New York: Columbia University Press, 2016).
5 M. Jackson, *The Age of Stress: Science and the Search for Stability* (Oxford: Oxford University Press, 2013).
6 See, for example: E. S. Watkins, 'Stress and the American vernacular: popular perceptions of disease causality', in D. Cantor and E. Ramsden (eds), *Stress, Shock, and Adaptation in the Twentieth Century* (Rochester, NY: University of Rochester Press, 2014), pp. 49–70; Jackson, *The Age of Stress*; A. Harrington, *The Cure Within: A History of Mind-Body Medicine* (New York: W. W. Norton, 2008).
7 On health education and marketing, see: V. Berridge, *Marketing Health: Smoking and the Discourse of Public Health in Britain 1945–2000* (Oxford: Oxford University Press, 2007); V. Berridge and K. Loughlin, 'Smoking and the new health education in Britain 1950s–1970s', *American Journal of Public Health*, 95:6 (2005), 956–64; A. Mold, 'Exhibiting good health: Public health exhibitions in London, 1948–71', *Medical History*, 62:1 (2018), 1–26.
8 N. Rose, *Governing the Soul: The Shaping of the Private Self* (London: Routledge, 1990); N. Rose, *Inventing Our Selves: Psychology, Power, and Personhood* (Cambridge: Cambridge University Press, 1998); P. Miller and N. Rose, 'On therapeutic authority: Psychoanalytical expertise under advanced liberalism', *History of the Human Sciences*, 7:3 (1994), 29–64.
9 E. Illouz, *Saving the Modern Soul: Therapy, Emotions, and the Culture of Self-Help* (Berkeley: University of California Press, 2008), pp. 4–5.

10. J. Secord, 'Knowledge in transit', *Isis*, 95:4 (2004), 654–72.
11. J. Hewitt, *Relaxation: Nature's Way with Tension* (Wellingborough: Thorsons, 1968), pp. 7–10.
12. Ibid.
13. For an analysis of how psychological knowledge and therapeutic strategies have modulated private suffering in the public sphere, see K. Wright, 'Theorizing therapeutic culture: Past influences, future directions', *Journal of Sociology*, 44:4 (2008), 321–36.
14. J. Williams, 'Health education by correspondence', *Health Education Journal*, 18:4 (1960), 173–80.
15. See Chapters 3, 4 and 5.
16. A. Karpf, *Doctoring the Media: The Reporting of Health and Medicine* (London: Routledge, 1988); A. Nathoo, *Hearts Exposed: Transplants and the Media in 1960s Britain* (Basingstoke: Palgrave Macmillan, 2009), pp. 33–56.
17. A *Woman's Hour* programme, 'Having a Baby in 1951', for example, featured an entire studio relaxation class by practitioner Joan Neville-Ness.
18. A similar approach was taken by Macdonald Wallace on *Woman's Hour* in the early 1960s, in a four-part series focusing on relaxing the muscles of the mouth, face, hands and arms.
19. C. Weekes (1977), audio recording. Uncatalogued archives of Relaxation for Living. *Nationwide* was a BBC 1 news and current affairs programme, broadcast between 1969 and 1985.
20. For example, 'Having a Baby: Preparation for Labour' (BBC1, 1965), which included a mother having her baby under hypnosis, and yoga programmes such as Sir Paul Dukes' 'Fatigue and Relaxation' (BBC TV, 1948) and practitioner Hazel Wills' contributions to the daytime television show *Pebble Mill at One* in the early 1970s.
21. Nathoo, 'Initiating therapeutic relaxation in Britain'.
22. J. Madders, *Relax: The Relief of Tension through Muscle Control* (London: BBC, 1973).
23. Ibid., p. 7.
24. S. Starker, *Oracle at the Supermarket: The American Preoccupation with Self-Help Books* (New Brunswick, NJ: Transaction, 1989); and J. Feather, *A History of British Publishing* (London: Routledge, 2006).
25. S. Newcombe, 'A social history of yoga and ayurveda in Britain, 1950–1995' (PhD dissertation, University of Cambridge, 2008), pp. 29–54; M. Singleton, 'Salvation through relaxation: Proprioceptive therapy and its relationship to yoga', *Journal of Contemporary Religion*, 20:3 (2005), 289–304; and Nathoo, 'Initiating therapeutic relaxation in Britain'.

26 J. Graves and V. Graves, 'The medical recording service and the medical audiovisual library', in J. Fry and R. Pinsent (eds), *A History of the Royal College of General Practitioners: The First 25 Years* (Lancaster: MTP, 1983), pp. 103–9.
27 I. Martin, 'Promoting differential relaxation', *Journal of the Royal College of General Practitioners*, 23:132 (1973), 485–94.
28 Ibid. Jacobson's original technique required months of intensive live training with a teacher in addition to home practice. Psychiatrist Joseph Wolpe (1915–97), a pioneer in behaviour therapy, developed a shortened version of Jacobson's relaxation teachings.
29 P. Lehrer, 'How to relax and how not to relax: A re-evaluation of the work of Edmund Jacobson', *Behavior Research and Therapy*, 20:5 (1982), 417–28.
30 C. Patel and British Holistic Medical Association, *Fighting Heart Disease* (London: Dorling Kindersley, 1987), p. 155.
31 While there is no single founder of the field of biofeedback, key innovators and populariser included Joe Kamiya, Elmer and Alyce Green, and Barbara Brown. For more on the history of the field see Harrington, *The Cure Within*, pp. 166–9 and E. Peper and F. Shaffer, 'Biofeedback history: An alternative view', *Biofeedback*, 38:4 (2010), 142–7.
32 Kroker, 'The progress of introspection in America, 1896–1938'.
33 P. Lehrer, 'Applied psychophysiology: Beyond the boundaries of biofeedback', *Applied Psychophysiology and Biofeedback*, 28:4 (2003), 297.
34 An educational film, *Relaxation and Biofeedback* (Arnold, c.1970), recorded at the Queen Elizabeth Hospital, demonstrated EEG biofeedback training for patients suffering from tension headaches and anxiety, and increased awareness of relaxation training among clinicians. It was available through the Graves Medical Audiovisual Library, and is currently held at the Wellcome Moving Image and Sound Collection.
35 This included, for example, the development of home pregnancy testing kits: J. Olszynko-Gryn, 'The feminist appropriation of pregnancy testing in 1970s Britain', *Women's History Review*, (2017), 1–26, doi: 10.108 0/09612025.2017.1346869; and tools for self-managing and monitoring diabetes: C. Sinding, 'Flexible norms? From patients' values to physicians' standards', in W. Ernst (ed.), *Histories of the Normal and the Abnormal: Social and Cultural Histories of Norms and Normativity* (London: Routledge, 2006), pp. 225–44. See also Chapter 2.
36 E. Jacobson, *You Must Relax: A Practical Method of Reducing the Strains of Modern Living* (New York: McGraw-Hill, 1934), p. 126.
37 Madders in *Under Pressure* (BBC Radio 4, 1982).

38 G. Harding, *Lying Down in Church: Stress in the City* (Worthing: Churchman, 1990), p. 33.
39 Weekes (1977), audio recording. Uncatalogued archives of Relaxation for Living.
40 Nathoo, 'Initiating therapeutic relaxation in Britain'.
41 J. Macdonald Wallace, *Relaxation: A Key to Better Living* (London: Max Parrish, 1965), p. 11.
42 On classes and books for men, see: C. Phillips, 'Coping with stress', *Industrial Management*, 75:10 (1975), 32–6; E. Jacobson, *Tension Control for Businessmen: How to Avoid Heart Attacks, Ulcers, Nervous Breakdowns, and Other Tension Disorders* (New York and London: McGraw-Hill, 1963); and N. Brierley, *Relaxation for Men: Tension in Modern Living* (London and Melbourne: Ward Lock & Co., 1965).
43 See J. Tomlinson, 'Inventing "decline": the falling behind of the British economy in the postwar years', *The Economic History Review*, 49:4 (1996), 731–57, for how notions of labour productivity became intimately linked to measurements of relative economic performance during wartime efforts to maximise labour force outputs. Prior to this, the Industrial Fatigue Research Board had also undertaken studies during the 1920s on the inclusion of 'rest pauses' in industry. See also Chapter 7.
44 Harding, *Lying Down in Church*, p. 9.
45 Ibid., pp. 9–10.
46 D. Dunne, *Deep Relaxation: The Yogism Technique Based on Relaxation of the Voluntary Muscles* (Surbiton, Surrey: School of Yoga, c.1950); D. Dunne, *Yoga for Everyman: How to Have Long Life and Happiness* (London: Gerald Duckworth & Co. Ltd, 1951).
47 G. Puri, *Yoga – Relaxation – Meditation: A Western-Trained Biologist Takes a New Look at an Age Old Eastern Science* (Liverpool: Self-published, 1974); Y. Sunita, *Pranayama Yoga: The Art of Relaxation* (West Midlands: The Lotus and The Rose Private Trust, 1971); and S. Newcombe, 'The institutionalization of the yoga tradition: "Gurus" B. K. S. Iyengar and Yogini Sunita in Britain', in M. Singleton and E. Goldberg (eds), *Gurus of Modern Yoga* (New York: Oxford University Press, 2014), pp. 147–67; Nathoo, 'Relaxation and meditation'.
48 Jacobson, *You Must Relax*, p. vii.
49 Ibid., p. viii.
50 This included German neurologist and psychiatrist Johannes Schultz's 'autogenic training', which developed at a similar time, and New Thought author Annie Payson Call's system of relaxation. Nathoo, 'Initiating therapeutic relaxation in Britain'; Nathoo, 'Relaxation and meditation'; Singleton, 'Salvation through relaxation'.

51 Macdonald Wallace, *Relaxation*, p. xi.
52 Phillips, 'Coping with stress', p. 35.
53 *Woman in Town* (Radio London, 1984).
54 L. Vines and M. Oakey, *The Heart that Has Truly Loved: The Memoires of Lorraine Vines*, 2nd edition ([S. I.]: Kathi Wyldeck, 2009), p. 280.
55 L. Mitchell, *Simple Relaxation: The Physiological Method for Easing Tension* (New York: Atheneum, 1979).
56 A. Meares, *Relief without Drugs: The Self-Management of Tension, Anxiety, and Pain* (London: Souvenir Press, 1968), p. 57.
57 J. Madders, 'Relaxation in the prevention of stress', presentation at 'Stress in Everyday Life conference', Royal Society of Health, London, 1974.
58 Relaxation for Living uncatalogued archives.
59 E. S. Watkins, 'An investigation into the medicalization of stress in the twentieth century', *Medicine Studies*, 4:1–4 (2014), p. 29.
60 R. Bivins, 'Histories of heterodoxy', in M. Jackson (ed.), *The Oxford Handbook of the History of Medicine* (Oxford: Oxford University Press, 2011), pp. 578–97.
61 Nathoo, 'Initiating therapeutic relaxation in Britain'.
62 I am grateful to Suzanne Newcombe for identifying this group in the personal archival collection of 1960s London yoga teacher Stella Cherfas.
63 K. Hay and J. Madders, 'Migraine treated by relaxation therapy', *Journal of the Royal College of General Practitioners*, 21:112 (1971), 664–9.
64 'Editorial: Meditation or Methyldopa', *British Medical Journal*, 1:6203 (1976), 1421–2.
65 C. Patel, M. Marmot and D. Terry, 'Controlled trial of biofeedback-aided behavioural methods in reducing mild hypertension', *British Medical Journal (Clinical Research Ed)*, 282:6281 (1981), 2005–8.
66 P. Parish, 'The prescribing of psychotropic drugs in general practice', *Journal of the Royal College of General Practitioners*, 21:92 Suppl 4 (1971), 1–77.
67 R. Cooperstock and H. Lennard, 'Some social meanings of tranquilizer use', *Sociology of Health and Illness*, 1:3 (1979), 331–47; A. Tone, *The Age of Anxiety: A History of America's Turbulent Affair with Tranquilizers* (New York: Basic Books, 2009); and A. Haggett, *Desperate Housewives, Neuroses and the Domestic Environment, 1945–1970* (London: Pickering & Chatto, 2012).
68 'Tacitin and Nobrium: New drugs for anxiety', *Drug and Therapeutics Bulletin*, 9:24 (1971), 93–4.
69 This film can be viewed at: https://publicdomainreview.org/collections/the-relaxed-wife-1957, accessed August 2019.

70 Meares, *Relief without Drugs*; S. Trickett, 'Withdrawal from benzodiazepines', *Journal of the Royal College of General Practitioners*, 33:254 (1983), 608.
71 Meares, *Relief without Drugs*; and Hewitt, *Relaxation*. See also J. Adams, 'Developing naturopathy in interwar Britain', in N. Gale and J. McHale (eds), *Routledge Handbook of Complementary and Alternative Medicine: Perspectives from Social Science and Law* (London: Routledge, 2015), pp. 63–73.
72 B. Parsons, *Understanding Childbirth* (London: Aurum, 1996), p. 61.
73 J. Macdonald Wallace, 'Health education and the control of stress', *Health Education Journal*, 35:3 (1976), 199–207.
74 Ibid.
75 Berridge and Loughlin, 'Smoking and the new health education in Britain 1950s–1970s'. See also Chapters 3 and 4 in this volume.
76 R. Paffenbarger, S. Blair and I. Lee, 'A history of physical activity, cardiovascular health and longevity: the scientific contributions of Jeremy N. Morris', *International Journal of Epidemiology*, 30:5 (2001), 1184–92.
77 D. Porter, 'The healthy body', in R. Cooter and J. Pickstone (eds), *Medicine in the Twentieth Century* (Amsterdam: Harwood Academic, 2000), pp. 201–16.
78 *Under Pressure* (BBC Radio 4, 1982).
79 Relaxation for Living uncatalogued archives.
80 Tomlinson, 'Inventing "decline"'.
81 G. Ives, 'Relax', *Journal of the Royal College of General Practitioners*, 28:188 (1978), 187.
82 C. Neil and British Medical Association, *Poise and Relaxation* (London: British Medical Association, 1958), p. 17.
83 Ibid., pp. 17–18.
84 Phillips, 'Coping with stress', p. 35.
85 Relaxation for Living uncatalogued archives.
86 Phillips, 'Coping with stress'.
87 Relaxation for Living uncatalogued archives.
88 H. Sears, *Do Something About Those Arteries* (London: Tandem, 1968), p. 128.
89 *Woman in Town* (BBC Radio London, 1974).
90 M. Karlins and L. Andrews, *Biofeedback: Turning on the Power of Your Mind* (London: Garnstone Press, 1973), inside cover.
91 Macdonald Wallace, 'Health education and the control of stress'.
92 Jacobson, *You Must Relax*, p. 126.
93 *Woman in Town* (BBC Radio London, 1974).
94 Mitchell, *Simple Relaxation*, p. 3.

95 M. Carruthers, *The Western Way of Death* (London: Davis-Poynter, 1974).
96 C. Cederström and A. Spicer, *The Wellness Syndrome* (Malden, MA: Polity Press, 2015), p. 3.
97 www.hannapickard.com/responsibility-without-blame.html, accessed August 2019.
98 A. Mold, *Patient Organisations and Health Consumerism in Britain* (Manchester: Manchester University Press, 2015).
99 S. Salmenniemi and M. Vorona, 'Reading self-help literature in Russia: Governmentality, psychology and subjectivity', *British Journal of Sociology*, 65:1 (2014), 43–62. See also Wright, 'Theorizing therapeutic culture', arguing for an acknowledgement of the positive and remedial effects of psychology and counselling in mid- to late twentieth-century Australia.
100 See Nathoo, 'Relaxation and meditation' on the relationship between the development of therapeutic relaxation and contemporary mindfulness-based interventions.

7

Pilot fatigue and the regulation of airline schedules in post-war Britain

Natasha Feiner

Introduction

On 13 March 1954, a British Overseas Airways Corporation (BOAC) Lockheed Constellation aircraft crashed at Kallang Airport, Singapore. Part way through a scheduled flight from Sydney to London, the aircraft struck a seawall on approach to runway six. The undercarriage was damaged and the integral fuel tank was disrupted. When the aircraft touched down on the runway the starboard wing broke off and the undercarriage collapsed. The aircraft came to rest eighty yards from the seawall, in flames. A number of crew members, including Captain T. W. Hoyle, managed to escape the burning wreckage through a glass panel in the cockpit, but the main cabin door and emergency exits could not be opened. Though attempts were made to rescue passengers through holes cut into the fuselage, these were, as one report commented following the accident, 'almost completely unsuccessful'.[1] Of the forty passengers and crew on board the aircraft, thirty-three were killed.

Following the accident, Singapore's Supreme Court conducted a public inquiry. On 16 November 1954 the inquiry commission published a forty-six-page report which detailed the causes and circumstances of the crash. The report drew attention to the 'undoubtedly long hours' worked by the crew and the limited availability of in-flight rest facilities.[2] The crew, it was found, had worked for a total of twenty-one and a half hours and, while rest facilities were available, the inquiry commission deemed these inadequate. The Constellation aircraft was not equipped with bunks and crew were required to rest instead on a mattress 'placed over the luggage'. The authors of the report noted that it seemed 'unlikely' this provided 'a very comfortable resting place'.[3] The report concluded that insidious fatigue might have affected Captain Hoyle's judgement in the last stages of the approach to landing. As the *Singapore Free Press* explained following the report's publication:

> The fact that his first point of touch down came closer to the threshold markings (at the seawall end of the runway) than he originally intended can probably be attributed to a degree of tiredness which he may or may not have been aware.[4]

Given the possibility that 'tiredness' might have affected Hoyle's performance and, in turn, caused the accident, the report published by Singapore's Supreme Court made two recommendations on the subject of crew fatigue: first, that crew fatigue be scientifically investigated; and, second, that the regulations controlling pilots' hours of work and rest be reviewed.

Though it is an international industry, in the twentieth century civil aviation was governed almost entirely by national regulations.[5] It was not, therefore, within the remit of Singapore's inquiry commission to produce directives in relation to the working practices of flight deck crew employed by British airlines. The recommendations outlined by the commission did, however, receive wide attention in Britain. In the days immediately following the report's publication a number of aviation associations in Britain publicly called for a review of pilots' hours of duty, in line with the recommendations of the Kallang inquiry. On 20 November 1954 Denis Follows, General Secretary of the British Airline Pilots Association (BALPA), penned an article for *The Times* in which he called for the introduction of a 'broad policy for maximum hours of duty for pilots' on a 'national scale'. 'The public has a right', Follows began, 'to expect that, whatever else may be the hazards of air travel, at least those which can definitely be eliminated by straightforward ministerial regulation should not be allowed to persist.' Since the close of the Second World War, he argued, commercial air transport had changed considerably. The 'social legislation', as Follows put it, that controlled the work and rest of pilots needed to be updated to reflect these changes.[6] It was important, he concluded, that long hours of continuous duty – the apparent cause of the Kallang crash – were limited wherever possible.

At the time of the 1954 accident, there were no statutory limitations governing flight times in Britain. The regulations that did exist were not obligatory, and laid the responsibility for establishing flight time limitations on operators.[7] The 1954 Air Navigation Order (ANO) required only that airlines produced flight time limitations in conformity with the permissive recommendations of the International Civil Aviation Organization (ICAO), which required simply that flight time limitations of some sort 'should be established such as to ensure safety'.[8] Airlines interpreted this rule in various ways, but in most cases imposed an upper limit on the number of hours pilots were permitted to fly in a month, in line with the principle of the operational limit employed by the Royal Air Force (RAF) during the Second World War.[9]

The Kallang crash was only one of many instances that called into question the safety of pilots' working practices in the 1950s. One year earlier a York aircraft en route from the Azores to Gander, Canada, crashed under similar circumstances. The accident report, published in January 1954, attributed the cause of the crash to pilot fatigue. It was found that the flight deck crew had worked continuously for twenty-three hours and, as such, the accident report recommended that 'the whole subject of crew fatigue [should] receive study'.[10] Prompted by this report, and increased public interest in flight safety following the air crash in Kallang, in the mid-1950s pilots' hours of work and rest were reviewed by national agencies, and in 1957 a new regulatory framework was introduced to control pilots' schedules.

Based on a model of fatigue that had its roots in the late nineteenth century, the concept of balance was implicit in these regulations from the outset. The notion of fatigue was vague and contested throughout the twentieth century. Attempts to find a biological marker for fatigue had failed, but by the mid-twentieth century there was broad agreement among researchers that fatigue was the result of bodily or psychological imbalance. In 1936 Howard E. Collier (1890–1953), a reader in Industrial Hygiene at the University of Birmingham, described fatigue as a state of 'unbalance'.[11] For Collier, fatigue occurred as a result of an 'absence of harmony' between 'the organism and its environment or between the various subordinate parts within the organism itself' or, more basically, between 'intake and output'.[12] Two decades later, physiologists based at the University of Leeds described fatigue in similar terms: as failure to maintain physiological 'equilibrium'.[13] In 1945 Adolphe Abrahams (1883–1967), a physician now considered the founder of British sports science, attributed chronic fatigue to an imbalance between work, rest and social activities.[14] Though opinion differed on the precise causes and manifestations of fatigue in humans, it was widely agreed by the middle decades of the twentieth century that if the dynamic equilibrium of the body was upset – by ill health, emotional stress or intensive working practices – fatigue would result. The notion that an imbalance of work and leisure time might cause fatigue (or what later became known as 'burnout') became increasingly commonplace as the twentieth century progressed. As these ideas spread, they shaped new norms about work, on the one hand, and 'life' (comprising all the activities pursued without financial reward, including education, leisure and consumption), on the other. In turn, these new norms informed and influenced the regulation of work and rest.

With a particular focus on post-war civil aviation, this chapter outlines how and why airline schedules were regulated in the post-war period. Though there were some attempts to harmonise regulations across Europe from the 1990s, full integration of flight time limitations in Europe by the European Aviation Safety Agency (EASA) only came to pass in February 2016.[15] The focus here is on national, rather than intergovernmental, regulation. Specifically, this chapter traces how the relationship between the British state, business and individual workers shifted in regulatory terms between 1954 and 1982, a period of significant political change, with state interventionism being replaced, by the 1980s, with widespread faith in market mechanisms and a retrenchment of the state under the Conservative governments of Margaret Thatcher. The chapter argues, however, that existing historiographical assumptions need to be re-evaluated. Though there are many examples of state interventionism in the post-war period, the picture is more complex than sometimes assumed. In the second half of the twentieth century, British governments consistently refused to formally control airline schedules.[16] Regulation and enforcement was, throughout the century, permissive and flexible. In order to highlight this complexity, the chapter traces three interconnected but distinct concepts through the post-war period: fatigue, the state and the self. Speaking to some of the core themes of this volume, it asks how and why new selves were constructed and regulated in the post-war period at the expense of structural adjustments to working environments, sets out a new timeline for twentieth-century subjectivity and historicises present-day concerns with work-life balance and the costs of overwork.[17]

Acute fatigue and the regulation of working hours, 1954–72

In the twentieth century overwork was under-regulated. In fact, many workers in post-war Britain were encouraged to stay on the job beyond their contracted working hours. Overwork, and the fatigue that this often entailed, were generally accepted where financial recompense was offered. There were, however, some instances where overwork was formally restricted. In the United Kingdom, regulations governing hours of work and rest stretch back to the nineteenth century. Many state regulations – including the 1844 and 1850 Factory Acts – had a social and moral imperative. They were intended to protect vulnerable groups from exploitation and to safeguard the health of workers.[18] From the early twentieth century, employers increasingly introduced more detailed regulations relating to working hours and rest periods, particularly for factory workers.[19] These regulations were often based on research produced by wartime and interwar research committees, such as the Health of Munition Workers Committee (HMWC) and the Industrial Fatigue Research Board (IFRB).[20] Workplace and laboratory studies carried out by these committees indicated that 'productivity was closely related to the health of the workers', and that longer hours – if these caused fatigue and ill health – did not necessarily entail greater output.[21]

Much useful historical literature has explored the regulation of work and rest in factory settings, but fatigue was also experienced and managed beyond the factory.[22] In nineteenth- and twentieth-century Britain fatigue was endemic in a number of industries, particularly those that required round-the-clock work, such as transportation, construction, agriculture, healthcare and other public services.[23] The regulation of working hours in these industries was inconsistent. For some, such as railway workers, hours of work had been controlled since the late nineteenth century.[24] For many others, though, there was no industry-specific regulation of work and rest. This trend was not specific to Britain. On the other side of the Atlantic, working hours were only regulated beyond the factory in certain circumstances. Alan Derickson

Pilot fatigue and regulation of schedules 195

has argued that working time regulation was limited to industries where 'sleeplessness posed a threat to the general welfare'.[25] In other words, working hours were controlled only in industries that were high risk – where the margin for human error was slim, and the results of error potentially catastrophic – and high responsibility – where the general public was likely to be involved or affected. In the twentieth century, American federal legislation was introduced to control the work and rest of train operators, long-haul truckers and commercial pilots. In some instances, further legislation was enacted on a state level. For example, in the 1980s New York State introduced restrictions on the number of hours postgraduate medical trainees could work.[26] In the post-war period the British government imposed comparable limitations on professional drivers and commercial aircrew.

As described above, detailed regulations governing pilots' hours of work were first introduced in the mid-1950s following a series of accidents that were attributed, in part, to crew fatigue. The regulations in place at that time were not obligatory, and laid the responsibility for establishing flight time limitations on operators.[27] The 1954 ANO simply required that airlines produced flight time limitations in conformity with the permissive recommendations of the ICAO: that limitations 'should be established such as to ensure safety'.[28] There was no specific guidance relating to maximum working hours and, given the long hours worked by the crews of the York in 1953 and the Constellation aircraft in 1954, the Ministry of Aviation felt it was important that the current system be re-examined. The Working Party on Operating Crew Fatigue and Flight Time Limitations (hereafter referred to as the Bowhill Working Party) was established to this end. Sir Frederick Bowhill (1880–1960), a well-known military figure who had acted as Commander-in-Chief of Coastal Command and later Transport Command during the Second World War, led the Working Party. Bowhill was joined by four others: E. A. Armstrong, the most experienced of the group in matters of civil aviation, had led the Civil Aviation Safety Group since 1953; Group Captain J. B. Veal and D. L. R. Halliday, formerly of the RAF; and Air Commodore J. D. Leahy, a medical officer at the Ministry of Transport.[29] The expertise of the Working Party was heavily weighted towards military flight. Though most of its members had some experience of civil aviation from a managerial or medical perspective, none had first-hand experience of operating commercial aircraft. This fact would influence the perspective, and subsequent recommendations, of the Working Party.

Unlike the industrial fatigue committees operating in the first half of the twentieth century, the Bowhill Working Party was not involved in the collection of original laboratory or observational data. No investigations were commissioned by the Working Party in either laboratories, simulators or operational aircraft. Instead, like the wartime surveys of flying stress and psychological disorder undertaken by the Flying Personnel Research Committee (FPRC), fatigue and its management were framed in terms of subjective opinion. The Bowhill Working Party consulted a number of medical specialists, all of whom agreed that fatigue could 'contribute to accidents'.[30] There was, however, no medical consensus on the apparent causes or physical manifestations of fatigue, so the Working Party chose to rely instead on evidence supplied by airlines and trade unions. Given this evidence base, economic, safety and social – rather than medical – concerns shaped the Working Party's understanding of aircrew fatigue.

The opinions of airlines and trade unions did not coincide. Operators argued that no more regulations were necessary or required, while trade unions made the case for specific statutory limits. The Bowhill Working Party recognised that neither operators nor trade unions considered the matter 'from an entirely fatigue point of view' – other matters were consistently brought up by both sides. As Bowhill noted after meeting with both parties in September 1954, 'the questions of operations, schedules, etc. loom very largely into the picture'. In this respect, he noted, operators had 'a dual capacity, one for the good of their aircrew and one for their good name', while trade unions were 'out to improve the conditions of the aircrew'.[31] Fatigue could not, as Bowhill's notes make clear, be considered in isolation as it related directly to issues of scheduling, working hours, rest time and time off. In other words, the financial, safety and social aspects of operating crew fatigue were inextricably linked. Apparent tensions between economic and safety considerations formed an important part of the Bowhill Working Party's final report, which concluded that:

> Any consideration of flight time limitations requires careful attention to be paid to the economic consequences. Every addition to the minimum operating crew of an aircraft means less pay load. Every additional stop

to enable crew to rest may mean adding to an operator's crew strength or slowing down a schedule. Bearing in mind the highly competitive nature of international air transport it will be necessary when determining limitations which ensure adequate safety standards to ensure that an operator's ability to compete successfully is not necessarily impaired.[32]

Though safety was paramount, for the Bowhill Working Party it was important that airlines were not financially 'impaired' by strict legislation.[33]

The Bowhill Working Party privileged the concerns of operators. Economic considerations were, its members believed, of greatest importance, and the apparent threat that flying fatigue posed to air safety was given little weight. Trade unions, the Working Party thought, had overstated the problems associated with pilot fatigue in order to justify their social aims. In December 1954 Britain's largest aviation union, BALPA, had submitted a memorandum to the Working Party in which it called for specific and detailed legislation to limit the working hours of pilots and to balance pilot workload within and between rosters. BALPA argued that the pattern of operations common in the post-war world – which included night-time and early morning flights – induced fatigue and had serious implications for flight safety. In previous decades, when operations had been limited to daytime, pilots were, the union reasoned, naturally protected against fatigue:

> This operational pattern had the effect of regulating to some extent the maximum hours of duty for the crews on the night-stopping services, but it had additionally an effect on the through services since it maintained the concept that the human body was pathologically designed to rest for a spell of some eight hours during darkness: hence the through services were run with the minimum violation of this then accepted rhythm and pilots were not usually required to sacrifice their rest during the hours of darkness more than on one occasion at a time.[34]

The turn to twenty-four-hour operations in the 1950s, BALPA concluded, had removed this 'natural protection' against fatigue.[35] The Bowhill Working Party, however, was not convinced by this argument. Its final report concluded that the union's allegations were 'unsubstantiated' and that there appeared to be 'truth to the operators' suggestion that the unions' object in making these allegations [was] to further their aim of using the problem of fatigue to achieve an industrial end'.[36]

These suspicions added weight to the Bowhill Working Party's position on working time regulation. In line with operators, the Working Party's members located responsibility for the management of fatigue with pilots, rather than with airlines or external agencies. 'There appears to be', Bowhill recorded following a meeting with airlines and trade unions in September 1954, 'a tendency to take away certain responsibilities from the captain of the aircraft and replace this by legislation.' 'Surely', he concluded, 'this is a wrong attitude.' For Bowhill, the captain of the aircraft 'must be responsible for the safety of his aircraft and in this safety factor fatigue must always be predominantly in his mind'. Though BALPA representatives had argued that pilots might be influenced 'by fear of [their] owners' or by 'being paid more' to continue work, after meeting with operators Bowhill decided that these positions 'very rarely, if ever' arose.[37] In the view of the Bowhill Working Party, then, responsibility for flight safety lay with the pilot. Pilots, the Working Party argued, should be able to demonstrate self-awareness and control. Like the mid-century explorers described in Chapter 8, pilots were expected to be conscious of their energy levels and able to self-manage fatigue in flight if necessary. Reflecting broader contemporary concerns about professional autonomy and masculine self-discipline, the Bowhill Working Party argued that pilots should not be divested of this responsibility by way of legislation.[38] This argument was predicated on a particular image of the post-war pilot. Pilots were, the Bowhill Working Party thought, trusted and skilled executives for whom professional autonomy was important. In this framework, pilots were envisioned as self-aware and self-sufficient, expected to be alert to mental and bodily changes and active in the management of fatigue.[39]

The reluctance of the Bowhill Working Party to impose strict limitations on pilots' hours of work and rest speaks to the uneasy relationship between the British state and industry in the post-war period. The immediate post-war years saw support for collectivist ideas and policies, the nationalisation of major industries, the birth of the National Health Service and economic management by the state.[40] Following the return of the Conservatives into government in 1951, though, this collectivist advance was stemmed.[41] High levels of public spending and taxation remained, but the idea of state intervention in economic and industrial matters was not universally popular.[42]

The Bowhill Working Party was uneasy about intervening in the operation of airlines but, given the apparent dangers of pilot fatigue, recommended that some limitations on flying hours should be introduced. Following the wartime RAF precedent, the report of the Working Party proposed that operators should set quantitative limitations on flying times to ensure that aircrews did not suffer from fatigue.[43] Operators, the Working Party suggested, should set these limits themselves. Although the Bowhill Working Party did not think operators should be left with too 'much discretion on a subject in which the effect on airline costs may come into conflict with safety requirements', it concluded that only operators were in a position to 'assess satisfactorily the nature and effects of the work falling on ... [their] operating crews'.[44] Based on the premise that fatigue was a short-term reaction to imbalanced working practices in a single day, the regulation of daily working hours was recommended above all else. The nature of civil flying in 1950s Britain – long hours of work followed by long hours of rest – caused, according to the Bowhill Working Party, acute rather than 'cumulative' fatigue.[45] As such, the Working Party's final report recommended that a daily limit on the number of hours pilots could work was the single most important countermeasure to fatigue. The report recommended a daily maximum of sixteen hours, but suggested that this could be extended to twenty-four consecutive hours 'to provide operators with reasonable flexibility in respect of slipping and rostering'.[46] Economic considerations, then, continued to loom large.

The recommendations of the Working Party formed the basis of a new ANO, which came into effect on 1 May 1957.[47] The regulations contained in the ANO 'fell far short' of trade union expectations.[48] BALPA argued that there was still 'too much discretion' for operators and that 'excessive flying' was still 'legally possible'.[49] Under the new ANO, long hours of work were still allowed in a single day. The flexible nature of the daily limit, BALPA representatives contended, entirely negated its existence. In addition, intensive and imbalanced rosters were not outlawed under the new ANO. No regulations were introduced in respect of rest periods and time off, as the Bowhill Working Party deemed these already adequate. As a result, BALPA argued that there was nothing to stop 'astute operators' exploiting 'loop-holes' to create intensive and imbalanced schedules.[50]

The regulations introduced by the Ministry of Transport in the 1950s set the tone for subsequent regulation of aircrew schedules. As in the 1957 ANO, later regulations tended to be permissive – to allow airlines discretion in terms of their implementation – to place the burden of responsibility for fatigue management on workers, and to conceptualise fatigue as a short-term rather than cumulative problem. This approach to flight time regulation was first challenged in the 1970s when, in response to growing concerns about the relationship between pilot workload and flight safety, the recently established Civil Aviation Authority (CAA) introduced new regulations that intended to balance the work and rest of pilots both within and between rosters, a framework that remained largely unchanged for almost half a century.

Cumulative fatigue and the balanced duty cycle, 1972–75

The 1970s marked a new, and increasingly complex, regulatory phase in Britain. While New Right ideologies gained momentum politically, in the same decade the most detailed statutory health and safety regulations to date were introduced under the 1974 Health and Safety at Work Act (HSWA).[51] Though more detailed and expansive than any prior regulatory framework, the HSWA constituted, as Christopher Sirrs has pointed out, an uncomfortable compromise between interventionism and voluntarism.[52] Premised on the ideal of self-regulation by industry, the HSWA situated the responsibility for workers' health outside the state, with employers and workers themselves.[53] The Act was intended to alleviate the need for piecemeal and industry-specific regulation, but it did not provide universal protections. Transport workers were explicitly excluded from coverage: transport safety was deemed too 'large' and 'difficult' an area to legislate on, so even after the introduction of the HSWA the transport sector was governed by industry-specific regulations.[54] Civil aviation, although not directly included under the purview of the HSWA, was influenced by the anti-legislative and self-regulatory sentiments contained in the 1974 Act, and the 1972 report on which it was based. This section sets out changes to the regulatory landscape of commercial flight in 1970s Britain. It will show that, though premised on new understandings of fatigue and pilot responsibility, the regulations introduced to minimise fatigue in 1975 marked a shift in principle rather than in practice.

As in the immediate post-war period, fatal accidents again prompted regulatory review of pilots' working practices. It was commonly acknowledged by contemporary commentators that 1972 was a bad year for the aviation industry. It was an especially bad year for air crashes: worldwide over 1,700 passengers and crew died in the space of twelve months.[55] The most widely reported accident in Britain, the Staines air disaster, killed 118 people. It was, by far, the worst ever accident in British aviation history. The Air Accidents Investigation Branch (AAIB) concluded following a public inquiry that the incident occurred as a result of poor crew coordination and pilot error caused by an 'abnormal heart condition'.[56] As in 1954, though, the British media focused on other issues. Much was made, for example, of the conditions of work commonly experienced by British European Airways (BEA) pilots prior to the accident. In November 1972, *The Times* published an article detailing the complaints made by Captain Stanley Key before his death. In the weeks preceding the incident, Key complained to others about the length of his working days and his 'lack of free weekends'.[57] The Staines air disaster was never formally attributed to fatigue, but the wide publicity afforded to Key's complaints following the crash raised concerns about pilot workload and morale, and flight safety that the CAA was keen to address.

The Bader Committee was established in response to these concerns. It was composed of six members: Group Captain Douglas Bader (1910–82), former military pilot, member of the CAA and chairman; Dr Walter Tye, expert in aviation medicine, member of the CAA, and deputy chairman; John R. Sidebotham, an operations director of a British airline; Laurie Taylor, a senior airline captain and BALPA representative; and Norman A. White and Michael Varley of the CAA.[58] The composition of the Committee was markedly different from that of the Bowhill Working Party two decades earlier. Some of its members had military backgrounds, but as a whole the Bader Committee had significant experience of commercial aviation. While the Bowhill Working Party made suggestions from outside the industry, the Bader Committee had relevant and varied expertise in matters of civil aviation and actively sought to co-create regulation with workers and airlines.

Though different in composition, the Bader Committee adopted a similar research strategy to its predecessor. Like the Bowhill Working Party, the Bader Committee disparaged medical and psychological models and measures of fatigue. Ambiguous and often only indirect, the medical offering was, in the Committee's view, not 'satisfactory'. On this basis the Committee concluded that 'assessment of fatigue' could only be undertaken subjectively.[59] This entailed the exclusion of evidence relating to circadian 'desynchronization'.[60] Tacitly recognised for centuries, the cyclical functions of the body were increasingly investigated in the twentieth century.[61] Extensive animal studies, and later experiments on humans in laboratories and workplaces confirmed early assumptions about biological periodicity.[62] Human and animal life, it was found, biologically oscillated over hours, days and weeks. No consensus existed on the precise mechanisms involved in the mediation of biological rhythms until later in the twentieth century, but by the early 1970s it was widely agreed that hormones excreted by the pineal gland played a role in synchronising biological rhythms. Though well-established anecdotally by the 1960s, medical discussion of circadian disruption in aircrew only began in earnest in the mid-1970s, after the Bader Committee had completed its regulatory review.[63] Medical and scientific models of biological rhythmicity did not inform the perspective or subsequent recommendations of the Bader Committee.

Like the Bowhill Working Party two decades earlier, the Bader Committee framed fatigue in terms of personal experience. Committee members collected the opinions of over 200 contributors – including medical experts, trade unions, airlines and flight deck crew – before publishing its final report in June 1973. The report recommended that existing legislation was simplified. The Committee admitted that, despite its collective knowledge and experience, members had difficulty 'disentangling the interconnected mass of rules, law, directions and guidance' about flight time limitations and the prevention of pilot fatigue.[64] The picture was, indeed, complex. By 1972 British civil aviation was subject to a number of national and international obligations. As a signatory to the Convention on International Civil Aviation held in Chicago in 1944, the UK had an obligation to comply with the international standards and recommended practices in the various annexes to the convention. The Bader Committee identified one annex that was particularly relevant to fatigue and flight time limitations – Annex 6, Part 1, 'The Operations of Aircraft', which stated that:

> An operator shall formulate rules limiting the flight time and flight duty periods of flight crew members. These rules shall also make provision for adequate rest periods and shall be such as to ensure that fatigue, occurring either in a flight or successive flights ... does not endanger the safety of the flight.[65]

Table 7.1: The basic limiting of flying duty periods for scheduling purposes, *Report of the Committee on Flight Time Limitations*, p. 8

Crew	ANO limit	Air Operators' Certificate limit
1 pilot	10	10
2 pilots	15	12
2 pilots and 1 flight navigator	15	13
2+ pilots	15	15
2+ pilots with sufficient bunks for in-flight rest	22	18

The guidance in Annex 6 was general in nature and did not provide any numerical values for rest or duty periods. A number of national requirements did, however, lay down explicit limitations on flying time, although these rarely matched up. There were, for example, disparities between the limits proposed by the 1972 ANO and the guidance material contained in the 1966 Air Operators' Certificate (see Table 7.1). Operators interpreted these guidelines inconsistently, and often set different internal limits on flying hours to those laid down by law as a result of industrial agreements with trade unions. There was also significant variation between airlines. Some airlines, such as BOAC, scheduled pilots right up to the legal 100-hour monthly limit, while others, such as BEA, imposed much more restrictive limits. Existing measures for the prevention of aircrew fatigue were, the Bader Committee concluded, complicated and disjointed. The Committee recommended that a new system of rules was introduced, 'preferably in one document', that simplified and clarified the limitations.[66]

Recommendations made by the Bader Committee were premised on the concept of a 'duty cycle' that included 'both duty and off-duty periods'.[67] The intention was to create a pattern of work for pilots 'akin to the normal manner of covering a like situation in other occupations and professions in industry and business'.[68] The model of work and rest common to office-based work – nine-to-five, Monday to Friday, with two days off at the weekend – offered workers, the Committee presumed, an appropriate work-life balance. Reflecting contemporary discussions about work-life balance, and the importance of home life for men as well as women, the Bader Committee argued that the 'home environment' was essential for the emotional health of pilots and was particularly important to mitigate the effects of personal stress 'leading to fatigue'.[69] Time at home had, the Bader Committee held, both physical and emotional benefits. To this end, pilot fatigue was transformed in regulatory discourse. Once framed in primarily physiological terms, by the 1970s the psychological and social pressures of commercial aviation were central to regulators' understanding of fatigue.[70]

In the early 1970s medical and social attitudes to work, and the emotional health of workers, were renegotiated. Moving away from strictly productivist arguments, a discourse of work-home interaction emerged that placed the health and well-being of the family centre stage. In this discourse the emotional health of workers was deemed important, not only for workplace safety and productivity, but also for the well-being of the nuclear family. 'When men are tired out', Michael Young and Peter Wilmott argued in 1973, 'they may bring home, if not the work itself, [then] some of its consequences'.[71] This, they suggested, had implications for the whole family. Medical practitioners were also concerned with the relationship between exhaustion and emotional resilience in this period. In 1974, German-born American psychologist Herbert J. Freudenberger (1926–99) conceptualised this as 'burn-out'.[72] These broader shifts in medical attitudes and social norms underpinned the recommendations of the Bader Committee. In its final report, the Committee suggested that proper attention be paid to the overall planning of the duty cycle and the time between consecutive duty cycles. This, the Committee argued, was the 'most appropriate framework for … preventing fatigue'.[73] Marking a break with previous regulatory trends, the Bader Committee argued that balance across the whole duty cycle was a better antidote to crew fatigue than limitations on single duty periods.[74]

The regulatory framework proposed by the Bader Committee in 1973 was premised on an understanding of fatigue far removed from that discussed by the Bowhill Working Party two decades earlier. Drawing on anecdotal evidence from flight deck crew, the Bader Committee reconceptualised fatigue as a cumulative, rather than acute, problem. Though fatigue might sometimes be acute, it was, members thought, often compounded by difficulty sleeping. For the Bader

Committee, fatigue became dangerous when pilots entered a cycle of acute fatigue and sleeplessness, often as a result of transmeridian travel. Though the Committee did not draw on the studies of circadian disruption carried out in laboratories and other workplaces since the 1960s, it did seek to recognise the problems associated with transoceanic travel – referred to as 'jet lag' by some – in its recommendations.

The Bader Committee suggested two solutions to the problem of aircrew fatigue: first, to balance work, rest and time off across and between duty cycles; and second, to impose limits on single duty periods that commenced very late at night and very early in the morning, which were likely to impinge on the 'normal hours of sleep'.[75] A sliding scale of duty period length was recommended. The length of duty periods should, the Committee proposed, depend on the time of day duty began and the number of sectors flown. It advised that the limitations in Table 7.2 'should be mandatory for scheduling purposes'.[76] However, the Committee recommended that this basic guide should be amended in a number of different circumstances. For flights that commenced away from base, for example, the Bader Committee recommended that flying duty periods should be modified to take into account the length of the preceding rest period and possible sleeplessness following transoceanic flight.

In an attempt to balance duty cycles, the Bader Committee proposed cumulative weekly, monthly and annual limits on flying hours, in addition to control of rest periods. The Committee's report recommended that weekly duty should not exceed fifty hours, monthly flying hours should not exceed 100 hours – although duty hours could be extended to 160, similar to the monthly hours the Bader Committee deemed 'normal' in other occupations – and set an annual limit of 900 flying hours.[77] Like the framework proposed for calculating the length of flying duty periods, the Bader Committee recommended a sliding scale for rest periods, ranging from twelve to eighteen hours, during which time crew were 'required' to rest.[78] Reflecting a wider contemporary discourse of therapeutic relaxation – which was 'best conducted lying down' – the Committee mandated that rest prior to flying should be at least eight hours in length, 'uninterrupted' and 'horizontal'.[79] Sleep was not a prerequisite, but was desirable.

The Bader Committee's report closed with a discussion of subsequent legislation and enforcement. It concluded that regulations should

Table 7.2: Flying duty period commencing at 'base'. *Report of the Committee on Flight Time Limitations*, p. 18

	Maximum length of flying duty period/number of sectors							
	1	2	3	4	5	6	7	8+
0801–1300	14	13.25	12.5	11.75	11	10.25	9.5	9
1301–1800	13	12.25	11.5	10.75	10	9.25	9	9
1801–2200	12	11.25	10.5	9.75	9	9	9	9
2201–0600	11	10.25	9.5	9	9	9	9	9
0601–0800	12.5	11.75	11	9.5	9.5	9	9	9

be easy to amend, given the constantly changing nature of the modern aviation industry. 'We believe', the Committee began, that a matter as 'technically complex, and in need of progressive review, as Flight Time Limitations does not lend itself to the processes involved in legislation ... We are not convinced of the need to provide rules in the form of legislation, the infringement of which renders either the individual or the operator liable to criminal proceedings.'[80] The Committee instead recommended a permissive system of control premised on voluntarism and self-regulation by industry. To this end, it proposed that subsequent regulations should be 'basic in form', so they could be applied to different circumstances.[81] The Committee recommended that the existing ANO be amended to offer more flexibility, and then supplemented by detailed guidance material in a Civil Aviation Publication (CAP).

Following the publication of the Bader Committee's report in June 1973, the CAA published a detailed guidance document in 1975, *The Avoidance of Excessive Fatigue in Aircrews*, more commonly referred to as CAP 371.[82] This publication closely followed the recommendations of the Bader Committee. The maximum permissible flying duty hours were lifted straight from the report: fourteen hours a day, 100 hours a month and 900 hours a year. Also on the recommendation of the Bader Committee, the CAA appointed an advisory Flight Time Limitations Board (FTLB), initially led by Douglas Bader, to advise the CAA on issues of flight safety, flight time limitations and associated legislation. The main function of the FTLB was to approve or disprove variations.

Under CAP 371 operators could submit a scheme with slight variations to the FTLB for consideration if compensatory factors meant that the overall scheme 'achieved an equivalent level of safety' to CAP 371.[83] Though formally titled a 'requirements document', the recommendations set out in CAP 371 had no legal standing but were, rather, a code of practice similar to the British Civil Airworthiness Requirements. Under CAP 371, airlines were allowed 'reasonable freedom' to apply the recommendations of the publication with 'commonsense.'[84] Deliberately flexible, it was hoped that, if airlines had scope to update flight time limitations in response to new technologies or demands, CAP 371 would be applicable for years to come.

However, the 'freedom' to interpret the regulations contained in CAP 371 in a way that suited the needs of operators left it open to manipulation.[85] In August 1973, shortly after the publication of its report, the Bader Committee discussed this potential problem. The Committee suspected that, particularly in the early stages of the new regulatory framework, there might be 'very large numbers of requests made for variations'. Widespread use of variations could, the Committee thought, 'debase the general level of protection' intended under CAP 371.[86] The Bader Committee's initial misgivings proved correct. By 1977 over 300 variations had been granted by the CAA, many with little or no regard for compensatory factors. Low-cost operator Dan-Air, for example, reduced some flying periods by just fifteen minutes – a cursory effort given that the airline had reduced rest periods following standby from eighteen to twelve hours.[87] The primary aim of CAP 371 – to balance work and rest within and between duty cycles – was undermined.

The flight time limitations introduced in 1975, then, marked a shift in principle but not in practice. Based on an understanding of fatigue as cumulative rather than acute, the 1975 limitations initiated a regulatory philosophy that attempted to balance work and rest across the duty cycle rather than limit single duty periods. But in practice, given the scope for variation and the extension of duty periods at the captain's discretion, it was still legally possible for operators to schedule imbalanced rosters. This became an increasing problem in the late 1970s, following economic deregulation and the increasing marketisation of civil aviation.[88] A number of new low-cost airlines entered the market in this period. Operating within often tight profit margins, many of these airlines were more commercially motivated than the traditional flag carriers. Employment of pilots was one of the major costs for airlines, after aircraft and fuel, and the new low-cost operators were keen to ensure a good return. Pilot utilisation and scheduling were key concerns, and increasing competition prompted some airlines to exploit the permissive nature of CAP 371 for commercial gain. In the decade following the introduction of CAP 371 low-cost airlines and inclusive tour operators, such as Dan-Air and Monarch, frequently scheduled pilots to work the maximum number of hours possible and rostered trips 'to the absolute limit of CAP 371'.[89] Ideally, operators should have made provision for minor delays, but charter airlines and low-cost operators – which tended to prioritise profitability above health and safety concerns – rarely observed this guidance. Within ever-tighter schedules, the slightest delay necessitated the use of the captain's discretionary power to extend the duty day.[90] Reminiscent of the intensive and imbalanced working practices that had first prompted regulatory intervention by the state in the 1950s, an article published in BALPA's membership magazine in 1982 claimed that the union had received 'extreme, but not infrequent' reports of pilots working for '24 hours or more without sleep'.[91]

The regulatory framework introduced by the CAA in 1975 did not protect flight deck crew from intensive and imbalanced rosters as it intended. The trends begun in the late 1970s were exacerbated in the early 1980s, following revisions to CAP 371 and the introduction of a new confidential reporting service. The second edition of CAP 371, introduced in 1982, was less detailed than its previous iteration. The general principle underpinning the publication – that work, rest and time off were balanced across and between duty cycles – remained intact, but the tone of the guidelines shifted. The language of the revised publication recognised the flexible and permissive nature of the limitations. It marked a pragmatic realisation by regulatory agencies that the framework of flight time limitations introduced in 1975 was negotiable: the updated guidelines recognised the pre-existing limitations of the regulatory framework, and clarified these for airlines and crew. In the same year the CAA also established a confidential reporting service, the Confidential Human Factors Incident Reporting Programme (CHIRP). Flight deck crew were encouraged to share concerns about scheduling, fatigue and sleeplessness with CHIRP. Housed at the RAF Institute of Aviation Medicine, CHIRP was formally separate from the CAA.

Rather than regulation, CHIRP's remit was to circulate pilots' concerns in incident reports, and provide advice on the self-management of fatigue in flight. 1982, then, marked a shift in regulatory policy. Though the framework of flight time limitations introduced in 1975 remained, pilot fatigue was reconfigured in collective terms; under the second edition of CAP 371 the avoidance of fatigue became a collective responsibility. Aircrew in the flight deck and the cabin were required to engage in collective self-regulation by reporting incidents about themselves and their colleagues to CHIRP. This updated regulatory framework echoed post-war public health approaches to disease management: pilots were framed both as individuals, but also as part of a broader collective. Tensions between individual and collective approaches to flying fatigue continued into the 1990s, but the pilot was formally repositioned in regulatory discourses following the introduction of mandatory Crew Resource Management training that emphasised the importance of crew-wide cooperation for air safety.[92] To this end, at the close of the twentieth century the 'self' was – finally – decentred in civil aviation.

Conclusion

The post-war era ushered in a 'new wave of state interventionism' in some respects.[93] The period is often defined as one of collective provision, with the nationalisation of industry, transport and healthcare cited as primary examples of this overarching trend.[94] As political historians are increasingly recognising, though, liberal values which stressed self-reliance rather than state intervention continued to influence policy throughout the post-war period.[95] The apparent shift from post-war settlement to neo-liberalism under Thatcher is an attractive but, as Peter Kerr has put it, 'ultimately misleading' picture of twentieth-century British social and economic policy.[96] As this chapter has shown, even in the immediate post-war period British governments were reluctant to extend their regulatory reach, and even when regulations were introduced the state did not put statutory systems of enforcement in place.

The regulatory framework to control airline schedules shifted somewhat across the twentieth century. The state initially demanded that airlines impose some form of limitation under the 1957 ANO, but in the 1970s these limits were quantified (although not standardised) in CAP 371. By the 1980s the permissive nature of these regulations was formally recognised. In this period, agencies involved in regulation multiplied and their focus shifted from command-and-control regulation of aircrew schedules towards surveillance on the one hand, and the collection and dissemination of information to workers on the other. In this framework the role of the state became limited to the facilitation of self-regulation by industry.

There was no fundamental shift in the approach or impact of flight time limitations in post-war Britain. Though premised on a new understanding of fatigue as cumulative rather than acute, the regulations introduced in 1975 marked a shift in principle rather than practice. The work and rest of pilots was more strictly regulated under CAP 371 than in any other industry in post-war Britain, but the responsibility for fatigue management clearly remained with pilots and airlines rather than state agencies. Reliant on a heroic understanding of flight centred on individuals, the regulatory frameworks introduced to minimise fatigue in the twentieth century envisioned commercial pilots as autonomous agents capable of self-awareness, governance and – ultimately – balance. A trusted professional, the post-war pilot was expected to balance health, safety and commercial concerns without the need for external intervention. Fatigue collapsed the distance between economics, biology and safety. It was identified as a modern hazard with obvious implications beyond the individual in the immediate post-war period, but the potential social consequences of pilot fatigue did not come to influence the regulatory frameworks designed to minimise its effects until the close of the twentieth century. For much of the post-war period flight safety, rather, relied on a rubric of personal responsibility, self-regulation and individualism.

Notes

1 Anon., 'The Kallang Inquiry', *Flight International*, 19 November 1954, p. 754.
2 The National Archives, London (hereafter TNA) BT/248/110, extract from the Kallang Accident Inquiry Report, 1954, p. 1.
3 Ibid., p. 1.
4 Anon., 'The pilot, not ridge gets blame', *The Singapore Free Press*, 16 November 1954, p. 1.

5 T. C. Lawton, 'Governing the skies: conditions for the Europeanisation of airline policy', *Journal of Public Policy*, 19:1 (1999), 91–112.
6 D. Follows, 'Duty hours of pilots: recommendations to minister', *The Times*, 20 November 1954, p. 7.
7 TNA BT 248/110, Ministry of Civil Aviation minutes, 26 November 1954, p. 19.
8 TNA BT 248/110, Report of the Working Party on Operating Crew Fatigue and Flight Time Limitations, 15 December 1954.
9 J. Terraine, *The Right of the Line: The Role of the RAF in World War Two* (Barnsley: Pen and Sword Military, 2010).
10 1954 accident report cited in TNA DR/13/4, Report of the Committee on Flight Time Limitations, June 1973, p. 42.
11 H. E. Collier, 'The recognition of fatigue, with special reference to the clinical diagnosis of morbid fatigue in industry', *British Medical Journal*, 2:3964 (1936), 1322–5, at p. 1323.
12 Ibid., p. 1323.
13 A. Hemingway, 'The physiological background of fatigue', in W. F. Floyd and A. T. Welford (eds), *The Ergonomics Research Society Symposium on Fatigue* (London: H. K. Lewis & Company, 1953), pp. 69–75.
14 A. Abrahams, 'Chronic fatigue', *Lancet*, 246:6371 (1945), 421–2. For a broader history of physiological research into balance and homeostasis, see: M. Jackson, *The Age of Stress: Science and the Search for Stability* (Oxford: Oxford University Press, 2013); and V. Heggie, *A History of British Sports Medicine* (Manchester: Manchester University Press, 2013).
15 Lawton, 'Governing the skies'.
16 The focus here is on the regulation of pilots' hours of work and rest, though cabin crew were also included in the regulatory framework described in the second part of this chapter.
17 R. Hayward, 'Busman's stomach and the embodiment of modernity', *Contemporary British History*, 31:1 (2017), 1–23.
18 C. Sirrs, 'Accidents and apathy: the construction of the "Robens philosophy" of occupational safety and health regulation in Britain, 1961–1974', *Social History of Medicine*, 29:1 (2016), 66–88.
19 V. Long, *The Rise and Fall of the Healthy Factory: The Politics of Industrial Health in Britain, 1914–60* (Basingstoke: Palgrave Macmillan, 2011).
20 S. Blayney, 'Industrial fatigue and the productive body: the science of work in Britain, c.1900–1918', *Social History of Medicine*, 32:2 (2017), 310–28.
21 A. J. McIvor, 'Manual work, technology, and industrial health, 1918–39', *Medical History*, 31:2 (1987), 160–89, at p. 167.
22 A. J. McIvor, 'Employers, the government, and industrial fatigue in Britain, 1890–1918', *British Journal of Industrial Medicine*, 44:11 (1987), 724–32; A. Rabinbach, *The Human Motor: Energy, Fatigue, and the Origins of*

Modernity (Los Angeles: University of California Press, 1992); A. K. Schaffner, *Exhaustion: A History* (New York: Columbia University Press, 2016); Blayney, 'Industrial fatigue and the productive body'.
23 A. Derickson, *Dangerously Sleepy: Overworked Americans and the Cult of Manly Wakefulness* (Philadelphia: University of Pennsylvania Press, 2014).
24 B. M. Hutter, *Regulation and Risk: Occupational Health and Safety on the Railways* (Oxford: Oxford University Press, 2001).
25 Derickson, *Dangerously Sleepy*, p. 27.
26 Ibid.
27 TNA BT 248/110, Ministry of Civil Aviation minutes, 26 November 1954, p. 19.
28 TNA BT 248/110, BALPA Flight Time Limitations Memorandum, 2 December 1954; TNA BT 248/110, Ministry of Civil Aviation minutes, 21 December 1954, p. 28.
29 TNA BT 248/110, Report of the Working Party on Operating Crew Fatigue and Flight Time Limitations.
30 Ibid., p. 6.
31 TNA BT 248/110, Working Party on Operating Crew Fatigue, meetings 2 and 3 September 1954, p. 1.
32 TNA BT 248/110, Report of the Working Party on Operating Crew Fatigue and Flight Time Limitations, pp. 7–8.
33 TNA BT 248/110, Report of the Working Party on Operating Crew Fatigue and Flight Time Limitations, p. 8; Chapter 8 (this volume) also speaks to the tension between practical considerations and the health of workers in the post-war period.
34 TNA BT 248/110, BALPA Flight Time Limitations Memorandum, p. 1.
35 Ibid., p. 2.
36 TNA BT 248/110, Report of the Working Party on Operating Crew Fatigue and Flight Time Limitations, p. 6.
37 TNA BT 248/110, Working Party on Operating Crew Fatigue, meetings 2 and 3 September 1954, p. 2.
38 On contemporary debates about the practical and ethical importance of professional autonomy in medicine, see: A. Seaton, 'Against the "sacred cow": NHS opposition and the Fellowship for Freedom in Medicine, 1948–72', *Twentieth Century British History*, 26:3 (2015), 424–49.
39 D. Armstrong, 'Actors, patients and agency: a recent history', *Sociology of Health and Illness*, 36:2 (2014), 163–74.
40 C. Muller, 'The Institute of Economic Affairs: undermining the post-war consensus', *Contemporary British History*, 10:1 (1996), 88–110.
41 A. Gamble, 'Privatization, Thatcherism, and the British state', *Journal of Law and Society*, 16:1 (1989), 1–20.

42 The idea of state intervention in industrial and economic matters was not universally popular in the immediate post-war period either. A rhetoric of planning permeated the political arena, but state intervention was subject to debate among economists, policy-makers and civil servants. For a history of post-war planning debates, see: J. Tomlinson, 'Planning: debate and policy in the 1940s', *Twentieth Century British History*, 3:2 (1992), 154–74; R. Toye, 'Gosplanners versus thermostatters: Whitehall planning debates and their political consequences, 1945–49', *Contemporary British History*, 14:4 (2000), 81–106.
43 Terraine, *The Right of the Line*.
44 TNA BT 248/110, Report of the Working Party on Operating Crew Fatigue and Flight Time Limitations, p. 6; TNA BT 248/110, Working Party on Operating Crew Fatigue, meetings 2 and 3 September 1954, p. 7.
45 TNA BT 248/110, Report of the Working Party on Operating Crew Fatigue and Flight Time Limitations, p. 7.
46 TNA BT 248/110, Working Party on Operating Crew Fatigue, meetings 2 and 3 September 1954, p. 8.
47 A. N. J. Blain, *Pilots and Management: Industrial Relations in the UK Airlines* (London: George Allen and Unwin, 1972).
48 A. T. Spooner, 'Flight time limitations', *The Log*, 42:5 (October 1982), 20–1, at p. 21.
49 TNA BT 248/111, note of meeting in Berkeley Square House, 28 September 1955, p. 1.
50 Ibid., p. 1.
51 B. Jackson, 'The think-tank archipelago: Thatcherism and neo-liberalism', in B. Jackson and R. Saunders (eds), *Making Thatcher's Britain* (Cambridge: Cambridge University Press, 2012), pp. 43–61.
52 Sirrs, 'Accidents and apathy'.
53 Lord Robens, *Safety and Health at Work: Report of the Committee 1970–72*, vol. 1, Cmnd 5034 (London: HMSO, 1972). There was widespread resistance to top-down regulation in this period, as Chapter 3 in this volume describes in relation to alcohol pricing.
54 Robens, *Safety and Health at Work*, p. xiv; Hutter, *Regulation and Risk*.
55 Blain, *Pilots and Management*.
56 Air Accidents Investigation Branch, *Trident I G-ARPI: Report of the Public Inquiry into the Causes and Circumstances of the Accident near Staines on 18 June 1972* (London: HMSO, 1973), p. 54.
57 Anon., 'Pilot gave warning of crash risk in using inexperienced crews "two hours before Trident take-off"', *The Times*, 29 November 1972.
58 TNA DR 13/4, Report of the Committee on Flight Time Limitations.
59 Ibid., p. 3.

60 J. Aschoff, 'Circadian rhythms in man', *Science*, 148:3676 (1965), 1427–32, at p. 1432.
61 For a broader view of physiological research in this period, see Jackson, *The Age of Stress*.
62 P. J. Taylor, 'Shift and day work: a comparison of sickness absence, lateness, and other absence behaviour at an oil refinery from 1962 to 1965', *British Journal of Industrial Medicine*, 24:2 (1967), 93–102; R. T. W. L. Conroy, A. L. Elliot and J. N. Mills, 'Circadian rhythms in plasma concentration of 11-hydroxycorticosteroids in men working on night shift and in permanent night workers', *British Journal of Industrial Medicine*, 27:2 (1970), 170–4. As Chapter 8 (this volume) makes clear, circadian disruption was also studied by scientists interested in human performance in extreme environments.
63 R. A. McFarland, 'Air travel across time zones', *American Scientist*, 63:1 (1975), 23–30.
64 TNA DR 13/4, Report of the Committee on Flight Time Limitations, p. 8.
65 Ibid., p. 8.
66 Ibid., p. 7.
67 Ibid., p. 15.
68 Ibid., p. 15.
69 F. Cooper, 'Medical feminism, working mothers, and the limits of home: finding a balance between self-care and other-care in cross-cultural debates about health and lifestyle, 1952–1956', *Palgrave Communications*, 2 (2016), article 16042, available at https://doi.org/10.1057/palcomms.2016.42, accessed 14 July 2016; TNA DR 13/4, Report of the Committee on Flight Time Limitations, p. 27.
70 Chapter 8 in this volume traces a similar shift. While early investigations of human performance in extreme environments focused almost exclusively on physiological adaptation, by the 1970s research interest centred on psychological and social factors.
71 M. Young and P. Wilmott, *The Symmetrical Family* (London: Penguin, 1973), p. 164.
72 H. J. Freudenberger, 'Staff burn-out', *Journal of Social Issues*, 30:1 (1974), 159–65.
73 TNA DR 13/4, Report of the Committee on Flight Time Limitations, p. 15.
74 This approach to working time regulation reflected the promotion of moderation in contemporary public health policy, as outlined in Chapters 3 and 4 in this volume.
75 TNA DR 13/4, Report of the Committee on Flight Time Limitations, p. 17.

76 Ibid., p. 12
77 Ibid., p. 8.
78 Ibid., p. 15.
79 A. Nathoo, 'Initiating therapeutic relaxation in Britain: a twentieth-century strategy for health and wellbeing', *Palgrave Communications*, 2 (2016), article 16043, p. 3, available at https://doi.org/10.1057/palcomms.2016.43, accessed 20 July 2016; TNA DR 13/4, Report of the Committee on Flight Time Limitations, p. 25.
80 TNA DR 13/4, Report of the Committee on Flight Time Limitations, p. 30.
81 Ibid., p. 26.
82 Civil Aviation Authority, *CAP 371: The Avoidance of Excessive Fatigue in Aircrews Requirements Document* (London: Civil Aviation Authority, 1975).
83 TNA DR 13/1, Flight Time Limitations Board, minutes of meeting, 13 November 1975, p. 1.
84 TNA DR 13/4, Report of the Committee on Flight Time Limitations, p. 32.
85 Ibid., p. 32.
86 Ibid., p. 3.
87 Ibid., p. 24.
88 For a broader history of financial deregulation and marketisation, see P. Addison, *No Turning Back: The Peacetime Revolutions of Post-War Britain* (Oxford: Oxford University Press, 2010).
89 R. Green and R. Skinner, 'CHIRP and fatigue', *The Log*, 48:5 (October 1987), 6–11, at p. 8.
90 Ibid.
91 T. Staples, 'Flight time limitations: is "up to a 14-hour day" really unacceptable?', *The Log*, 43:6 (1982), 19.
92 R. Flin, P. O'Connor and K. Mearns, 'Crew resource management: improving team work in high reliability industries', *Team Performance Management*, 8:3/4 (2002), 68–78.
93 G. Eghigian, A. Killen and C. Leuenberger, 'The self as project: politics and the human sciences in the twentieth century', *Osiris*, 22:1 (2007), 1–25, at p. 22.
94 Addison, *No Turning Back*.
95 N. Rollings, 'Cracks in the post-war Keynesian settlement? The role of organised business in Britain in the rise of neoliberalism before Margaret Thatcher', *Twentieth Century British History*, 24:4 (2013), 637–59.
96 P. Kerr, *Postwar British Politics: From Conflict to Consensus* (London: Routledge, 2001), p. 5.

Part III
Reconfiguring balance

8

Extreme acts: narratives of balance and moderation at the limits of human performance

Vanessa Heggie

Introduction

The highest and coldest regions of the earth might seem an unpromising choice of location to find studies of balance and moderation; but throughout the twentieth century physiologists and other biomedical scientists used extreme environments as forms of 'natural laboratory' to study not only the limits of human performance and survival, but also the ways in which normality and balance were maintained, and altered, in the face of extreme external pressure – both physical and mental. Indeed, some of the earliest historians of the concept of homeostasis were themselves physiologists who worked on human and animal adaptation.[1]

This chapter investigates notions of balance in the 'natural laboratories' of extreme physiology – specifically the high Arctic, Antarctica and high altitude in South America and the Himalaya. Physiologists and other biomedical scientists celebrated these sites as spaces in which many varieties of *im*balance could be studied. Here I will concentrate on three different kinds of balance: moderation, physiological homeostasis and psychological stress responses. Through these case studies extreme environments emerge as sites where, firstly, notions of balance could be debated and reconstituted, and secondly where the white adult male's body became established as the norm for such research. This unquestioned centralisation of a very specific kind of body as a standard measure in balance research – particularly as it was a body not indigenous to extreme environments – had consequences for the practices of both science and exploration.

That the choice of norms and benchmarks in balance research can have deep socio-political consequences is well established through the other chapters in this volume. In the case of extreme physiology the focus on sea-level-born white scientists not only obscured the fact that there were multiple ways of adapting to altitude, but also led to a backlash by South American researchers who began to refigure the 'Andean man' as the baseline normal for studies.[2] More broadly, extreme physiology's centralisation of the white European body and its problems was one pillar that maintained ideas of white supremacy at a moment when theories about the origins and evolution of the human race were shifting.[3] It also acted as a self-reinforcing tautology that impeded women's access to extreme spaces and prevented them benefiting from the lessons of the physiological work done there.[4]

Clearly, then, however remote or exotic the sites of extreme physiology appear, they were part of broader research networks. As an example, the first physiological expedition to Antarctica (INPHEXAN, discussed in more detail below) explicitly set out to study what the physiologists broadly called 'stress' – although caused by the external pressures of an extreme environment and isolated conditions, this was an '*internal* physiological or psychological [process] generated by environmental pressure'.[5] The American researchers involved concentrated on hormonal and biochemical responses to cold, isolation and physical labour, reflecting, and feeding into, the pervasive endocrine focus of mid-century stress research. Meanwhile, the British researchers studied metabolism, fat deposition, nutrition, fatigue and desensitisation to cold – all markers of earlier twentieth-century stress research, but also themes that would become absorbed into later studies of stress which figured it as part of a complex of lifestyle disorders that included obesity and heart disease.[6] Such work contributed to the development of psychomedical standards for astronaut recruitment (finding balanced personalities), to the design of improved (nutritionally balanced) rations for military forces, but also to everyday lives as part of studies that established the 'ideal' (read: balanced and normal) temperature for office buildings and factories.

Of course extreme physiology fieldwork also had characteristics that distinguished it from research in laboratories or more temperate locations, most notably the fact that it was interested in two kinds of adaptation – not just the immediate failure of adaptive bodily or behavioural systems which made up Hans Selye's famous formulation of 'stress' in the mid-1930s, but also much longer-term processes, happening over lifetimes and generations, which would gradually evolve human bodies adapted to their environmental conditions.[7] Would the conditions of high altitude, extreme heat or cold, create new 'normal' bodies? Such questions, when posed in a context of Western scientific work, often contrasted the skills and abilities of indigenous and non-indigenous peoples: was the superior climbing ability of the Sherpa peoples evidence of physiological acclimatisation – which Western climbers could simulate in their own bodies – or was it evidence of long-term hereditary change – which Western climbers were denied (but could perhaps replicate with drugs or other assistive technologies)?[8]

Extreme physiological research therefore exposes the connections between balance in micro and macro worlds – from the minute and rapid biochemical changes in individual haemoglobin molecules, to million-year histories of the balance between human bodies and changing environmental pressures. Focusing predominantly on fieldwork emphasises these connections. The physiologists and biomedical researchers supporting expeditions worked to 'rebalance' the explorer's body, using behavioural changes and technological interventions. In so doing they explicitly recognised the mismatch between reductive studies of isolated bodily systems and the clearly holistic reality of the homeostatic/balance systems in the human body.[9] They consistently argued for the value of whole-body, field-site studies as the only way to consider the multi-factorial issues of stress, fatigue and imbalance; indeed, as I have outlined elsewhere,[10] these researchers created complex spaces for knowledge production, blurring the boundaries other scholars have described between laboratory and fieldwork.[11] This process included turning sites of sport, as well as of exploration, into 'natural laboratories', particularly for (more) extreme sports such as the marathon (discussed below), or major international events held at altitude or in non-temperate countries.[12] Further, the researchers discussed in this chapter dealt with the difficulty of balancing different working practices and political aims (for example, civilian and military researchers routinely worked alongside one another), while these collages of laboratory, clinical and field researches were created to test and disrupt homeostatic mechanisms. This chapter will start with the laboratory understanding of human balance, and spread out, via blood, breath and psychological stresses, to consider the field study of balance at the extremes of human survival.

Finding the balance: early work on extremity and homeostasis

Despite the later focus on the field, the history of extreme physiology tends to build from laboratory studies in the middle of the nineteenth century; the apparent conflict between findings 'in the field' and the laboratory – part of ongoing debates about whether artificial models were good scientific representations of 'the real world' – led to a focus on expeditionary fieldwork as a form of 'reality testing' for laboratory concepts.[13] As a consequence it was the *male* body that became not only normalised, but also effectively universalised as the only body about which we had either observational or experimental knowledge when it came to balance and imbalance in extreme conditions.

French physiologist Claude Bernard (1813–78) coined the term *milieu intérieur* in the 1870s to describe the complex, self-regulating system of the animal body; he also promoted a reductive, experimental approach to studying this system, whereby artificially induced disruption (e.g. placing an animal in a barometric chamber, removing an organ or severing a nerve) sought to isolate individual parts and understand their role in the living, holistic whole.[14] It was in this context that French physiologist Paul Bert (1833–86) created a simplified laboratory model of mountain sickness, in deliberate emulation of Bernard's laboratory-prioritising experimental ideology.[15] Thus the lived phenomena of fatigue, headaches, disorientation and nausea experienced by climbers, explorers and soldiers at altitude was specifically defined as an imbalance in the *milieu intérieur* – eventually identified as a problem with the regulation of respiration and oxygen levels (a mechanism which alongside 'water … temperature and chemical reserves' had formed the touchstones of Bernard's research).[16] Based on extensive barometric studies in the 1870s, Bert created a reductive, single-cause explanation for mountain sickness, turning it into 'altitude sickness'. Simply speaking, the reduced oxygen partial pressure at high altitude caused a deficit in inhaled oxygen, an inadequacy for which the homeostatic responses of the body attempted to compensate. While this was usually successful at medium altitudes, the extremity of Everest and other high-altitude sites pushed beyond the human body's ability to adapt. The extreme 'milieu extérieur' pushed the *milieu intérieur* to the point of collapse, but this could be fixed with a simple rebalance – the addition of supplementary oxygen.

What was easy in the laboratory was a 100-year challenge on the mountainside. Away from the simplified conditions of the barometric chamber, altitude sickness was a more unpredictable beast – climbers might experience bouts of it on one expedition, but not another, and it might manifest at a variety of altitudes. The first compressed oxygen cylinders were produced (for medical purposes) in 1868, and by the late nineteenth century contained breathing systems (designed for diving and mining as well as respiratory therapy) were sufficiently light and robust to take on an Alpine climbing trip.[17] But oxygen was used with very mixed success as a form of emergency medicine in these circumstances; altitude sickness was treated as an acute-onset disease for which the usual treatment was a retreat down the mountain. When oxygen was given it was prescribed as if it were a medication, on the onset of symptoms, and for only as long as the symptoms lasted. Its most famous failure was the death of Dr Etienne Jacottet on Mont Blanc in 1891, and ongoing scepticism about the usefulness of oxygen to climbers meant that Bert's hypothesis about the altitude-oxygen link was not established as fact until the beginning of the twentieth century.[18]

One of the staunchest critics of the altitude sickness-oxygen link was Italian physiologist Angelo Mosso (1846–1910). Otherwise one of the leading scientists working on fatigue, extreme physiology and mountaineering around the turn of the century, Mosso specifically used Jacottet's death as a case study proving his theory that it was a deficiency of carbon dioxide, rather than oxygen, that caused mountain sickness.[19] Having studied under organic physicist Carl Ludwig (1816–95), Mosso was influenced by reductive laboratory methodologies but, unlike Bert, used a mixed system of research in his studies, combining the barometric chamber with field study; indeed he was in part responsible for the construction of the world's first mid-altitude laboratory, the Capanna Regina Margherita, built first as a shelter on Punta Gnifetti (Monte Rosa) c.4,559 m above sea level.[20] The Margherita hut was opened in late 1893; in 1894 proposals were made to add further rooms for scientific work, and the building was gradually expanded and developed into a multi-room research facility. It remained in almost continuous use until the 1930s, but after the Second World War only a few trips were made there, until the facility was entirely rebuilt by the Italian Alpine Club in 1980. The Margherita hut is significant to this story because research into altitude physiology became a robustly *field*-based specialism in the twentieth century: although barometric chambers and (especially around the two world wars) aeroplanes were used as alternatives, the seminal studies on high altitude, blood and respiration were predominantly those that involved mountain expeditions. So while contemporary altitude physiologists look to Bert – and his theory about oxygen balance – as the 'father' of their professional field, it was Mosso who best models the actual research practices of physiologists interested in human limits and homeostasis.[21]

Scientists repeatedly referred to the sides of mountains, and, too, to the Arctic and Antarctic regions, as their 'natural laboratories'; while more attention has been paid to the astronomical and physical sciences in these spaces, recent scholarship has shown that these were important places for biological research too.[22] While ecologists considered these natural laboratories as spaces to consider other kinds of balance (for example the ways in which the processes of evolution 'fitted' organisms for their ecological niches, or the 'balance' of specific ecosystems),[23] for the physiologist, doctor and psychologist high altitude, the polar regions and similar 'natural laboratories' were spaces in which the human body was exposed to extreme conditions: extremes of temperature, altitude, fatiguing physical work and mental strain, and extreme isolation. Here, as in the barometric chamber, the *milieu extérieur* could force the *milieu intérieur* to the very limits of its capacity to adapt – that is, to the point at which it became irreparably unbalanced. This imbalance explains the attractiveness of these spaces to scientists, and opens up another form of balance and moderation for consideration: the limits of ethical and reasonable experiments on human beings. There is an interlacing of the legal experiments conducted on mountaineers and explorers, the potentially exploitative studies that used military recruits and the clearly abusive work done using the bodies of prisoners and concentration camp victims – this will be picked out later in this chapter. But one of the advantages of studying explorers and sportsmen (and this was exclusively men until the middle of the twentieth century, a bias that existed in civilian as well as military research) was that they were willing to put themselves into environments, and carry out activities, that 'normal' human guinea pigs would not tolerate, or which would not be considered safe and ethical by review boards.[24] This is not a situation limited to the pre-Nuremberg research past: when the American Medical Research Expedition to Everest gained funding from The National Heart, Lung and Blood Institute and the American Thoracic Society for their 1981 expedition, the death rate for summiteers on Everest was around one in fifteen; it is extremely doubtful whether any laboratory or clinic-based research practice would have been approved if it offered such a significant risk of morbidity, let alone mortality, for young, healthy, adult male participants.[25]

Sportspeople of all kinds were useful not just for their willingness to enter uncomfortable environments, but also to deliver extreme, reliable and repeated physical efforts. Almost as soon as the marathon became a regular sporting event, doctors and physiologists crowded the start line in order to study the effects of the race on participants. Effectively invented as an event at the 1896 revival of the modern Olympic Games, marathons began to be run elsewhere, the first in Boston in 1897. Boston immediately became a site for physiologists as well as runners, with the first studies (concentrating on cardiovascular work) published in 1899.[26] Where else, after all, could a physiologist find not just one, but many human guinea pigs willing to run twenty-six miles non-stop? As the Nobel prize-winning British physiologist A. V. Hill put it in 1927, the advantages of experimenting on athletes were that 'athletes themselves, being in a state of health and dynamic equilibrium, can be experimented on without danger and can repeat their performances exactly again and again'.[27]

The use of explorers and elite sports performers as subjects had a significant effect on the study of extreme physiology, as it reinforced the erasure of the female body. Even where scientists acknowledged that women's physiology was poorly understood, they made little effort to rectify their ignorance. For example, in 1959 a major symposium on Polar Medicine in Cambridge, with an all-male speaker list, concluded that 'the time had come to observe the reaction of women as well as of men', but none of the attendees went on to design field studies that would include women in extreme environments.[28] Studying men was not just an intellectual default, it was the easiest option; women's participation in elite sport was extremely limited in the first half of the century, and they were effectively barred – through legal means, soft power and social pressure – from routinely accessing sites at high altitude or Antarctica until the last decades of the twentieth century.[29] That is, Western European and North American *white* women were excluded; 'Sherpani' and other female porters were routinely used as part of long treks in mountainous regions, and of course women had been living in the Arctic for millennia. But few of these women participated in Western scientific experiments as subjects, and none ran the experiments themselves.[30] Therefore the narratives of balance and moderation at extremes explicitly framed the white adult male body as the standard form: theirs was the 'normal' homeostasis, which was disrupted by extreme environments; theirs were the 'normal' physiological reactions that responded to this disruption.

Moderate gentlemen and scientific ethics

These earliest investigations into human adaptation – that is, *r*ebalancing – to altitude discovered that altitude caused an apparently universal, 'normal' physiological reaction in the blood. Significant changes, outlined below, appeared rapidly in the blood profile of those who moved from sea level to mid-altitude; attempts to manipulate these processes to improve performances in extreme environments provoked questions not only about the balance of the homeostatic system, but also about moderation and fairness – the ethics of sport and of science.

The immediate homeostatic responses of the human body to altitude – those that occur within hours or days – mostly involve the cardiorespiratory system, increasing breathing rates, increasing heart rate and so on. The next stage of response, after several days or weeks, is the development of polycythaemia – a higher red blood cell count per millilitre of blood than is considered 'normal'. As with so many of the body's balance systems, there are two counterbalanced ways to 'concentrate' the blood – either increase the production rate of red blood cells, or decrease the amount of fluid (plasma) in the blood. Early research into this phenomenon was complicated by the fact that mountaineers were often dehydrated, which meant their bodies might be responding to the lack of fluids by reducing plasma. It was therefore difficult to prove experimentally how the polycythaemia was produced – whether it was a response to altitude or to dehydration, or a combination of both.

In 1906, two French physiologists, Paul Carnot and Clotilde-Camille Deflandre, developed a theory that a hormone might stimulate the red blood cell production process, and they named this theoretical signalling hormone 'hémopoïétine'. Renamed erythropoietin, it was eventually specifically identified and isolated by Eugene Goldwasser and his team in the late 1950s and 1960s.[31] By the early twentieth century, then, it was clear that it was *possible* that altitude polycythaemia was due to active hormone-stimulated cell production, rather than being a side effect of dehydration.[32]

This offered another potential solution to the problem of mountain sickness and climbing fatigue: as well as being able to supplement the respiratory system with oxygen, perhaps it would also be possible to create a state of polycythaemia artificially. This 'blood packing' could either be used to 'pre-acclimatise' someone to altitude, so that they did not have to wait the week or more for their body's systems to respond; or it could be pushed further, to create a state of super-polycythaemia, giving an individual an advantage over their 'natural' level of red blood cell production. By the end of the twentieth century this theory had become a reality, and it became the basis of 'blood doping' systems used by athletes; but in the first half of the century it remained only a theory and a rumour – there were whispers in the British climbing community in the 1950s that the Germans had tried blood transfusions during their attempts at the high Himalaya in the 1930s.[33]

While the British focused their efforts on Everest in the 1920s and 1930s, the Germans looked to Nanga Parbat, the ninth highest mountain in the world, and in an area to which, unlike Everest, the Germans could negotiate access. The German teams did conduct physiological research on the mountain, but the technology for blood transfusions was nowhere near effective and safe enough in the 1930s for blood doping to be a realistic prospect at high altitude, and transfusions of blood long before the expedition were unlikely to aid climbing. It is probable that the British rumours of the 1950s were fuelled by a misunderstanding of research into polycythaemia that was done on Nanga Parbat, particularly that by Ulrich Luft (1910–91).[34] Luft was a doctor and research physiologist with a particular interest in the respiratory system and in respiratory distress, which involved suffocation, low oxygen pressure responses and so on. As a keen climber, he managed to get himself on the 1937 expedition to Nanga Parbat, led by the physiologist and mountaineer Karl Wein.[35] Early in the expedition Luft was left behind at Base Camp to do some routine observations while the rest of the team, seven German climbers and nine Sherpa porters, went on to set up camps higher up the mountain; they created Camp IV at about 6,100 m, and began preparing the way to Camp V. Three days later Luft and five porters resumed the climb, intending to go on to Camp IV – except that they could not find it. Where Camp IV should have been there was nothing but fresh, flat snow. They dug, and found three rucksacks belonging to members of the team, but the snow was too hard and packed for further digging without the right tools. A new climbing team was flown out and, with Luft, dug up the tents and the crushed remains of the entire expedition – wiped out in a single massive avalanche. They retrieved the bodies of five of the German climbers (finding that their smashed wristwatches recorded the time of the disaster as just after midnight), and carefully collected as much of the scientific work, in the form of notebooks and equipment, as was possible.[36]

Because of his research interests, Luft was recruited into the Luftwaffe to work on anoxia, oxygen systems and aviation. The significant exchanges between military and civilian research are exemplified by the crossover between mountaineering and aviation, not least because they demonstrate that the relationship was clearly a two-way street, and included important crossovers in the study of mental, as well as physical, stress.[37] As I have explored elsewhere, altitude physiology also highlights occasions when military aviation experience was dismissed as irrelevant or unhelpful by civilian explorers.[38] At the end of the war, Luft was targeted and extracted by the Americans during Operation Paperclip, again because of his research expertise.[39] While other German scientists from this project went to work on the atomic bomb and rocket science, Luft went to the National Aeronautics and Space Administration, translating his expertise in extreme survival physiology to designing systems to test and support astronauts.[40] As a beloved teacher and widely admired scientist he was celebrated in his lifetime, and immediately after his death in 1991, with honours and buildings named after him; but with the opening of East German archives, documents were discovered suggesting that his expertise in what happened to human bodies exposed to extreme conditions had come from work done by others in the Nazi concentration camps.[41] While there is no

Balance at the limits of human performance

evidence of him as an active participant, it is clear that he knew about and profited from the hypothermia experiments in Dachau, and possibly the murder of 'undesirables' in decompression chambers.[42]

Ironically then, the study of homeostasis, extreme physiology, and thus balance in human biology, inevitably raises questions of balance in research ethics – not just in the design and regulation of new experiments, but also the balance between the potential to save current lives (or win important political space races) and the ethical problems of using data from murderous experiments of the past. Expeditionary science is a risky form of scientific practice, and therefore one of its significant advantages is that its participants have been willing to enter environmental situations and engage in physical practices that offer a small but serious risk of physical harm, and even death. In terms of high-altitude science, the first death on a British expedition to Everest was a doctor – Alexander Kellas, a pioneer of oxygen systems in the very early twentieth century, who died from dysentery on the trek to Everest in 1921. Famously, George Mallory and Sandy Irvine died somewhere near the summit in 1924, bringing to an end the expeditions of the 1920s; less famously, seven Sherpa porters had fallen to their deaths on the British expedition in 1922, largely due to an error of judgement by Mallory. The involvement of Sherpa people was a matter of concern to the Europeans who relied on them in the high Himalaya. It was Kellas who first popularised the use of local people at high altitude (as opposed to bringing Alpine porters), and, yet again, we find a fine balance necessary in the discussion of indigenous support. On the one hand, more than sixty Sherpa porters and guides have died while assisting foreign climbers on Everest in the twentieth century, and climbers themselves have asked whether it was fair to use financial bribes to persuade people to undertake this risk for the benefit of their own sporting, imperial or scientific goals (goals which, arguably, brought little benefit or credit to the Sherpa). On the other hand, the attitude of early climbers to their Sherpa guides was undeniably paternalistic and patronising (including the suggestion that the Sherpa were like children and did not fear death), and so ethical concerns could sometimes be framed in a condescending way that denied local people agency.[43]

It is important to recognise that the Sherpa participants in high-altitude expeditions were also participants directly in the science, not just the exploration. They appeared as human guinea pigs in various published and unpublished experiments on fatigue, respiration and other elements of exercise physiology. Some of these practices certainly pushed the boundaries of acceptable research practice, most notably the testing of performance-enhancing drugs on Everest. The 1953 British expedition was trying a new route up the mountain, tackling the Lohtse Face. This was, overall, a longer route than had been used by the rival Swiss expedition in 1952, but had the advantage of a stepped ascent, allowing for more camps and depots of equipment to be laid. This in turn required a lot of to-and-fro trips by the Sherpa porters to set up the camps – all of which had to pass through the extremely technically challenging Khombu Icefall. The expedition leader John Hunt feared this would tire the porters, and in the second week of May the team doctor, Mike Ward, ran a test of the amphetamine Benzedrine as an anti-fatigue medication. Two (unnamed) Sherpa participants 'volunteered', and took it while carrying food, tents, fuel and other supplies between camps. Several of the team were familiar with the use of amphetamines as a stimulant – it had been used by allied military forces, particularly by pilots – and there were two highly qualified doctors in the climbing team, which controlled the risks; but without consent forms, without any record of what the Sherpa porters were told, it is difficult to understand how this negotiation of risk and reward occurred, if it occurred at all.[44] Luckily, no harm was done, and as the two participants reported back that the drug merely cured one Sherpa's headache and made the other sleepy, the team seem to have decided it would not be useful to repeat the dosing further up the mountain.[45]

The use of amphetamines and other performance-enhancing substances is obviously a topic of heated debate in the sporting world. Most of the European high-altitude climbing teams had amphetamine and/ or cocaine derivatives in their medical kits, and this use of stimulants and tonics may initially seem to conflict with the 'gentlemanly amateur' identity of the early twentieth-century climbing elite.[46] In fact, attitudes towards such performance enhancers were much more relaxed prior to mid-century – George Mallory himself offered to secure for the teams of the 1920s a stimulant 'similar to caffeen [sic] and kola, but much better and absolutely innocuous' from his Cambridge colleague J. B. S. Haldane.[47] This fact leaves historians with an apparent puzzle relating to debates about supplemental oxygen in the 1920s, 1930s and 1950s. Typically, at least for the British case, these debates have been represented as an 'oxygen controversy', a face-off between modern scientific rationalism (oxygen is necessary) and old-fashioned gentlemanly amateurism (oxygen is 'cheating').[48] In that context it is not obvious why the boost given by an amphetamine should be morally acceptable, if attempts to rebalance a homeostatic disturbance by using oxygen were considered ethically dubious; but as I have shown elsewhere, this puzzle is solved when we see this representation as at best a partial story, and at worst a misunderstanding of the debate.[49] Far more important than the issue of ethics in the 'controversy' was the fact that early oxygen systems did not work as well as they might, and there were serious scientific and experimental reasons to wonder whether heavy oxygen canisters and respiration-restricting masks might actually hinder a climber more than they helped him.

What this 'oxygen controversy' – and, indeed, many of the debates about technology in exploration science – demonstrates is that even if there was a clear scientific consensus on theories of balance and homeostatic regulation in the laboratory, it still took a great deal of work to turn solutions *in theory*, such as supplemental oxygen, into solutions *in practice*. Blood packing is another example of this process: although by the 1930s it was reasonable to believe that rival climbing teams might be trying the technology, the reality was that blood transfusions remained difficult and dangerous even in advanced medical facilities at sea-level locations. Attempts to increase the concentration of red blood cells in human subjects continued in laboratory-based experiments, but it seems to have taken another two or three decades before the technology was seriously used to improve sporting performance, and even then in the relative safety of training rooms and motels,[50] rather than on icy mountain slopes.

While elite sportspeople began to take blood packing seriously as an enhancement technology (before it was banned in the mid-1980s), German mountaineers began to consider the exact opposite: haemo*dilution*. In the early 1980s, the American Medical Research Expedition to Everest applied to the American Lung Association for money to study haemodilution on their planned expedition in 1981, because:

> the Germans have been fooling with this, but they have done no really scientific, controlled studies. The Germans state that hemodilution is great – makes you feel like a million and enables you to climb like the wind. We're interested in seeing if this is so, and also because the findings will have implications for managing patients with hypoxic disease at sea level.[51]

This practice might seem counterintuitive – how could both increasing *and* decreasing the concentration of red blood cells in a climber's blood improve their performance? The answer lies in the concept of balance, or rather homeostasis, where for every adjustment there is a counter-adjustment. One of the healthy human body's responses to increased altitude is, it turns out, to create polycythaemia by up-regulating the production of red blood cells; this increases the oxygen-carrying capacity of the blood, which means that when there is less oxygen in the atmospheric air, and therefore less in the lungs on each breath, the red blood cells are capable of capturing as much of that scarce oxygen as possible and transporting it around the body. But this response does not come without its own side effects, the most pernicious of which is that increasing the number of cells in a millilitre of blood makes that blood more viscous. This thicker, stickier blood travels with much more difficulty around the capillaries and the areas of microcirculation in the body, which results in an increasing risk of losing circulation in the peripheries of the body, and of suffering from the results of blockages and clots. Further, the process is exacerbated by another alteration in the body's homeostatic balance: the 'right shifting' of the oxygen-haemoglobin dissociation curve. This curve describes the chemical response of red blood cells to lower-than-normal oxygen concentrations, which is to have more affinity to oxygen – that is, to bind to oxygen more strongly.[52] At the lungs this is a positive trait, allowing even more of the oxygen in the lungs to be 'captured' by the blood instead of being exhaled, and therefore 'wasted'. But this is counterbalanced – as are so many bodily processes – by a negative, as the red blood cells are also more resistant to releasing their oxygen where it is needed in the body. The more oxygen is transferred away from blood cells as they travel around the body the lower the oxygen concentration is in the blood, until a point is reached, usually in the peripheries and small capillaries, where the red blood cells' attachment to their oxygen is so strong that they cannot 'do their job' and deliver it. This exacerbates the challenges that thicker blood poses to the microcirculation, and compounds the risk of loss of circulation in some parts of the body.

One of the crucial lessons of extreme physiology is this realisation that the compensatory mechanisms of the body can only go so far, and that at the limits of adaptation they may become maladaptive, or cause harm to other bodily systems, or make bodily processes less efficient. This facet of adaptation was also, inadvertently, the spur that motivated the foundation of some of the world's most important and productive research centres into extreme physiology, when, as we will see below, due to the slippage between 'blood', 'race' and 'ethnicity', a Peruvian researcher interpreted a British researcher's statement about homeostasis as a national slur.

Blood and race

Western physiologists working in the nineteenth century maintained a long-standing, Eurocentric assumption that the ideal environment for humans was the temperate zone. While the (white) body might be able to survive in extreme environments, there would inevitably be a biological price to pay, both in an individual sense and also a racial one, evidenced by the fears of mortality and morbidity for civilians and soldiers in the 'White Man's Grave', and by anxieties that tropical environments would lead to the hereditary degeneration of more long-term colonial settlers.[53] The classic early twentieth-century restatement of this belief came from Joseph Barcroft (1872–1947), the British chemist and physiologist who researched extensively into respiration, circulation and altitude. In his seminal 1925 book, *The Respiratory Function of the Blood*, he suggested that '[a]ll dwellers at high altitude are persons of impaired physical and mental powers'.[54]

In context, this statement anticipated demonstrations of the rightshifted curve of oxygen affiliation – that is, the situation described above where animals, including humans, adapt to altitude by forcing their haemoglobin to bind more strongly to oxygen – good at the lung, but potentially disastrous at the extremities. More generally it was a statement about acclimatisation and adaptation: homeostatic responses of the body sometimes come at a price, especially at the extremes of adaptation. It was read, however, by the Peruvian physiologist, Carlos Monge Medrano (1884–1970), as a specific and racialised insult against midaltitude populations – mostly those of South America. Barcroft's work drew on his 1921 expedition to Cerro de Pasco in Peru, a mining town that, at 4300 m above sea level, was thought at the time to be the highest permanent human settlement.[55] So, in the following decade, Monge Medrano arranged a rival expedition to study the exercise capacity of such high-altitude residents to specifically rebuff Barcroft's insistence that residents at altitude were 'impaired' – indeed, Monge Medrano suggested that the eminent scientist must himself have been befuddled by altitude sickness to have made such a mistake of interpretation.[56]

As the director of the Instituto de Biología y Patología Andina, Monge Medrano instituted a concerted programme of research into altitude physiology, which included collaborations across national boundaries; South America became a powerhouse of research into this area, in part due to its ability to provide convenient field sites, but also because of local scientific and biomedical expertise.[57] Monge Medrano himself contributed to new understandings of mountain sickness and adaptation, and later in his career developed a much broader interpretation of the consequences of altitude physiology, one which attempted to write what we would now term an environmentally determinist account of South American history. He wrote about what he called 'climatic aggression', which was the damage done on the one hand to people who failed to adapt to new environments and, on the other, to those who were perfectly adapted but then uprooted from their 'natural' homes.[58] This theory has obvious resonances with earlier nineteenth-century fears about white racial degeneration in the tropics, and with late nineteenth- and twentieth-century concerns about the potential 'extinction' of indigenous people, expedited by their removal from native lands as well as by the interference of Western civilisation – from alcohol to fatty foods and tuberculosis.

There was, however, a significant contextual difference between Monge Medrano's 'climatic aggression' and the degeneracy fears of colonial late Victorians, because ideas of the *natural* human body, in terms of adaptation and origin, had moved from the temperate zone to the tropics. This is of course also echoed in broader research into stress, neurasthenia and other related disorders, which increasingly from the end of the nineteenth century highlighted the conditions of modern life – overcrowding, mechanical work, 'unnatural' life rhythms – as a cause of sickness and decline.[59] As work elsewhere in this volume shows – particularly Chapter 4 on anti-obesity campaigns, Chapter 3 on 'problem' drinking and Chapter 10 on the renegotiation of 'normal' in the treatment of Parkinson's Disease – public health programmes in Western countries increasingly framed challenges to human health as the products of 'civilization'. What extreme physiology shows us is that the same assumptions were built into our study of even the most basic environmental difficulties people faced: heat, cold and altitude. Therefore, while the white body had, in 1880, been perfectly adapted to the temperate zone and therefore at risk in the tropics, in the mid-twentieth century the naked (thus 'natural') primitive human form was considered to be perfectly organised for survival in hot and humid climates. Logically, then, our ability to survive outside the temperate zone was a matter of *technology*, not *biology*; we wore clothes, built shelters, mined coal to keep ourselves warm (processes which then, as forms of civilisation, placed new pressures on our physical and mental health). The origins of this shift from the temperate zone to the tropics are too complex to be detailed here, but came from multiple sources from around 1880 to the middle of the twentieth century: anthropologists and archaeologists reconsidered the path of human origins; race scientists and geneticists reconsidered the relationships between ethnic groups, and the age of the human race; physiologists actively studied a range of different ethnic groups and their responses to cold, heat, deprivation and disease.[60]

This shift in understanding of the normal *natural* human body had significant consequences for physiological research into homeostasis and balance. First, it maintained a racial hierarchy, despite disrupting the centrality of the temperate zone; as adaptations to heat and altitude were biological, they were primitive, while adaptations to cold (which included the whole temperate zone, if we assume that the tropics were the 'normal' site for human life) were technological, innovative, inventive and civilising.[61] Or, to put it another way, studying adaptations to heat or altitude was physiology; studying adaptations to cold was bioprospecting for technology. This presumption was confirmed by early studies into cold adaptation, which proved difficult, contradictory and inconclusive through the 1930s and 1940s, and which by the 1950s seemed to be creating a consensus that most people did not significantly *biologically* adapt to cold (that is, they do not have as strong a physiological defence mechanism for cold climates as they do for increasing altitude or heat), with the possible exception of local adaptations in the bodily peripheries: hands, feet and face.[62]

The move away from studies of cold adaptation is most obvious in large-scale projects. As an example, the International Biological Programme, which was founded in 1964 (in emulation of the International

Geophysical Year), included from the start a 'Human Adaptability' theme. But among this research, studies of cold adaptation were a minority, and physiologists of the Poles instead turned their attention to issues of daylight and isolation – circadian rhythms, sleep and the psychology of exploration.[63] Indeed, at the first International Symposium on Polar Human Biology in 1972, attendees did not even mention the only large physiological expedition to the Antarctic – the INternational PHysiological EXpedition to ANtarctica (INPHEXAN) in 1957–58.[64] INPHEXAN was an Anglo-American expedition, timed to coincide with both the International Geophysical Year and the late stages of (Sir) Edmund Hillary (1919–2008) and (Sir) Vivian Fuchs's (1908–99) attempt to cross Antarctica as part of the Commonwealth Trans-Antarctic Expedition. Dr Lewis Griffith Cresswell Evans Pugh (1909–94), the physiologist in part responsible for the British success on Everest in 1953, was the lead British researcher and, as outlined above, the team conducted very varied work into cold adaptation, metabolism, cold injury and stress.[65] By the time of the next physiological expedition to Antarctica – a full twenty years later in 1977–78 – the focus had clearly shifted; the 1970s International Biomedical Expedition to the Antarctic did consider adaptation to cold, but only as part of a psychological as well as physiological analysis.[66] Consequently, the Arctic and Antarctic were figured as useful 'natural laboratories' to study 'freak' phenomena such as human responses to 24-hour daylight; the question of human adaptation to cold was, by the 1970s, no longer a pressing *physiological* research issue.

The 'rebalancing' of the 'natural' human environment to a tropical, rather than temperate, base meant that the inhabitants of warmer countries remained a focus of *both* physiological and anthropological fascination. Studies through the middle of the twentieth century still used terms such as 'primitive' to describe the indigenous people of the tropics, and their study was racially coded, as they were used (and are still used) as 'proxies' for earlier stages of human adaptation. Studies of homeostasis, of the natural balance of the human body, were marked by complicated webs of assumptions about racial science, indigenous rights and human evolution. So, for example, early twentieth-century studies of Australian Aboriginal peoples were shaped by concerns about 'White Australia'; while some thought Aboriginal people would be the victims of racial decline, and eventually 'die out', others wondered at their ability to survive harsh environments that decimated settler colonies. By the middle of the twentieth century, one of the most prominent researchers into environmental physiology was arguing that, while better adapted than the white populations, Aboriginal peoples showed adaptation to hot *humid* climates, not the hot *dry* climate of central Australia – evidence of a migration (the date of which was in great dispute) from the tropical islands of South East Asia.[67] This meant that both their physiology, and what were considered 'primitive' customs – such as organising societies around water sources – were in fact useful lessons for Europeans also trying to survive in the harsh Australian interior; this was an argument that proved difficult for physiologists, and politicians, to accept.[68]

Even in the later work of the International Biological Programme, adaptation physiology routinely used a methodology that compared tropical and subtropical indigenous populations to white incomers (such as 'white' and 'negro' sharecroppers and American soldiers, or Balan and Chaamba Arabs versus French servicemen).[69] While temperate and Arctic peoples were largely thought to have adapted to their environment using ingenuity and technology, those in tropical and subtropical areas were still depicted as surviving as a result of biology and superstitious, or at least irrational, custom. In this way, research into extreme physiology managed to maintain an imbalance – namely an established hierarchy of civilisations.

Making a 'balanced team': finding the right *men*

In addition to balance constituting a literal property of the human body, the term balance also carried metaphorical weight, providing ways of understanding the world and shaping the nature of research programmes and expeditionary teams. In particular, there were parallels between the ecosystem of the body and that of the research group. Expeditions in spaces such as Everest or the South Pole functioned with a fixed set of resources – whether it was rations, person hours or gasoline – and therefore all functions of the team were elements in a zero-sum game: resources spent on scientific work were not available to be spent on travel, exploration or survival. At every stage of planning and execution issues of balance were in question, from the design of ration boxes (more fat or more carbohydrates, or more calories at the expense of more weight) to the loading of aeroplanes and Sno-Cats.

When it came to the human component of an expedition, leaders, whether explorers or scientists, tended to use the term 'harmony' rather than 'homeostasis' or 'balance'. Here the concern is not only to maximise the skill sets available across the chosen group, but also to ensure that the team worked together efficiently in dangerous, isolated conditions. As with bodily homeostasis, it could be challenging to compensate for extreme changes in circumstances, such as the death or serious illness/disablement of a team member, which may lead to evacuation, premature ending of the expedition, or in the worst case scenarios further deaths. For 'milder' disturbances, leaders hoped that their choice of team members would be able to compensate for temporary absences from work or other unexpected disruptions. While it was theoretically easy to ensure balance of skills on paper, ensuring *harmony* in terms of interpersonal relationships proved to be a much greater challenge.

In the first half of the twentieth century, and in many cases well into the 1970s and 1980s, the major technique for picking reliable expedition members was to rely on experience. Above all other factors, personal experience of a potential recruit by the expedition leader or a trusted colleague appears to have been crucial to their engagement on an expedition. This could even outweigh specific experience of the environment in question; for example, successful participation in high-altitude mountaineering could be taken as evidence of suitability for an Antarctic expedition. Attempts were made from the mid-1960s to put this experiential practice on a more empirical footing by studying the psychological factors that correlated with successful overwintering and teamwork, and resilience in the face of environmental challenges and isolation.[70] But, echoing the experience of attempts to create 'scientific' and objective personnel selection tests in the military, psychological questionnaires, physiological stress tests and other interventions functioned either as an adjunct to, or a refinement of, the more informal and 'gut instinct' processes of selection and role allocation on expeditions throughout the twentieth century.[71]

As a consequence, extreme physiology – at least in the Anglophone world – tended to be a closed shop, based around cliques, either those

Balance at the limits of human performance 239

centred on individuals (such as Edmund Hillary) or organisations (such as the Royal Geographical Society). This process undoubtedly created well-bonded and successful expeditionary teams; but it also reduced the diversity of such work, and in particular acted as yet another barrier to female participation. Women routinely applied to be parts of such expeditions. In 1935, Kathleen M. Taylor (then living in Nanking, China) wrote to ask to be included in the British expedition to Everest. As evidence of her capability she claimed two solo ascents of Mount Fuji ('It is a very easy mountain, but you start at sea level, and do the whole 13,000 ft. in one night'), and many other climbs with a pack weighing 'not less than 20lbs'. The response letter said she had applied too late to be considered.[72] In 1957, a female geologist, Dawn Rodley, succeeded in persuading not only her male expedition colleagues, but also their wives, that she would be a good colleague. Unfortunately the US Navy refused to transport her to Antarctica; as a site of military activity, Antarctica was forbidden to women from 1956, until the US Congress removed its ban in 1969.[73]

While there were no laws banning women from British bases, Fuchs, head of the British Antarctic Survey from 1959 to 1973, emphatically opposed female participation on the grounds that they would disrupt the 'harmony' of Antarctic stations.[74] Here, 'balance' and 'harmony' were key; routinely throughout the twentieth century women were figured as a disruptive influence – even their letters from home, let alone their physical presence, could bring unwanted emotional stress to a closed homosocial homeostatic universe. There is an irony here that the desire for 'balance' (or 'harmony') results in extremely *un*balanced research teams – and, consequently, extremely disrupted patterns of physiological research. Almost all physiology practised in Antarctica or Everest – and other extreme environments – was self-experiment and 'citizen science', with the bodies of the explorers themselves functioning as human subjects. By excluding women from this practice, not only were they unable to gain the 'experience' that was so crucial to future inclusion in expeditionary teams, but the bodies of women were systematically ignored in research projects. This imbalance fed back into laboratory studies; even though these occurred in 'safe' sea-level locations, women were not a focus of serious interest until the 1970s, when some early studies seemed to suggest women actually adapted more efficiently to altitude than men.[75]

This is not to say that women were not involved in research into extreme physiology. As I have shown elsewhere, they have participated in extreme physiology, but often in unacknowledged roles. Indeed, it was not until a female 'computer' was hired that a major part of the INPHEXAN data could be analysed, showing the lack of adaptation to cold.[76] And, of course, none of the European trips to the high Himalaya could have been undertaken without women; among the thousands of porters hired to carry vital survival gear, food and scientific equipment were many Sherpani. Their double invisibility – not only women, but non-white women – is a stark illustration that our histories of expeditionary science remain unbalanced.

Conclusion: balancing *which* 'self'?

Through the first two-thirds of the twentieth century – perhaps until the International Biological Programme began significantly reshaping research practices – biomedical experimentation in extreme environments was frequently experiment, literally and metaphorically, on the *self*; it was conducted by white Western men, on the bodies of white Western men – often their own bodies. Physiologists and expedition doctors took samples of their own blood and breath, encouraged their children and laboratory assistants into pressure chambers and onto treadmills, and recruited colleagues and co-explorers into experimental studies of the effects of cold, heat, fatigue and low oxygen pressure.[77] While this use of the self and of close colleagues as experimental organisms might seem a rational response to spaces like Antarctica where the potential experimental population is small, or to those like Everest where access is expensive and limited, there was obviously also extensive use of self- and colleague experimentation in temperate zone laboratory studies – for example, at the Harvard Fatigue Laboratory, or earlier studies of gas poisoning by J. S. Haldane on his son J. B. S. Haldane.[78] This chapter can only gesture to the possibility that such 'heroic' self-experimentation, whether on a treadmill or a glacier, might be related to notions of the self that connect scientific experimentation with exploration, with ideas of robust masculinity, science as conquest over feminine nature and the value of personal testimony and experience in generating truth about a complicated natural world.[79] What it has more extensively laid out is how those practices reinforced, if not necessarily created, a normalised, homeostatic, balanced (sea-level and temperate) white adult male body, which was read as the standard – the ideal – from which others deviated. While this is not a novel argument for histories of medicine, what is apparent is how broadly the notion of balance could be applied, and how extraordinarily self-reinforcing it was – to stretch the metaphor, it is itself a homeostatic mechanism, which prioritised certain kinds of self, and created practices and assumptions that functionally excluded other kinds of bodies, and even personalities, from the creation and application of standards. When other selves were included, such as the use of Sherpa guides to test amphetamines or of Inuit peoples to study physiological adaptation using radioactive tracers, their inclusion was often on an unequal, and sometimes exploitative basis.[80] Women's bodies, identified as disruptive or inadequate to the task, were simply not studied; at the same time as adaptational physiology asserted the difference of women, it failed to recognise this difference as a potential source of research findings.

The balanced self in an extreme earthly environment possesses a set of moral and behavioural characteristics, as well as a specific, scientifically defined, body. The ability to respond to environmental stressors is a question not only of metabolism, body chemistry and inherited capacity, but also personality: team spirit and self-reflection are necessary for a climber or explorer to recognise, for example, when they are overtired or suffering from anoxic mental fog and beginning to pose a risk to their team; sportsmanship and honesty are necessary to know when it is and is not acceptable to use a technological or pharmacological supplement to aid a sporting goal; stoicism and a strong stomach are necessary for an explorer to eat sufficient calories for survival, even when that is presented as unpalatable blocks of pemmican or hard biscuit. These practices are gendered and racialised in such ways that it is not always possible for all 'selves' to successfully engage in them.[81] They also highlight the ways in which responsibility for self-balance could be divided between teams, leaders and individuals: explorers were expected to demonstrate self-awareness, to spot fatigue or hunger before they could cause problems; to judge whether illness or injury were serious or not; to act in prompt, preventative ways to situations such as mild frostbite or anoxia. And, again, the belief that this sort of self-responsibility and self-regulation was a particular property of the white male was part of the justification for excluding other people – particularly women – from expeditionary teams. It was also sometimes an excuse for using manipulative or misleading approaches to try to get non-white participants to 'volunteer' for studies: writing as late as the 1970s, one researcher examining adaptation and physiology among Inuit people complained of the challenge of using even standard exercise tests as 'there are difficulties in motivating primitive and non-competitive people to perform an all-out effort' – while the sporting, competitive, *civilised* white man offered no such challenge to scientific experiment.[82]

Despite their exotic nature, then, extreme environments emerge from this account as prime 'natural laboratories' for the study of human balance – mental and physical. In part, this is because of the strong military interest in topics of cold and low-oxygen survival, which has provided funding and – when self-experiment was not sufficient – human guinea pigs for studies of adaptation and acclimatisation. Relatedly, it is also in part to do with issues of consent and performance – it is 'nature' that is causing the real physical risk and discomfort, not the scientists, which has appeared to allow experimentation that might not otherwise find volunteers or ethical clearance. But the Arctic, Antarctic and sites at high altitude have also been able to function as spaces to explore all kinds of balance. It is no coincidence that the focus of adaptational studies shifted over the mid-twentieth century away from physiological adjustments to cold, and towards more psychosocial aspects such as circadian rhythm studies, isolation and depression; this reflects a more general direction in human physiological, psychological and stress research, which increasingly took seriously the 'pressures of civilization' – shift work, jet lag, overcrowding, overstimulation – as sources of disruption in the *milieu extérieur*. Hard physical labour, lack of daylight and cramped, impoverished living conditions could be the lot of the low-paid shift worker in Detroit, or the mechanic doing a rotation at an Antarctic base.[83] Extreme environments prove to be useful for the historian of science, just as they have been for the scientist, because they were spaces in which all the pressures on the human being – both wild and civilised – could be studied.

Notes

1 University of Adelaide special collections, W. V. Macfarlane Papers 1947–1985 (MS0006). See, for example, F12/2 containing multiple letters relating to the animal and human physiologist Macfarlane's research on

the history of homeostasis, and further papers on the development of his manuscript 'Homeostasis: machinery for living free'.
2 V. Heggie, 'Blood, race and indigenous peoples in twentieth century extreme physiology', *Studies in the History and Philosophy of the Life Sciences*, 41 (2019), doi: 10.1007/s40656-019-0264-z.
3 E. Kern, *Out of Asia: A History of the Global Search for the Origins of Humankind* (forthcoming).
4 V. Heggie, *Higher and Colder: A History of Extreme Physiology and Exploration* (Chicago: Chicago University Press, 2019).
5 M. Jackson, *The Age of Stress: Science and the Search for Stability* (Oxford: Oxford University Press, 2013), p. 145, my emphasis.
6 For a broader take on stress as one of many 'diseases of civilization', see C. E. Rosenberg, 'Pathologies of progress: the idea of civilization as risk', *Bulletin of the History of Medicine*, 72 (1998), 714–30.
7 Jackson, *The Age of Stress*, p. 18. See also the explicit formulation of 'acclimatization versus tolerance' in the extensive mid-century bibliography put together for the US Air Force in the context of space flight and aviation research: J. T. Celentano, H. B. Kelly Jr and W. L. Lilley, *Acclimatization Versus Tolerance to Stress: An Annotated Bibliography*, report no: SAM-TR-67-95-VOL. I and VOL. II (Texas: USAF School of Aerospace Medicine, September 1967).
8 M. F. Wisemann, 'Unlocking the "Eskimo secret": defence science in the Cold War Canadian Arctic, 1947–1954', *Journal of the Canadian Historical Association*, 26 (2015), 191–223.
9 Heggie, *Higher and Colder*.
10 V. Heggie, 'Higher and colder: the success and failure of boundaries in high altitude and Antarctic research stations', *Social Studies of Science*, 46 (2016), 809–32.
11 R. E. Kohler, 'Labscapes: naturalizing the lab', *History of Science*, 40 (2002), 473–501; R. E. Kohler, *Landscapes and Labscapes: Exploring the Lab–Field Border in Biology* (Chicago: University of Chicago Press, 2002); H. Kuklick and R. E. Kohler, 'Science in the field: introduction', *Osiris*, 11 (1996), 1–14.
12 V. Heggie, '"Only the British appear to be making a fuss"; the science of success and the myth of amateurism at the Mexico Olympiad, 1968', *Sport in History*, 28 (2008), 213–35.
13 This continued well into the twentieth century: on 'reality testing' see P. W. Clements, *Science in an Extreme Environment: The 1963 American Mount Everest Expedition* (Pittsburgh, PA: University of Pittsburgh Press, 2018).
14 W. Coleman, 'The cognitive basis of the discipline: Claude Bernard on physiology', *Isis*, 76 (1985), 49–70.

15 W. Rostène, 'Paul Bert: homme de science, homme politique', *Journal de la Société de Biologie*, 22 (2006), 245–50.
16 Jackson, *The Age of Stress*, p. 65.
17 J. M. Leigh, 'The evolution of oxygen therapy apparatus', *Anaesthesia*, 29 (1974), 462–85, at p. 465.
18 For this and other examples of the uselessness of oxygen, see Chapter XIII in A. Mosso, *Life of Man on the High Alps*, trans. E. Lough Kiesow, 2nd edition (London: Taylor Unwin, 1898).
19 P. Felsch, *Laborlandschaften: Physiologische Alpenreisen Im 19. Jahrhundert*, Wissenschaftsgeschichte (Göttingen: Wallstein, 2007).
20 A. Cogo et al., 'Italian high-altitude laboratories: past and present', *High Altitude Medicine & Biology*, 1 (2004), 137–47.
21 J. B. West, *High Life: A History of High-Altitude Physiology and Medicine* (New York: Published for the American Physiological Society by Oxford University Press, 1998) – see in particular chapter two, which ends with a subsection titled 'Paul Bert: the father of modern high-altitude physiology and medicine', p. 62.
22 Pace claims by G. E. Fogg, *A History of Antarctic Science* (Cambridge: Cambridge University Press, 1992), p. 377, that little systematic physiology was done in the Antarctic, see V. Heggie, 'Why isn't exploration a science?', *Isis*, 105 (2014), 318–24; H. R. Guly, 'Bacteriology during the expeditions of the heroic age of Antarctic exploration', *Polar Record*, 49 (October 2013), 321–7; H. R. Guly, 'Human biology investigations during the heroic age of Antarctic exploration (1897–1922)', *Polar Record*, 50 (April 2014), 183–91. Arctic research is much better represented in the historiography – for example M. Farish, 'The lab and the land: overcoming the Arctic in Cold War Alaska', *Isis*, 104 (2013), 1–29.
23 E. Aronova, K. S. Baker and N. Oreskes, 'Big science and big data in biology: from the International Geophysical Year through the International Biological Program to the Long Term Ecological Research (LTER) Network, 1957–present', *Historical Studies in the Natural Sciences*, 4 (2010), 183–224.
24 M. Jackson, 'Men and women under stress: neuropsychiatric models of resilience during and after the Second World War', in M. Jackson (ed.), *Stress in Post-War Britain, 1945–85* (London: Pickering and Chatto, 2015), pp. 111–30.
25 Mandeville Special Collections, University of California San Diego [hereafter UCSD] West archive, MSS 444, Box 79, folder 11, AMREE Newsletter.
26 H. Williams and H. D. Arnold, 'The effects of violent and prolonged muscular exercise upon the heart', *Transactions of the American Clinical and Climatological Association*, 15 (1899), 267–85; H. Williams and H. D. Arnold,

'The effects of violent and prolonged muscular exercise upon the heart', *The Philadelphia Medical Journal*, 3 (1899), 1233–9.
27 A. V. Hill, *Muscular Movement in Man: The Factors Governing Speed and Recovery from Fatigue* (New York and London: McGraw-Hill, 1927), p. 3.
28 Anon., 'Polar medicine', *Lancet*, 274 (7 November 1959), 786–7, at p. 787.
29 The first all-women climbing teams in the Himalaya went out in the late 1950s; for Antarctica, see below.
30 With the exception of some Inuit women who were enrolled onto physiological and other biomedical trials – although even here, as some of the research was kept confidential or secret, the extent of their participation is uncertain. See Farish, 'The lab and the land'.
31 J. Rhee and T. Erickson, 'Erythropoietin stimulation and other blood doping methods', in D. G. Barceloux (ed.), *Medical Toxicology of Drug Abuse: Synthesized Chemicals and Psychoactive Plants* (Hoboken, NJ: Wiley, 2012), pp. 306–25.
32 J. S. Windsor and G. W. Rodway, 'Heights and haematology: the story of haemoglobin at altitude', *Postgraduate Medical Journal*, 83 (2007), 148–51, at p. 149.
33 UCSD: MSS 491 Pugh Papers. Box 39, Folder 1, Letter Pugh to JS Horn 14th July 1953.
34 Ulrich Luft, 'Die Höhenpassung', *Ergbnisse der Physiologie, biologischen Hemie und experimenteilen Pharmakologie*, 44 (1941), 256–314; H. Hartmann, G. Hepp and U. C. Luft, 'Physiologische Beobachtungen am Nanga Parbat 1937/1938', *Luftfahrtmedizin*, 6 (1942), 1–44.
35 G. W. Rodway, 'Ulrich C. Luft and physiology on Nanga Parbat: the winds of war', *High Altitude Medicine & Biology*, 10 (2009), 89–96.
36 Various, 'The disaster on Nanga Parbat, 1937', *Alpine Journal*, 49 (November 1937), 210–27.
37 L. Shaw Cobden, 'The nervous flyer: nerves, flying and the First World War', *British Journal for Military History*, 4 (2019), 121–42.
38 V. Heggie, 'Experimental physiology, Everest and oxygen: from the ghastly kitchens to the gasping lung', *British Journal for the History of Science*, 46 (2013), 123–47. See also Chapter 7.
39 Rodway, 'Ulrich C. Luft'.
40 A. Jacobson, *Operation Paperclip: The Secret Intelligence Program that Brought Nazi Scientists to America* (Boston: Little, Brown, 2014).
41 P. Weindling (ed.), *From Clinic to Concentration Camp* (London: Routledge, 2017); on the range and numbers of experimental abuses, see P. Weindling, A. von Villez, A. Loewenau and N. Farron, 'The victims of unethical human experiments and coerced research under National Socialism', *Endeavour*, 40 (March 2016), 1–6.

42 H. Hoebusch, 'Ascent into darkness: German Himalaya expeditions and the National Socialist quest for high-altitude flight', *International Journal of the History of Sport*, 24 (2007), 520–40.
43 S. B. Ortner, *Life and Death on Mt Everest: Sherpas and Himalayan Mountaineering* (Princeton, NJ: Princeton University Press, 1999).
44 D. H. Robinson, *The Dangerous Sky: A History of Aviation Medicine* (Seattle: University of Washington Press, 1973), p. 187.
45 W. Noyce, *South Col: One Man's Adventure on the Ascent of Everest* (London: Reprint Society, 1955), p. 198.
46 H. Guly, 'Use and abuse of alcohol and other drugs during the heroic age of Antarctic exploration', *History of Psychiatry*, 24 (2013), 94–105; J. C. Anthony, *Hoosh: Roast Penguin, Scurvy Day, and Other Stories of Antarctic Cuisine* (Lincoln, NE: University of Nebraska Press, 2012), p. 9.
47 Royal Geographical Society, London [hereafter RGS] RGS/EP/EE/22/1/8 Baldrey to Colonel Bruce, 22 Nov. 1923.
48 At least one member of the 1953 team expressed the opposite opinion – that he felt his tube of Benzedrine was somehow 'cheating', but recognised this was irrational since he did not feel the same way about oxygen. Noyce, *South Col*, p. 197.
49 Heggie, 'Experimental physiology, Everest and oxygen'.
50 Infamously, the US Olympic cycling team admitted to transfusions of blood to 'blood dope' in the 1980s: Anon., 'Editorial: sports medicine – is there lack of control?', *Lancet*, 332 (10 September 1988), 612.
51 UCSD: West Papers, Box 81, folder 6, Letter West to AMREE team, 17 Nov. 1980.
52 H. Chiodi, 'Respiratory adaptations to chronic high altitude hypoxia', *Journal of Applied Physiology*, 10 (1957), 81–7; F. Kreuzer and Z. Turek, 'Influence of the position of the oxygen dissociation curve on the oxygen supply to tissues', in W. Brendel and R. A. Zink (eds), *High Altitude Physiology and Medicine* (New York: Springer-Verlag, 1982), pp. 66–72.
53 This sense of anxiety and displacement lasted into the twentieth century: see P. D. Curtin, '"The white man's grave" image and reality, 1780–1850', *The Journal of British Studies*, 1 (1961), 94–110, at p. 94; and M. Harrison, *Climates and Constitutions: Health, Race, Environment and British Imperialism in India, 1600–1850* (Delhi and Oxford: Oxford University Press, 1999), esp. pp. 102–8.
54 J. Barcroft, *The Respiratory Function of the Blood, Part I: Lessons from High Altitudes* (Cambridge: Cambridge University Press, 1925), p. 176.
55 J. Barcroft, C. A. Binger, A. V. Bock, J. H. Doggart, H. S. Forbes, G. Harrop, J. C. Meakins et al., 'Observations upon the effect of high altitude on the

physiological processes of the human body, carried out in the Peruvian Andes, chiefly at Cerro de Pasco', *Philosophical Transactions of the Royal Society of London. Series B, Containing Papers of a Biological Character*, 211 (1 January 1923), 351–480; J. Barcroft, 'Recent expedition to the Andes for the study of the physiology of high altitudes (BAAS Section of Physiology)', *Lancet*, 200 (23 September 1922), 685–6.
56 C. Monge Medrano, *Acclimatization in the Andes* (Baltimore: Johns Hopkins Press, 1948), p. xiii.
57 S. Tracey, 'The physiology of extremes: Ancel Keys and the international high altitude expedition of 1935', *Bulletin of the History of Medicine*, 86 (2012), 627–60.
58 Monge Medrano, *Acclimatization in the Andes*.
59 R. Porter, 'Diseases of civilization', in W. F. Bynum and R. Porter (eds), *Companion Encyclopaedia of the History of Medicine* (London: Routledge, 1993), pp. 585–600.
60 Heggie, *Higher and Colder*.
61 M. Adas, *Machines as the Measure of Man* (Ithaca, NY: Cornell University Press, 2015).
62 This hierarchy of cold to warm did not mean that Inuit peoples were considered racial or cultural equals by the white and Western explorers or scientists who worked among them. The use of their technology by late nineteenth- and early twentieth-century explorers, and their role in military studies of adaptation (including potentially harmful radiation experiments) demonstrates a deeply ambivalent, and sometimes exploitative relationship. See Heggie, *Higher and Colder*; Farish, 'The lab and the land'; S. Pickman, 'Dress, image, and cultural encounter in the heroic age of polar exploration', in P. Mears (ed.), *Expedition: Fashion from the Extreme* (New York: Thames & Hudson, 2017), pp. 31–56. See also Wisemann, 'Unlocking the "Eskimo secret"'.
63 These interests – in fatigue, sleep patterns and the psychology of workers in extreme conditions – are of course reflected in other situations, most obviously in the research that fed into regulations controlling flight crew's working hours – see Chapter 7.
64 Held in Cambridge, England and co-sponsored by the Scientific Committee on Antarctic Research (SCAR), the International Union of Physiological Sciences (IUPS) and the International Union of Biological Sciences (IUBS). O. Edholm (ed.), *Polar Human Biology* (London: William Heinemann Medical Books, 1973).
65 Bancroft Library, University of California Berkeley. Smith Hughes, Sally. 'Interview Transcript: Will Siri', 1980; UCSD: Pugh papers, Box 39, Folder 10, Antarctic Studies Programme.

66 I. A. McCormick, A. J. W. Taylor, J. Rivolier and G. Cazes, 'A psychometric study of stress and coping during the International Biomedical Expedition to the Antarctic (IBEA)', *Journal of Human Stress*, 11 (December 1985), 150–6; A. J. W. Taylor and I. A. McCormick, 'Prediction of performance on the International Biomedical Expedition to the Antarctic (IBEA)', *Polar Record*, 22 (1985), 643–52; A. J. W. Taylor and I. A. McCormick, 'Human experimentation during the International Biomedical Expedition to the Antarctic (IBEA)', *Journal of Human Stress*, 11 (December 1985), 161–4.
67 University of Adelaide special collections, W. V. Macfarlane Papers 1947–1985 (MS0006). WV Macfarlane, 'Water, Salt and Food for Tropical Medicine', n.d.
68 Such use of the colonial and post-colonial 'other' as a subject is echoed in research into chronic diseases too: see M. Moore, 'Harnessing the power of difference: colonialism and British chronic disease research, 1940–1975', *Social History of Medicine*, 29 (May 2016), 384–404.
69 For a survey of this work, see R. H. Fox, G. M. Budd, P. M. Woodward, A. J. Hackett and A. L. Hendrie, 'A study of temperature regulation in New Guinea people', *Philosophical Transactions of the Royal Society of London B: Biological Sciences*, 268 (1974), 375–91.
70 Psychological screening and 'attitude testing' was part of the selection process for Antarctic personnel from 1963, although at first this meant adaptations of standard military psychological profiling: E. K. Gunderson, 'Psychological studies in Antarctica', in E. K. Gunderson (ed.), *Human Adaptability to Antarctic Conditions*, Antarctic Research Series, vol. 22 (Washington: American Geophysical Union, 1974), pp. 115–31; McCormick et al., 'A psychometric study of stress'. See also the psychological studies conducted as part of the 1963 American Mount Everest Expedition: Clements, *Science in an Extreme Environment*.
71 Jackson, 'Men and women under stress'.
72 RGS: Box 53, Letter Taylor to RGS, 28 Dec. 1935.
73 This despite the fact that two American women – Jackie Ronne and Jennie Darlington – were probably the first to spend an entire year in Antarctica, when they accompanied their husbands in the late 1940s. E. Chipman, *Women on the Ice* (Melbourne: Melbourne University Press, 1986); C. Bull, 'Behind the scenes: Colin Bull recalls his 10-year quest to send women researchers to Antarctica', *The Antarctic Sun*, 13 November 2009, available at https://antarcticsun.usap.gov/features/contentHandler.cfm?id=1955, accessed June 2017. See also: the interview with Colin Bull by Brian Shoemaker as part of the Polar Oral History Programme (2007), available at http://hdl.handle.net/1811/28580, accessed July 2017; M. Seag, 'Women

need not apply: gendered institutional change in Antarctica and outer space', *The Polar Journal*, 7 (2017), 319–35.
74 F. Aston, 'Women of the White Continent', *Geographical*, 77 (September 2005), no pp.
75 J. A. Wagner et al., 'Maximal work capacity of women during acute hypoxia', *Journal of Applied Physiology*, 47 (1 December 1979), 1223–7.
76 Heggie, *Higher and Colder*.
77 For much more on the enclosed experimental world of extreme physiology see: ibid.
78 L. K. Altman, *Who Goes First? The Story of Self-Experimentation in Medicine* (Berkeley: University of California Press, 1986), p. 225.
79 B. Hevly, 'The heroic science of glacier motion', *Osiris*, 11 (1996), 66–86; M. Dettelbach, 'The stimulations of travel: Humboldt's physiological construction of the tropics', in F. Driver (ed.), *Tropical Visions in an Age of Empire* (Chicago: University of Chicago Press, 2005), pp. 42–58; Altman, *Who Goes First?*
80 Farish, 'The lab and the land'.
81 Jackson, 'Men and women under stress'.
82 R. J. Shephard, 'Work physiology and activity patterns of circumpolar Eskimos and Ainu: A synthesis of IBP data', *Human Biology*, 46 (1974), 263–94.
83 R. W. Scheffler, 'The fate of a progressive science: the Harvard Fatigue Laboratory, athletes, the science of work and the politics of reform', *Endeavour*, 35 (2011), 48–54.

9

Self-help, marriage guidance and the making of the midlife crisis

Mark Jackson

Introduction

In 1965, the Canadian-born psychoanalyst and social scientist Elliott Jaques introduced a term – the midlife crisis – that continues to structure Western experiences and expressions of love and loss in middle age. Jaques's early work, carried out at the Tavistock Institute of Human Relations during the 1940s and 1950s, had focused primarily on the ways in which social systems operated as forms of 'defense against persecutory and depressive anxiety' among their members, as well as a mechanism for protecting the integrity of the system itself.[1] During the following decades, Jaques became an influential figure in studies of bureaucracy, managerial accountability and leadership, as well as human capacity, work and social justice, introducing terms such as 'corporate culture' and 'requisite organisation' into discussions of occupational hierarchies and working practices. Jaques's contributions bridged a number of academic domains – including sociology, psychology, economics and applied research – but his theories of the interrelations between individual, institutional and social behaviour were connected through his preoccupations with time, creativity and trust.[2]

Although Jaques's sociological and psychological writings were plainly patterned by his empirical studies of organisations such as factories, churches and health services, they were also affected by his training and practice as a psychoanalyst and by the theories of Sigmund Freud, Melanie Klein and Wilfred Bion. These influences are particularly evident in his formulation of the midlife crisis. Jaques had begun to think about the concept in 1952 – at the age of 35 – during a period of personal reflection on the challenges of midlife. When he first presented the paper to the British Psychoanalytical Society in 1957 it generated only a muted response, and it was not published in the *International Journal of Psycho-Analysis* until eight years later.[3] In the article, Jaques argued that during the middle years of life growing awareness of personal death precipitated a depressive crisis, masked by a manic determination to thwart advancing age:

> The compulsive attempts, in many men and women reaching middle age, to remain young, the hypochondriacal concern over health and appearance, the emergence of sexual promiscuity in order to prove youth and potency, the hollowness and lack of genuine enjoyment of life, and the frequency of religious concern, are familiar patterns. They are attempts at a race against time.[4]

Jaques's formulation of the midlife crisis emerged primarily from studying what he referred to as 'a random sample' of over 300 'creative artists' – such as Mozart, Raphael, Rossini, Bach and Shakespeare – who had either died in their mid- to late thirties or whose work had changed radically in volume or mode of expression during that period of their lives.[5] Stimulated by contemporary interest in the physical, psychological and spiritual dimensions of ageing and death – evident in the emergence of geriatrics as a medical speciality on both sides of the Atlantic and in the proliferation of self-help guides to retaining the vitality of youth – biographical and autobiographical studies of 'the curve of life' were not unusual in the mid-twentieth century.[6] In the 1920s, the American psychologist Granville Stanley Hall – renowned for his studies of both adolescence and old age – had substantiated his theory of a 'dangerous age' by recounting the emotional disturbances evident in the lives of middle-aged men as they faced the 'bankruptcy of some of their youthful hopes'.[7] Indeed, in a series of mini case studies that prefigured Jaques's approach, Hall referred directly to 'the middle-age crisis' experienced by Nietzsche in his thirties.[8] Similarly, Jung's central concept of individuation (or integration of the self), with its emphasis on development across the second half of life, was assembled by juxtaposing case histories, notions of an archetypal life course and reflections on his own midlife struggles to balance conflicting facets of his personality.[9] What Jaques added to these earlier, largely descriptive accounts was a psychoanalytical framework that provided a basis for not only explaining, but also mitigating, the 'emotional impoverishment' and psychological imbalance that appeared to be characteristic of midlife crises.[10]

According to Jaques's wife and co-researcher, Kathryn Cason, it took twenty-five years for her husband's 'work on midlife crisis to be accepted'.[11] Although there is some, admittedly rather raw, evidence to support Cason's view that usage of the term only reached a peak in the 1990s,[12] it is nevertheless clear that Jaques's model of midlife as a tipping point in the life course soon captured the attention of psychologists, sociologists, self-help authors and journalists. From the late 1960s, it began to guide clinical approaches to understanding and resolving what became known as the 'search for meaning' that was thought to typify the midlife identity crisis.[13] It also became a notable motif in the work of American researchers, who were developing a variety of ethnographic and survey techniques to evaluate the impact of life transitions on personal identity, health and well-being.[14] The sense of inevitable crisis and decline that Jaques's concept was thought to carry was often contested, however, particularly by feminist authors who were keen to invert the negative connotations of the midlife crisis and focus instead on the potential for growth and self-fulfilment in women after midlife.[15] In Britain, the perceived impact of midlife crises on marriage shaped efforts to address the personal, familial and social consequences of rising levels of divorce,[16] and inflected the psychoanalytical approaches to resolving marital tensions adopted by Henry V. Dicks and his colleagues at the Tavistock Clinic in London.[17] The notion of crisis carried wider resonance as a tool for articulating the anguish of ageing. Jaques's depiction of the 'defensive fantasies', embraced by middle-aged men in particular, to forestall the effects of growing old, figured strongly in post-war literary and cinematic treatments of love and loss around midlife.[18] In the novels of John Updike, Sloan Wilson, Simone de Beauvoir and Joseph Heller, or in Ingmar Bergman's film *Scenes from a Marriage*, the emotional turbulence of middle age provided the plot line for explorations of the interrelations between personal, marital and social crises.[19]

There have been some historical studies of the reception and diffusion of Elliott Jaques's psychoanalytical formulation of the midlife crisis, particularly in the context of subsequent feminist critiques of contemporary preoccupations with men at midlife.[20] So far, however, historians have rarely focused on how Jaques's work drew on, and gained purchase from, earlier studies of the challenges of middle age written by the authors of self-help manuals and marital advice literature during the interwar and immediate post-war years. Although self-help and marriage guidance differed in many ways – one focusing largely on self-fulfilment, the other on marital or relational fulfilment – they also had much in common. Both were strongly gendered. According to self-help authors and some proponents of psychoanalytical approaches to marriage guidance, men's crises were primarily the product of psychological anxieties about work and death; by contrast, women's difficulties at midlife were interpreted as an inability to cope with, or to see beyond, menopause and the empty nest. In addition, self-help literature and marriage guidance both responded to, and helped to reconstitute, interwar and post-war pressures to restore political order and social stability in the face of economic recession, global conflict, failing marriages and the apparent disintegration of conservative norms and values. Effective social reconstruction, like the resolution of personal and marital tensions at midlife, demanded the realignment of individual, domestic, occupational and social selves and a reconfiguration, or rebalancing, of the needs of self and others in a climate of aggressive individualism.[21] Self-help books and marriage guidance literature also reveal how the boundaries of middle age and the parameters of the midlife crisis were fluid and ambiguous, constructed by shifting configurations of the life course and prominent Western emphases on the correlation between personal prosperity, social harmony and economic productivity.

Ambiguities of midlife

According to Elliott Jaques, the midlife crisis was typically encountered by men and women in their mid-thirties. This critical age, he argued, constituted a pivotal, if equivocal, moment in the life course: 'The paradox is that of entering the prime of life, the stage of fulfilment, but at the same time the prime and fulfilment are dated. Death lies beyond.'[22] Jaques's identification of 35 as the age at which the future began to be eclipsed by the weight of the past and overshadowed by the spectre of death relied on a strict scriptural calibration of life expectancy. His normalising narrative of creativity and despair was informed by the opening stanzas of Dante's *Divine Comedy*, in which the narrator revisits an encounter with death that occurred precisely halfway along the biblical life span of three score years and ten.[23] The 'beautiful lines' at the start of *Inferno*, wrote Jaques shortly before his death in 2003, 'melded with my own inner experiences of the midlife struggle with its vivid sense of the meaning of personal death'.[24] Pictured as a fulcrum situated midway between birth and death, or at the onset of middle age, Jaques's notion of the midlife crisis folded personal experience, literary metaphor and lessons from his psychoanalytical practice into a predictive model of psychological health across the life course.

In spite of Jaques's temporal precision, it is clear that the boundaries of middle age – and by inference the timing of the midlife crisis – were unstable. In an article on 'America's unknown middle-agers' published in the *New York Times* in 1956, the Chairman of the Joint Legislative Committee on Problems of the Aging, Thomas C. Desmond, explored the 'much misunderstood period' of middle age. Reversing contemporary emphases on 'decay and decline' through midlife, he argued, required creating a distinct medical speciality of 'mediatrics' – analogous to paediatrics and geriatrics – to 'blossom forth to care for middle-aged folks'.[25] As Desmond and others recognised, however, there was a major challenge involved in establishing a dedicated field of scientific and clinical enquiry of this nature: there was no single definition or agreed meaning for the term 'middle age'.[26] For some, middle age constituted a fixed period between 40 and 60;[27] for others it signified not a precise time period, but a set of life-course experiences – and often crises – related to balancing work, family and leisure and characterised by fatigue, discontent and boredom; for yet others, it constituted a phase of life in which mental vigour and flexibility began to deteriorate and the body's recuperative powers were increasingly compromised.

The cultural complexities and ambiguities of midlife and the relative invisibility of middle age, indicated in the writings of Desmond and others, have shaped the historiography of ageing. Just as mid-twentieth-century scientists, clinicians and governments were more interested in the very young and the elderly than those in middle age, which was arguably the 'last portion of the life span to be discovered',[28] so too historians have been slow to historicise midlife on its own terms, rather than as the silent sequel to youth or merely a prelude to old age. Recently, however, a number of key studies have begun to expose the social, cultural and political determinants of shifting representations of midlife and to open up questions about the diversity of experiences of middle age according to class, race and gender across the nineteenth and twentieth centuries. John Benson, Kay Heath, Patricia Cohen and Steven Mintz have done much to direct scholarly attention to the middle years of life and to expose many of the myths of ageing through adulthood, in both the past and present.[29] The anthropological and cultural studies of Margaret Lock and Margaret Morganroth Gullette have also challenged beliefs in the biological inevitability of decline through the middle years, highlighting the ways in which narratives of ageing are themselves cultural fictions.[30]

Although they adopt distinct perspectives, historical, sociological and anthropological studies reveal the ways in which middle age has been measured and experienced variably in temporal, biological and social terms. Modern Western approaches to ageing have been dominated by chronology, characteristically distinguishing different life stages in terms of boundaries or years lived. In the late nineteenth century, censuses regarded those between 30 and 50 years old as middle-aged but, as Benson has shown, increasing life expectancy and cultural resistance to the inevitability of decline helped to shift the lower limit of middle age from 30 to 40.[31] In 1920, a report in the *Lancet* suggested that much 'misery and ill-health' could be avoided by compulsory medical examination for those around the age of 40, that is 'half-way through what we all hope will be our span of life'.[32] During subsequent decades, considerable advertising space was dedicated to selling products to people struggling to counter the 'middle-aged spread' associated with complacency and self-indulgence and to alleviate their fear of reaching 40 – or 'forty-phobia' (see Figure 9.1).[33] At the same time, the upper limit of middle age was stretched to 60 or 65. This framing of middle age as the years between 40 and 65 was not incompatible with Jaques's subsequent chronology of life transitions: a midlife crisis occurred characteristically in the mid to late thirties at the onset of middle age and was followed by another crisis at 'full maturity around the age of sixty-five.'[34]

The passing of time was not the only measure of ageing, although it was perhaps the most commonly used across the twentieth century. As

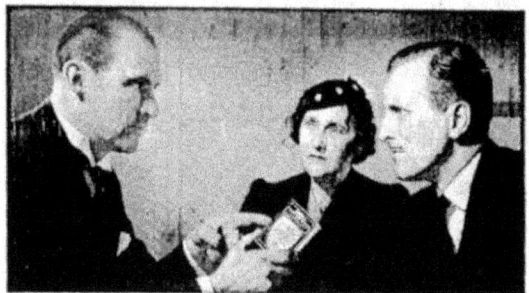

9.1 'Forty-phobia (fear of the forties)', *The Times*, 28 April 1938, p. 19

some historians have indicated, the end of middle age in particular was often read in biological terms, particularly in women, whose middle years were reckoned by the ticking of a biological clock and whose later years were thought to be dominated, and in some cases disrupted, by the hormonal imbalances, physical changes and emotional unsteadiness associated with menopause.[35] Men were also thought to experience a male menopause or climacteric, typified by declining virility and a range of psychological problems, but its more muted and extenuated character rendered it a less obvious determinant of midlife crises.[36] However, the timing and experiences of biological transitions or crises across the life course were mediated by social and cultural norms. Margaret Lock, Judith Houck and Elizabeth Siegel Watkins have revealed how the manifestations of ageing and the 'change of life' in women and men were experienced, narrated and medicalised in line with culturally specific gendered notions of domestic duties and occupational aspirations and achievements. In women, the upper limit of middle age was marked not merely by menstrual changes, but also by the departure of children from the home (the 'empty nest syndrome'), or in some cultures by the transition from mother to grandmother.[37] In men, by contrast, the boundaries of middle age were more often measured in terms of the onset, rhythms and cessation of working life and were largely bureaucratic conveniences associated with taxation, retirement and pension rights.[38]

The writings of Margaret Morganroth Gullette and others remind us that experiences of middle age are 'culturally patterned' and linked to a Western market economy that is dependent on sustaining the political and economic power of individuals across the life course.[39] They also suggest that conceptualisations of midlife as a time of crisis presuppose certain constructions of selfhood. Margaret Lock's comparative studies of menopause in America and Japan indicate that Western accounts of ageing have tended to emphasise individual uniqueness and to valorise the pursuit of self-empowerment and personal agency.[40] Indeed, twentieth-century models of midlife transition articulated by Carl Jung, Erik Erikson, Elliott Jaques, Daniel Levinson and Gail Sheehy focused on the ways in which crises could be harnessed to sculpt new identities, new healthier forms of 'self', although in doing so they generated fresh opportunities for conflict between competing individualities and temporalities within relationships and families.[41] In contrast, Japanese models of socialisation towards maturity focused traditionally not on 'learning how to maximize one's own interests', but on becoming 'social and moral beings'.[42] At least before the gradual encroachment of Western family structures and values and the rise of individualism, Japanese narratives of midlife – which differed temporally between men and women – conveyed an alternative model of the self, one that was 'created and recreated in daily life, beyond and within the confines of the body, through committed participation in social life and through self-reflection' rather than self-interest.[43] It was precisely the challenge of balancing the welfare of self and others, as well as coping with shifting experiences of time and identity across the life course, that preoccupied mid-twentieth-century authors of self-help and marriage guidance literature for the middle-aged.

Life begins at 40

In his early twentieth-century studies of 'senescence', or the last half of life, Granville Stanley Hall cited the work of the Danish author Karin Michaëlis as the origin of the term 'a dangerous age', which Hall took to mean the point in life when men were 'prone to weigh themselves in the balance' as death approached.[44] What is interesting about Hall's appropriation of the term, given his almost exclusive emphasis on the creative crises of ageing men and shaped partly by his own experiences during middle age and on retirement in his seventies,[45] is that Michaëlis's novel, *The Dangerous Age* – which was first published in Danish in 1910 and translated the following year into English – comprised letters and fragments from the diary of a 42 year-old woman, Elsie Lindtner. In narrating the emotional traumas of solitude and divorce in middle age, Michaëlis drew attention to the painful 'years of transition' in women between 40 and 50: 'The time is gone by', Lindtner reflects in one journal entry. 'Life is over.'[46] According to Michaëlis, *The Dangerous Age* generated 'storms of abuse from the ranks of the radicals all over Europe', and the text also attracted a combination of acclaim and disapproval from American journalists.[47] Contemporary outrage, particularly among suffragists, was partly triggered by Michaëlis's insistence that middle-aged women were unfit for office because of their biological limitations. From Michaëlis's perspective, the 'distressing enigmas of feminine psychology', which included a propensity for women to lie more often than men, stemmed from physiological imbalances and crises dictated not by their social status but by nature.[48]

There were, of course, alternative narratives of crises in the lives of women. In 1921, for example, the English novelist Rose Macaulay stressed the social, cultural and economic factors that shaped women's capacities to cope across the life course, not just at midlife. In what was regarded at the time as a riposte to Michaëlis's work, Macaulay's account of the lives of four women at different stages of the life cycle – written when she was in her late thirties – suggested that the absence of full voting rights and the lack of financial or professional independence meant that all ages were dangerous for women.[49] Nevertheless, it is clear that the notion that midlife constituted a particularly critical stage of life gained considerable purchase immediately before and after the First World War. In *Midstream*, an autobiography published in 1914 when he was 35, the American author Will Levington Comfort referred to 'the restlessness and agony' experienced by many women at midlife when they realised that they had become strangers to their husbands and children.[50] In men, a similar crisis was thought to be triggered by the tedium of working life: 'when twenty years of toil have come and gone', wrote Pastor Newell Dwight Hillis in *Good Housekeeping Magazine* in 1912, 'the work grows stale, the labor mechanical and meaningless, and the months become an endless round of hopeless repetition'. During this 'dangerous age', he continued, both men and women turned to new sources of excitement, such as betting, gambling and reading sensational fiction, to combat the monotony of their lives.[51]

Widespread acceptance of the notion of a dangerous age was expedited by its use as a metaphor to capture the causes and consequences of global conflict and economic crisis. Citing H. G. Wells's prescription for salvaging Western civilisation from the wreckage of the First World War, Hall suggested that the human race had 'passed its prime' and that a 'new social consciousness' was required to steer the world into a healthier old age.[52] American entry into the war had also provided the context for the emergence of more affirmative narratives of middle and old age, narratives that encouraged women and men actively to address and redress incipient physical and mental decline not merely for their own sake, but for the sake of their country. In an interview in *The Pittsburgh Press* published in April 1917, Mrs Theodore Parsons, the widow of an army officer, implored American women to 'train for the duties that war time may bring.'[53] Drawing on a wide range of evidence, including the work of Hall and her own experiences training pupils in schools and colleges, Parsons had for some years been advocating a particular form of 'New Education' that emphasised the role of physical exercise in developing the brain and balancing the emotions.[54] In 1917, she argued that preparing for war duties was analogous to preparing for 'wifehood and motherhood' and demanded the same attention to physical training. Her comments were directed particularly at 'the adipose woman of forty' who had neglected to care for herself:

> 'It is a paradox of life,' Mrs. Parsons continued, 'that we do not begin to live until we begin to die. Death begins at thirty, that is, deterioration of the muscle cells sets in. Most old age is premature, and attention to diet and exercise would enable men and women to live a great deal longer than they do to-day. The best part of a woman's life begins at forty.'[55]

Although applied explicitly to women in relation to wartime exigencies, Parson's phrase – 'life begins at 40' – was adopted as a catchphrase by American self-help authors hoping to check the loss of health and vitality associated with the stress of living through periods of economic depression. In 1932, Walter B. Pitkin, Professor in Journalism at Columbia University and author of numerous self-help guides between the 1920s and 1940s, used the phrase for the title of a popular book that promised readers an antidote to the seemingly inevitable downward curve of life after 40.[56] Enticing his audience with a vision of the excitement, joy and riches on offer in the 'Machine Age', which had reduced the 'hours of toil' and increased opportunities for leisure, Pitkin's prescription for happiness exploited belief in the American dream – the notion of freedom, upward mobility and self-made prosperity that had been articulated by James Truslow Adams in 1931 and subsequently translated into liberal capitalist commitments to self-governance and self-fulfilment.[57]

Although contemporary faith in self-improvement through material consumption had already been satirised in Sinclair Lewis's novel of 1922, *Babbitt*,[58] the key message in Pitkin's work – that modern populations could now progress from 'making a living' to 'living' – proved attractive to aspiring middle-class middle-agers keen both to generate wealth and to display their well-earned capacity for leisure. Pitkin accepted that metabolism and energy decreased with age and that midlife transitions might be the result of 'some obscure shift in the endocrine balance'.[59] But he insisted that biological limitations need not prevent people from living more contentedly as they aged. The increased capacity to afford goods, pursue leisure activities and make the most of their time allowed the middle-aged to attain the 'emotional poise which underlies enduring happiness'.[60] 'Happiness', Pitkin argued, 'comes most easily after forty.'[61]

Pitkin's invocation to spend time and money wisely across the life course in order to prolong health and happiness was not merely a disinterested form of self-help; it was also a prescription for social stability and recovery from the Great Depression. Austerity and automation, he argued, had limited opportunities for young people to work and adversely affected their capacity to purchase either 'goods and services for simple subsistence' or those which helped 'towards self-improvement both vocational and cultural'.[62] His manifesto for personal fulfilment in older age, along with the mantra that 'life begins at forty', was therefore underscored by a belief that economic growth depended primarily on harnessing the spending power, managerial capacities and wisdom of the middle-aged in order to expand employment prospects for the young, encourage independence and self-sufficiency, enable more people to work part-time, promote longer lives in better health and provide greater opportunities for leisurely 'self-realization'.[63]

In 1965, Pitkin's son, Walter Pitkin Jr, reflected on the impact of his father's work. By focusing popular and professional attention on '*the subjective, or inner life* of the middle-aged and aging person', he argued, *Life Begins at Forty* had encouraged readers to believe that life could be creative, happy and challenging after the onset of middle age, in the process launching 'a whole industry' of inspirational self-help literature for the middle-aged.[64] As his son suggested, Pitkin was by no means the only writer of lifestyle manuals during the middle decades of the twentieth century.[65] Books on diet, relaxation and yoga were sometimes marketed directly at those over 40 years of age to help them counter the effects of stress, tension, poor diet, lack of exercise, excessive work and inadequate rest that were thought to lead to nervous breakdowns and premature death.[66] The belief that a 'full and happy life is a balanced one' figured strongly in these self-help texts.[67] In their 1938 discussion of the merits of relaxation in a frenzied world where few could 'attain equilibrium', the British physician E. J. Boome and speech therapist M.

A. Richardson emphasised the role of relaxation in achieving equanimity: 'The balance and stability which can be obtained by the practice of relaxation', they suggested, 'enables a man to face and deal fearlessly with responsibility and trouble instead of trying to evade them.'[68] The advice of the German-born American nutritionist Gayelord Hauser similarly focused on the manner in which readers could ensure good health across the life course, not only by adopting balanced diets, but also by balancing their personality, mind, activity, emotions, recreation, friends, budget and marriage.[69]

Arguments for prioritising leisure and relaxation as routes to happiness, or as mechanisms for balancing life in order to improve health across the life course, were restated by contemporary commentators on both sides of the Atlantic during the middle decades of the twentieth century. In a paper published in the American journal *Marriage and Family Living*, for example, Nadina R. Kavinoky, a Swiss-born gynaecologist and the first female president of the American National Council on Family Relations, claimed that individual and family mental stability depended on an appropriate mix of work, rest and recreation, a formula for health that also influenced post-war debates about safety and efficiency in transport industries.[70] Recreation in particular, she argued, facilitated the rehabilitation of 'men wounded in body and spirit' and enhanced the capacity of couples and their children to cope with the physical and emotional demands of modern living.[71] Yet, there were alternative approaches to healthy ageing that valorised work rather than leisure. Tom Lutz has pointed out that during the 1920s work was portrayed by American physicians and novelists as a solution to boredom and ennui, a means of invigorating mind and body, controlling or 'working through' emotions and realising the self. Men employed outside the home and housewives both needed work in order to foster feelings of self-worth: while for men satisfaction came from the office or factory, for women their 'real work was not the monotony of cleaning but the more significant, ennobling job of raising a family'.[72]

Guidance about how to age well at midlife, and how to balance the competing demands of work, family and leisure, was therefore modulated by normative notions of gender. Although self-help authors framed their advice as if it applied equally to men and women, they nevertheless singled out for separate discussion the specific challenges faced by women, challenges that were partly linked to their distinctive domestic duties and social roles. The importance of achieving or maintaining a balanced life clearly structured recommendations for women's self-fulfilment in later life, as well as dictating debates about paid employment for women.[73] According to the older Pitkin, wives and mothers whose children had left home and whose husbands were 'sunk deeply in the miry ruts of their own business offices' needed to identify educational and career opportunities that made use of their skills and experience in order to prevent boredom, unhappiness and periods of personal crisis.[74] By contrast, college women – those educated in 'spinster factories' – needed to temper their commitment to work with more opportunities for play.[75] Balancing their lives in these ways, Pitkin argued, would enable women in their forties and fifties to achieve a greater sense of utility and fulfilment in later years.

Although contemporary writers recognised the domestic and occupational determinants of well-being, interwar and post-war advice literature for middle-aged women, particularly in Britain, often focused on the biological changes associated with the menopause, which was thought to occur generally between the ages of 40 and 55. Self-help approaches to the menopausal years varied, not only in terms of weighing the physiological against the situational causes of menopausal difficulties, but also in terms of their empathy for middle-aged women. In a short book intended to reveal to both men and women the 'facts and fallacies of middle age', Joan Malleson, a clinical assistant in the Obstetric Unit at University College Hospital, explained that, although many menopausal symptoms were shaped primarily by hormonal imbalances – and in that sense might require treatment – popular accounts of 'the change' often exaggerated the sense of disruption, leading to unnecessary anxiety.[76] Malleson's advice, like other studies of housewives and mothers experiencing menopausal anxieties, was aimed at reducing the impact of age-related biological and psychological changes on the health and self-esteem of the woman herself. Indeed, Malleson believed that the menopause need not constitute a crisis, or dangerous age, at all.[77]

In contrast to Malleson's emphasis on normalising menopause in order to minimise the personal distress of middle-aged women themselves, Kenneth C. Hutchin, the author of numerous self-help books written under the pseudonym 'A Family Doctor', drew attention to the negative impact of menopause on other members of the household:

'The woman who makes the most of her symptoms', he wrote in 1963, 'can turn the climacteric into a time of misery for the whole family ... Whether it is in family life or in married life, women in the climacteric should try not to take things too seriously.'[78] Hutchin's flippancy betrayed long-standing beliefs in the responsibility of wives and mothers to subjugate their own health concerns for the welfare of their families. His argument that menopause constituted a dangerous age not only for a wife and mother, but also more importantly for her husband and children, was not unusual, and was often repeated on both sides of the Atlantic.[79] In the context of widespread concerns about rising levels of divorce and the breakdown of conventional social values before and after the Second World War, it was the potential for marriages and families to undergo a crisis that provided the framework for another form of mid-century lifestyle guidance that foregrounded relational, rather than individual, dimensions of midlife transitions.

Fractured families

In their wonderful study of the 'collision of interests between love, family and personal freedom', Ulrich Beck and Elisabeth Beck-Gernsheim argued that, in the twentieth century, 'deep cracks' appeared 'across the picture of the family'.[80] Situating the apparent 'chaos of love' in the context of new opportunities and pressures to 'break free and discover one's true self', Beck and Beck-Gernsheim regarded the midlife crisis as a marriage crisis, one made possible by the coincidence of three factors: 'individualization in general, female individualization in particular and increased life expectancy'.[81] Although, like Jaques, they considered the midlife crisis to be analogous to the adolescent pursuit of identity, Beck and Beck-Gernsheim understood the challenge of middle age not in terms of a growing awareness of personal death, but as a struggle for two individuals 'to survive within a shared life'. By disrupting the sense of stability and identity previously made possible by traditional gender roles and normative notions of the nuclear family, individualisation was encouraging men and women to escape from what were seen as the constraints of 'marital symbiosis'.[82]

The image of fractured families was apt. Before the Second World War, no more than 7,000 couples were divorced in England and Wales annually. After the war, however, the number of divorces rose rapidly

Table 9.1: Number of divorcing couples in England and Wales, 1945–85

Year	Number of divorces
1945	15,634
1950	30,870
1955	26,816
1960	23,868
1965	37,785
1970	58,239
1975	120,522
1980	148,301
1985	160,300

(Source: Office for National Statistics)

in Britain, reaching 37,785 by 1965 (see Table 9.1).[83] A similar pattern emerged in North America, where a perceived crisis in marriage and family was regarded, already by the late 1930s, as equally serious as the crisis in the 'economic system and political order'.[84] A report on marriage and divorce statistics in the United States, published in 1973, highlighted a gradual rise in divorce across the first half of the twentieth century, a sharp peak immediately after the Second World War, and then another steady increase through the 1960s (see Figure 9.2).[85]

Contemporary commentators offered numerous reasons for these trends. The rise in divorces immediately after the war was explained as a 'symptomatic feature of the disturbance brought about by war in the field of family relations': extramarital affairs on the part of both men and women during long periods of separation and the challenges of readjusting to domestic life and civilian work created the conditions for the breakdown of relationships and families.[86] But, as a number of government enquiries and commissions indicated, other factors may have contributed to the steady increase in rates of divorce across the post-war decades, particularly among those aged between 35 and 49. According to the British 1946 Denning Committee on Procedure in Matrimonial Causes, it was the exhausting 'mechanics of everyday life' that were reducing women's marital satisfaction and happiness in particular.[87] Ten years later, the widely discussed Royal Commission on Marriage and Divorce suggested that friction between husbands and

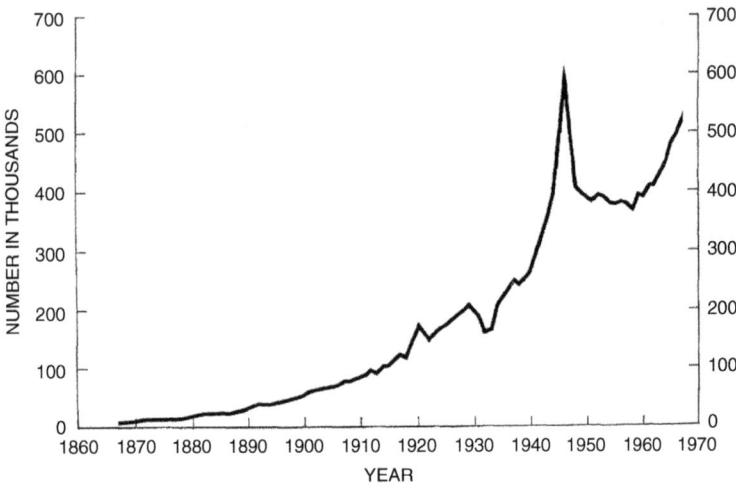

9.2 Divorces in the United States, 1867–1967 (Source: US Department of Health, Education and Welfare, *100 years of Marriage and Divorce Statistics: United States, 1867–1967* (Rockville, MD: Health Resource Administration, HRA 74-1902, 1973), p. 8

wives, and any resultant family instability, could be traced to socioeconomic factors such as 'the housing shortage, the earlier age of marriage, the higher standard of living, the transformation in the social position of women, and the change in attitudes towards non-marital sexual relations'.[88] The rapid increase in divorce rates was therefore regarded by some as an 'index of domestic decay' and the product of greater divorce-mindedness among post-war couples.[89] Although many post-war British commentators, including Denning, emphasised the need for state-sponsored marriage guidance rather than easier divorce for couples struggling to 'deal with the post-marital causes of unhappiness',[90] the Divorce Reform Act 1969 (and similar legislation in America and Canada) signalled a more permissive and less punitive approach to marital breakdown, leading to further dramatic increases in the number of divorces.

Divorce was also linked to the manner in which partnerships were supposedly being weakened by the 'atomistic tendencies of modern life',[91] most notably 'the propensity to regard the assertion of one's own individuality as a right, and to pursue one's personal satisfaction, reckless of the consequences for others'.[92] As Beck and Beck-Gersheim's work demonstrates, contemporary focus on the role of individualism and self-realisation in promoting 'divorce-mindedness' has attracted the interest of scholars keen to explain the breakdown of relationships in terms of the internalisation of neo-liberal, consumer ideologies. However, any simplistic historical, sociological or economic emphasis on the threat posed to family stability by the rise of individualistic values can be contested. Jane Lewis's study of changing patterns of marriage and cohabitation suggests that selfish individualism, supposedly manifested in women's increased employment outside the family and in men's 'flight from commitment', has been assumed rather than demonstrated both in contemporary discussions of marriage and divorce and in historical accounts of changing family structures and values.[93]

Lewis's contention that historians need to challenge ungrounded assertions about the sources of individualism and more carefully contextualise its impact on relationships is certainly valid. At the same time, overemphasis on the structural determinants of divorce or the macro-politics of Western individualisation fails to recognise fully the relational and family traumas associated with midlife marital tensions, or to appreciate the narrative devices and norms employed by marriage guidance counsellors and their clients to make sense of and alleviate the pain of betrayal, separation and divorce. Whether they were offered by state-supported marriage counsellors or by psychoanalysts at the Tavistock Clinic (initially funded privately, but later incorporated into the National Health Service), marriage guidance and couples counselling immediately before and after the Second World War were shaped by a recognition that the collapse of established relationships could be traced to a combination of family stresses, personality traits and ill health in middle age, as much as to the pursuit of self-fulfilment. Equally, routes to the resolution of marital differences or the reconfiguration of broken homes were not only fashioned by national campaigns for more effective regulation of marriage and divorce in order to rebuild family life and restore social stability after the Second World War; they were also determined by locally contingent strategies for mitigating the impacts of life transitions on the physical and emotional health of parents and children.[94]

The Marriage Guidance Council was founded in Britain by David Mace and his colleagues in order to 'promote successful marriage and parenthood' in the face of what Mace referred to, in deliberately sensationalist terms, as a 'marriage crisis'.[95] Although the initial idea for an organisation to ease 'marriages in trouble' had been formulated in 1938, the Council was formally established in 1942 and the first Marriage Guidance Centre opened in London the following year.[96] Mace's belief in the importance of marriage in generating and maintaining social cohesion, and his conviction that divorce 'was nearly always the end of a long and sad story' that could have been avoided, were not the first articulations of a perceived need for effective marriage guidance.[97] In a number of books published widely during the 1920s and 1930s, well before divorce rates began rising in Britain, Marie Stopes had offered marital advice not only to couples at the start of their relationships, but also to those in middle age whose marriages had become tinged by a 'common sadness'.[98] Rejecting contemporary fears that declining happiness within marriage was inevitable, Stopes advised readers on how to overcome the various physical and psychological obstacles to 'enduring passion' and lifelong contentment, framing her guidance in the relatively new language of endocrinology: women were vulnerable to disruptions to the 'harmony of the hormones' during menopause; and alterations in 'glandular secretions' could generate emotional crises in middle-aged men.[99] In neither case, however, was it inevitable that 'the change' (or what Stopes also referred to as a 'critical period' or 'dangerous time') would prevent health and satisfaction in later life.[100]

Stopes regarded crises across individual life courses and in marriages as products of maladjustment and ignorance triggered by the 'artificiality of civilisation', a pessimistic refrain commonly articulated in the interwar years.[101] In response, her prescription for promoting healthy ageing prioritised effective communication as a means of countering melodramatic media accounts of decline in middle and older age.[102] While interwar advice literature focused primarily on individual strategies for self-fulfilment, Stopes approached marriage difficulties from a relational perspective, foregrounding the necessity for couples to learn about and help each other through troubled times. Similar arguments for recognising the needs of others permeated psychological understandings of marital difficulties in the interwar years. In 1938, William Brown, Director of the Institute of Experimental Psychology at the

University of Oxford, suggested that successful adjustment to marriage – and indeed to middle age – required individuals to surrender 'the very pronounced degree of narcissism which we all have in our earlier years' and see life from the perspective of their partners.[103]

For marriage guidance counsellors – who included probation officers, social workers, nurses, occupational therapists and doctors – it was also the marital dyad that provided the principal focus for analysis and intervention. Indeed, some post-war counsellors explicitly acknowledged Stopes's relational approach: Mary Macaulay, a marriage counsellor in Merseyside, thanked Stopes (as well as Joan Malleson and David Mace) in the preface to her 1952 book *The Art of Marriage*, in which she argued that middle-aged couples needed to study and respond to 'each other's interests' if they were to avoid apathy and infidelity.[104] The clearest example of the practical approaches to marital disharmony adopted by marriage counsellors – whose work was sometimes dismissed as a 'technique in search of a theory'[105] – can be found in a study by J. H. Wallis and H. S. Booker, whose 1958 description of the National Marriage Guidance Council's work included the tabulation and analysis of the problems faced by couples, mostly middle-aged and middle class, who had consulted counsellors for help between 1952 and 1954. The significance of the couple was clear. Even when counsellors were approached by only one partner at a time of crisis, they were to remember that 'in marriage counselling there are no problems independently of the marriage, independently of husband and wife'.[106] After one or more individual consultations, counsellors were expected to invite the other partner to join them.[107]

The second section of Wallis and Booker's study illustrated the range of factors precipitating requests for help from the Marriage Guidance Council and situated marital problems in relation to the duration of marriage, the number of children and the ratio of wives to husbands who first sought guidance (57.5 per cent women; 37.5 per cent men; and 5 per cent together in 1952). The study also traced the outcomes of counselling, including the marriage difficulties being overcome (19 per cent), the relationship being improved (16.5 per cent) or showing no improvement (31.5 per cent).[108] Wallis and Booker identified a variety of causes of crisis, including ill health, personal defects (such as selfishness, especially of the husband), parental interference, sexual difficulties and known or suspected infidelity, more often, but by no means exclusively, on the part of the husband.[109] Marital difficulties experienced by couples were illustrated by abbreviated case studies that provided alternative perspectives on the critical period of middle age and marriage to those presented by self-help authors. As in Stopes's work, it was the relational and familial dimensions of crisis that emerged in condensed narratives of marital disharmony, revealing the assumptions and expectations that counsellors imported into encounters with clients. Descriptions of thirty-seven cases of infidelity of the husband and fifteen of the wife, often after many years of marriage, highlight the ways in which blame was apportioned and success measured in terms of continuation of the marriage. In one case, a marriage of thirty-one years and four children had ended when the husband left his wife to live with 'a third party', citing his wife's lack of affection and her tendency to talk 'like a parrot, never ending'. Another couple had been 'happy for fifteen years' before the husband – who was described as overbearing and cruel – had begun 'an affair with the widow of a friend'.[110]

In 1963, Wallis drew further on his experiences of helping clients and their partners struggling with the challenges generated by 'the uncertainty of middle age'.[111] Like Jaques two years later, Wallis prefaced his work with the opening lines of Dante's *Divine Comedy*, equating the turbulence of midlife to the physiological and emotional transformations, as well as the defiant and narcissistic tendencies, associated with adolescence.[112] Reflecting on how men and women coped during midlife with changes at home and work, with altering relationships and parenthood, and with the tensions involved in establishing and maintaining a partnership between two individuals (the 'Us' of marriage), Wallis set out what he regarded as one of the key symptoms and triggers of upheavals in middle age, whether within or outside marriage: 'The most startling is the sudden compulsive infidelity that not infrequently comes the way of the counsellor.'[113] The abandoned partner, or 'the innocent party' in the eyes of the divorce laws, he explained, was shocked, bewildered and desolated by the loss of what had previously appeared to be a 'happy, normal, stable marriage'.[114] In a discussion that captured many mid-century anxieties about middle age, Wallis suggested that the psychological determinants and behavioural manifestations of the accompanying 'emotional typhoon', evident in both partners, constituted a 'middle-age crisis'.[115]

Self-help and the making of the midlife crisis 271

The focus of marriage guidance counsellors on couples rather than individuals stemmed directly from the contemporary commitment of the state, as well as the Catholic and Anglican churches, to reinvigorating family life and restoring social order by strengthening marriage: marital stability was a precondition for national stability.[116] According to the National Marriage Guidance Council, successful marriage, achieved only through 'unselfish love and self-discipline', was vital to social well-being.[117] By contrast, as the Royal Commission on Marriage and Divorce had pointed out with concern in 1956, psychodynamic approaches to marital and midlife difficulties tended to ignore the significance of existing family relationships; instead, they focused on promoting self-expression and self-fulfilment through a process of prolonged individual psychoanalysis of the type used by Elliott Jaques to reveal the unconscious drivers of the midlife crisis.[118] Yet not all psychotherapists neglected the relationship between partners or the dynamics of the family in seeking to resolve marital tensions, whatever their cause. One of the features of the social casework carried out by staff at the Family Discussion Bureau of the Tavistock Clinic was its emphasis not only on the dynamics of individual personality development, but also on the 'disturbances of emotional equilibrium' between two partners.[119]

Drawing on a combination of methods adapted from psychoanalysis, child guidance and the work of Michael Balint, caseworkers at the Bureau developed a team approach that focused not on 'the individual but the marriage, and behind it the family'.[120] Although caseworkers did see clients individually, particularly in the initial consultation or if a partner was reluctant to attend, emphasis on the couple as a single analytical unit prioritised involving both parties in addressing marital problems. The published, anonymised narratives of marital tensions presented by members of the Bureau were more detailed and more vivid than those provided by the National Marriage Guidance Council, but similarly revealed the web of norms and assumptions that structured couples therapy as well as the marital problems that it was designed to mitigate. Case reports of the Bureau's work with particular clients stretched over several pages, aiming to connect and make sense of the couple's family backgrounds, their courtship and marriage and the birth of their children, and to articulate current problems within the relationship from the perspective of each partner. As staff at the Bureau pointed out in an introduction to their techniques published in 1955, the purpose of discussing such issues openly was to enable the couple to address 'the vicious circles of intolerance and resentment' and to establish in their place a 'beneficent spiral' that ideally enabled the satisfaction of both husband and wife and facilitated the well-being of what the Bureau referred to as the 'primary family unit'.[121] Staff at the Bureau measured success in terms of improvements in marital and other relationships and in the adjustment of individuals to personal circumstances.

The value of joint, rather than merely individual, psychotherapy at the Tavistock was most forcefully articulated by Henry V. Dicks, whose study of marital tensions, published in 1967, set out the analytical principles and practices of marital therapy. Although Dicks criticised David Mace for his 'reliance on clichés', his analysis was similarly shaped by contemporary truisms about the importance of investigating 'disturbed marriages' in order to address the 'trail of unhappiness' generated by 'broken homes' after the Second World War.[122] Dicks's approach, however, was more clearly structured by an understanding of the complex interrelations between cultural norms, social expectations, emotional growth and what he termed 'marital pathology'.[123] Drawing on the findings from a pilot study initiated in 1949 and first published in 1953, Dicks developed a strategy for diagnostic interview and joint therapy that moved well beyond the dyadic approach advocated by marriage guidance counsellors.[124] For Dicks, effectively working through and remedying relational tensions required establishing a novel system of joint interview and joint therapy involving both partners and two therapists.[125] Over time, this 'four-person relationship', Dicks suggested, would allow couples, whether married or not, to uncover and address conflicts generated by disappointed role expectations, the power of past identifications and the projection of one partner's repressed needs or characteristics onto the other.[126]

Dicks acknowledged that factors other than those linked to personality and emotional immaturity impacted on marital harmony: marriages could become strained under the influence of in-laws, economic and housing difficulties, and clashes of culture. In addition, he argued, marriages contracted under certain forms of stress – such as 'a child on the way, the rebound from another affair, or as a desperate remedy for social loneliness' – were often doomed from the start.[127] Such situational pressures were, of course, understood by marriage guidance counsellors such as Wallis to be key drivers of marital tensions, and often framed medical and popular advice to couples struggling to cope with the social and biological effects of ageing, the climacteric, emotional isolation and infidelity. Particularly poignant in this context are the stories of women on both sides of the Atlantic who sought to escape from domestic boredom, economic constraints and unhappy marriages by going out to work.[128] However, unlike much marriage guidance literature aimed at the middle-aged, Dicks insisted that social circumstances still needed to be understood primarily along psychoanalytical lines – that is, 'in terms of the meaning they have for the two intrapersonal worlds'.[129] Given his commitment to reading both individual and dyadic development in psychoanalytical terms, it is not surprising that Dicks was one of the first writers on marital stress and divorce among the middle-aged to cite Elliott Jaques's emphasis on understanding midlife transitions in terms of 'bio-psychological crisis points' triggered by an awareness of death.[130]

Conclusion

In *The Normal Chaos of Love*, Ulrich Beck and Elisabeth Beck-Gernsheim insisted quite rightly that 'the mid-life crisis is a *social*, not a natural event'.[131] During the middle decades of the twentieth century, breaking free to discover one's true self might have been posited by self-help authors as an individual journey of discovery, a path to happiness that necessitated sacrificing certain social commitments for personal biological and psychological fulfilment. But the pursuit of self-realisation at midlife and its manifestations in infidelity and marital disruption also conformed to 'a general imperative': the symptoms and social significance of marital decay were dictated by the contrasting domestic and occupational expectations of middle-aged men and women, by concerns about the fragmentation of families and its impact on social stability and cohesion, and by a competitive labour market that prioritised mobile and productive individuals across the life course, sometimes at the expense of stable family relationships.[132] Individual and collective, private and public strategies for realising selfhood, sustaining marriages and coping with crises at midlife were interwoven and bounded by political, economic and cultural contingencies.

The publication of Elliott Jaques's article in 1965 is often regarded as the moment of conception of the midlife crisis, as if it emerged *de novo* from Jaques's psychoanalytical practice and biographical study of creative artists. But, as this discussion of self-help literature and marriage guidance suggests, many of the key ingredients of Western narratives of middle age were well established by the early 1960s. Jaques's articulation of the emotional turbulence associated with the midlife search for meaning in the face of death was made possible by narrative traditions – focusing on the tensions between individual freedom, marital harmony and social stability – already evident during the interwar and immediate post-war years. Similarly, academic acknowledgement of Jaques's ideas, and their incorporation into literary and cinematic sources during the 1970s and 1980s, was facilitated by widespread acceptance of the biological and psychological dimensions of midlife and marital crises that self-help authors and marriage counsellors had been addressing for some decades.

There were clear similarities between self-help and marriage guidance on both sides of the Atlantic, not only in terms of their scope and purpose, but also in terms of the ways in which their formulations of midlife and marriage often drew – like Jaques's work – on personal experiences of ageing. Both genres were also framed by shifting and contested notions of crisis, balance and selfhood, concepts that gained considerable social and cultural traction in the unstable years of economic depression, global conflict and social reconstruction before, during and after the Second World War. Yet, there were also differences between self-help and marriage guidance. Unlike the authors of advice literature for the middle-aged, who promoted self-realisation and self-fulfilment, those involved in marriage guidance preferred to regard narcissism as an obstacle, rather than a pathway, to personal and conjugal happiness in later life. Coping with crises required adults to learn how to live together in a society supposedly weakened by individualisation and to effectively balance the needs of self and others, including not only partners but also children.[133]

In some cases, these seemingly contradictory messages – one focusing on balancing the self, the other on balancing the family – were juxtaposed in a single exposition of the route to health and happiness. In 1950, Gayelord Hauser's 'passport to a new way of life' included advice to readers to balance their diet, activity, mind and emotions at an individual level in order to achieve health and longevity; it also emphasised the need to 'give and take' in marriage, to recognise that, particularly in later years, marriage should be based on sharing 'mutual interests, mutual accomplishments, as well as mutual affection.'[134] Here, in a single text, Hauser had not only defined one of the central challenges of middle age in terms of the interactions between individual and social behaviour – a theme that ran through Elliott Jaques's work throughout the post-war years; he also articulated what had become a key paradox for those attempting to restore social and marital stability after the Second World War, namely how to balance – without eliding – the competing interests of the individual, the family and the state.

Acknowledgements

The research on which this chapter is based was generously funded by a Wellcome Trust Senior Investigator Award, 'Lifestyle, health and disease: changing concepts of balance in modern medicine', Grant No. 100601/Z/12Z. I would also like to thank Martin Moore for his astute comments on the first draft. As always, I am grateful to Siobhán, Ciara, Riordan and Conall for their love and support through my own midlife – and other – crises.

Notes

1 E. Jaques, *The Changing Culture of a Factory* (London: Tavistock Publications, 1951); E. Jaques, 'Social systems as a defence against persecutory and depressive anxiety', in M. Klein, P. Heimann and R. E. Money-Kyrle (eds), *New Directions in Psychoanalysis* (London: Tavistock Publications, 1955), pp. 478–98.

2 E. Jaques, *The Form of Time* (London: Heinemann, 1982); E. Jaques, 'On trust, good, and evil', *International Journal of Applied Psychoanalytic Studies*, 2 (2005), 396–403. Overviews of Elliott Jaques's life and work were published shortly after his death in a special issue of *International Journal of Applied Psychoanalytic Studies*, 2 (2005). See also S. Long, 'Organizational defenses against anxiety: what has happened since the 1955 Jaques paper', *International Journal of Applied Psychoanalytic Studies*, 3 (2006), 279–95.

3 D. Kirsner, 'The intellectual odyssey of Elliott Jaques from alchemy to science', *Free Associations*, 11 (2004), 179–204. Kirsner's account draws heavily on conversations with Jaques.
4 E. Jaques, 'Death and the midlife crisis', reproduced in E. Jaques, *Work, Creativity, and Social Justice* (London: Heinemann, 1970), pp. 38–63, at p. 59.
5 Ibid., pp. 39–45.
6 C. Bühler, 'The curve of life as studied in biographies', *Journal of Applied Psychology*, 18 (1935), 405–9. On the history of ageing, geriatrics and anti-ageing therapies, see: S. Ottoway, 'Medicine and old age', in M. Jackson (ed.), *The Oxford Handbook of the History of Medicine* (Oxford: Oxford University Press, 2011), pp. 338–54; J. Stark, 'The age of youth', *Lancet*, 388 (2016), 2470–1; and K. Heath, *Aging by the Book: The Emergence of Midlife in Victorian Britain* (New York: State University of New York Press, 2009).
7 G. Stanley Hall, 'The dangerous age', *Pedagogical Seminary*, 28 (1921), 275–94. See also G. Stanley Hall, *Senescence: The Last Half of Life* (New York: D. Appleton and Company, 1922).
8 Hall, 'The dangerous age', p. 290.
9 For Jung's theory of individuation, see: C. G. Jung, *Modern Man in Search of a Soul* (London: Kegan, Paul, Trench, Trubner and Co., 1933); C. G. Jung, *The Integration of the Personality* (London: Kegan, Paul, Trench, Trubner and Co., 1940).
10 Jaques, 'Death and the midlife crisis', p. 59.
11 Cason is cited in Jaques's obituary in *Business Wire* (14 March 2003), available at www.businesswire.com/news/home/20030313005534/en/OBITLeading-Psychologist-Century-Dr.-Elliott-Jaques-Dies, accessed 21 July 2017.
12 See, for example, the rising frequency of references to the midlife crisis in English language books through the 1980s and 1990s in Google NGram Viewer, available at https://books.google.com/ngrams/graph?content=midlife+crisis&year_start=1800&year_end=2000&corpus=15&smoothing=3&share=&direct_url=t1%3B%2Cmidlife%20crisis%3B%2Cc0, accessed 21 July 2017.
13 E. Sherman, *Meaning in Mid-Life Transitions* (New York: State University of New York Press, 1984), p. 221.
14 B. Fried, *The Middle-Age Crisis* (New York: Harper and Row, 1967); G. Sheehy, *Passages: Predictable Crises of Adult Life* (New York: E. P. Dutton, 1974); H. Schreiber, *Midlife Crisis: Die Krise in der Mitte des Lebens* (Munich: C. Bertelsmann, 1977); G. E. Vaillant, *Adaptation to Life* (Boston MA: Little, Brown, 1977); H. Still, *Surviving the Male Mid-Life*

Crisis (New York: Thomas Y. Crowell, 1977); N. Mayer, *The Male Mid-Life Crisis: Fresh Starts After Forty* (New York: Doubleday, 1978); D. J. Levinson, *The Seasons of a Man's Life* (New York: Alfred A. Knopf, 1979); R. A. Segalla, *Departure from Traditional Roles: Mid-Life Women Breaking the Daisy Chains* (Ann Arbor, MI: UMI Research Press, 1979); J. Conway and S. Conway, *Women in Midlife Crisis* (Wheaton, IL: Tyndale House, 1983); A. Lawson, *Adultery: An Analysis of Love and Betrayal* (New York: Basic Books, 1988).

15 S. Schmidt, 'The feminist origins of the midlife crisis', *Historical Journal*, 61 (2018), 503–23. As Schmidt shows elsewhere, the feminist perspective on midlife transitions was also contested and often unfairly dismissed by psychologists: S. Schmidt, 'The anti-feminist reconstruction of the midlife crisis: popular psychology, journalism and social science in 1970s USA', *Gender and History*, 30 (2018), 153–76.

16 D. R. Mace, *Marriage Crisis* (London: Delisle, 1948).

17 H. V. Dicks, *Marital Tensions: Clinical Studies towards a Psychological Theory of Interaction* (London: Routledge and Kegan Paul, 1967), pp. 223–5.

18 M. M. Gullette, *Safe at Last in the Middle Years: The Invention of the Midlife Progress Novel* (Berkeley: University of California Press, 1988).

19 For post-war literary formulations of crises across the life course, some of which refer directly to the midlife crisis and most of which explore love, infidelity and betrayal in middle age, see: J. Updike, *Rabbit, Run* (New York: Alfred A. Knopf, 1960); J. Updike, *Rabbit Redux* (New York: Ballantine Books, 1971); J. Updike, *Rabbit is Rich* (New York: Ballantine Books, 1981); J. Updike, *Rabbit at Rest* (New York: Ballantine Books, 1990); S. Wilson, *The Man in the Gray Flannel Suit* (New York: Simon & Schuster, 1955); S. Wilson, *The Man in the Gray Flannel Suit II* (New York: Arbor House, 1984); S. de Beauvoir, *The Woman Destroyed* (New York: G. P. Putnam's Sons, [1967] 1979); I. Bergman, *Scenes from a Marriage* (AB Svensk Filmindustri, 1973). On American cinematic treatments of the aspirations and disappointments of middle-aged men and women, see J. Levinson, *The American Success Myth on Film* (Basingstoke: Palgrave Macmillan, 2012).

20 Schmidt, 'The feminist origins of the midlife crisis'; Schmidt, 'The anti-feminist reconstruction of the midlife crisis'.

21 Or what Ulrich Beck and Elisabeth Beck-Gernsheim have referred to as an 'ego epidemic': U. Beck and E. Beck-Gernsheim, *The Normal Chaos of Love* (Cambridge: Polity Press, 1995), p. 4.

22 Jaques, 'Death and the midlife crisis', p. 48.

23 The opening stanza has been variably translated, but Jaques's version read: 'In the middle of the journey of our life, I came unto myself in a dark wood where the straight way was lost.' See E. Jaques, *The Life and Behavior of Living Organisms: A General Theory* (Westport, CT: Praeger, 2002), p. 3. Dante was in his late thirties when he wrote this passage, and elsewhere referred to the normative biblical lifespan of seventy years – see R. M. Durling (ed.), *The Divine Comedy of Dante Alighieri, Volume I: Inferno* (Oxford: Oxford University Press, 1996), p. 34.
24 Jaques, *The Life and Behavior of Living Organisms*, p. 3.
25 T. C. Desmond, 'America's unknown middle-agers', *New York Times*, 29 July 1956, pp. 5, 42–3.
26 See, for example, D. B. Bromley, 'Middle age: an introduction', in R. Owen (ed.), *Middle Age* (London: BBC, 1967), pp. 7–21.
27 The notion of a 'fixed period' drew partly on William Osler's belief that great advances were only made between the ages of 25 and 40, that men over 40 were comparatively useless, and that men above 60 should retire – W. Osler, 'The fixed period', in *Aequanimitas* (Philadelphia: P. Blakiston's Son and Co., 1910), pp. 389–411. Osler's work formed one of the starting points of G. Stanley Hall's studies of ageing – Hall, 'The dangerous age'.
28 M. Lock, 'Deconstructing the change: female maturation in Japan and North America', in R. A. Schweder (ed.), *Welcome to Middle Age! (And Other Cultural Fictions)* (Chicago: University of Chicago Press, 1998), pp. 45–74, at p. 45.
29 J. Benson, *Prime Time: A History of the Middle Aged in Twentieth-Century Britain* (Harlow: Addison Wesley Longman, 1997); Heath, *Aging by the Book*; P. Cohen, *In Our Prime: The Invention of Middle Age* (New York: Scribner, 2012); S. Mintz, *The Prime of Life: A History of Modern Adulthood* (Cambridge, MA: Belknap Press, 2015).
30 M. Lock, *Encounters with Aging: Mythologies of the Menopause in Japan and North America* (Berkeley: University of California Press, 1993); M. M. Gullette, *Declining to Decline: Cultural Combat and the Politics of the Midlife* (Charlottesville: University Press of Virginia, 1997); M. M. Gullette, *Aged by Culture* (Chicago: University of Chicago Press, 2004).
31 Benson, *Prime Time*, pp. 8–12. For contemporary reference to middle age as the years between 35 and 50, see Active 54, 'The middle-aged man and the war', *Lancet*, 184 (5 September 1914), 667–8.
32 'A medical survey at middle age', *Lancet*, 195 (1 May 1920), 974. A correspondent to the same journal agreed that 'the downward curve of life' began after the age of 35 or 40 – Aetas, 'Age and pensions', *British Medical Journal*, 1 (12 February 1921), 249–50.

Self-help and the making of the midlife crisis 279

33 Phyllosan promised readers that they would 'feel younger as they grow older' – 'Forty-phobia (fear of the forties)', *The Times*, 28 April 1938, p. 19. For a discussion of advertisements and the growing use of terms such as 'middle-aged spread', see Benson, *Prime Time*, pp. 9–10, 17–18.
34 Jaques, 'Death and the midlife crisis', p. 38.
35 On the medicalisation of menopause, see: Lock, *Encounters with Aging*; J. A. Houck, *Hot and Bothered: Women, Medicine, and Menopause in Modern America* (Cambridge, MA: Harvard University Press, 2006); L. Foxcroft, *Hot Flushes, Cold Science: A History of the Menopause* (London: Granta, 2009).
36 E. Siegel Watkins, 'The medicalisation of the male menopause in America', *Social History of Medicine*, 20 (2007), 369–88; H.-G. Hofer, 'Medicine, aging, masculinity: towards a cultural history of the male climacterium', *Medizinhistorisches Journal*, 42 (2007), 210–46; H.-G. Hofer, 'Men in the critical age: Kurt Mendel and the controversy over the male climacteric', *Urologist*, 50 (2011), 839–45.
37 Lock, *Encounters with Aging*; Houck, *Hot and Bothered*; Watkins, 'The medicalisation of the male menopause'.
38 According to the American psychologist Bernice Neugarten, men perceived 'a close relationship between life-line and career-line' – B. L. Neugarten, 'The awareness of middle age', in B. L. Neugarten (ed.), *Middle Age and Aging: A Reader in Social Psychology* (Chicago: University of Chicago Press, 1968), pp. 93–8, at p. 96. For discussion of definitions of age in terms of the bureaucratic processes involved in distributing government pensions, see C. Port, '"Ages are the stuff!": The traffic in ages in interwar Britain', *NWSA Journal*, 18 (2006), 138–61.
39 R. A. Schweder, 'Introduction: welcome to middle age', in Schweder (ed.), *Welcome to Middle Age!*, pp. ix–xvii.
40 Lock, 'Deconstructing the change'.
41 On the inevitability of collisions created by competing individualities in relationships, making love 'more difficult than ever', see Beck and Beck-Gernsheim, *The Normal Chaos of Love*, pp. 52–6. For a discussion of divergences between individual, family and historical time, see T. K. Hareven, 'Family time and historical time', *Daedalus*, 106 (1977), 57–70.
42 Lock, 'Deconstructing the change', p. 60.
43 Ibid., pp. 60–1, 65–8.
44 Hall, 'The dangerous age', pp. 275, 287.
45 T. R. Cole, 'The prophecy of *Senescence*: G. Stanley Hall and the reconstruction of old age in America', *Gerontologist*, 24 (1984), 360–6.
46 K. Michaëlis, *The Dangerous Age: Letters and Fragments from a Woman's Diary* (New York: John Lane, 1911), available on the Project Gutenberg

website, www.gutenberg.org/files/14187/14187-h/14187-h.htm, p. 25, accessed 16 September 2016.
47　A. Tridon, 'Author of the latest "daring" novel is in America', *New York Times*, 16 July 1911, Magazine Section, p. 9.
48　K. Michaëlis, 'Why are women less truthful than men?', *Munsey's Magazine* (May 1913), pp. 185–8; K. Michaëlis, 'Why are women less truthful than men?', *Munsey's Magazine* (June 1913), pp. 343–5. Michaëlis continued to enrage American women in particular with her views on their 'selfish, vain and arrogant' personalities – 'Insults American women: articles by Mme. Michaëlis called "international scandal"', *New York Times*, 2 August 1914, p. 11. According to Hall, Michaëlis was regarded 'as a traitor to her sex' – Hall, *Senescence*, p. 29.
49　R. Macaulay, *Dangerous Ages* (London: Collins, 1921). For a discussion of Macaulay's work, see Port, '"Ages are the Stuff!"'.
50　W. Levington Comfort, *Midstream: A Chronicle at Halfway* (New York: George H. Doran, 1914), p. 293. Helen Keller, an American author and political activist, used the same metaphor to narrate her life: H. Keller, *Midstream: My Later Life* (New York: Doubleday, Doran and Co., 1929).
51　N. D. Hillis, 'The dangerous age in man', *Good Housekeeping Magazine*, 54 (1912), 537–40. The peculiar challenges of middle age also figured in medical commentaries exploring the role of diet and exercise in maintaining health through midlife. See: 'Middle age and old age', *British Medical Journal*, 2 (10 July 1915), 57–8. The article was reviewing S. Taylor, *Health for the Middle-Aged* (London: Methuen, 1915).
52　Hall, *Senescence*, pp. 30–1, citing H. G. Wells, *The Salvaging of Civilisation: The Probable Future of Mankind* (London: Cassell, 1921). Contemporaries also used the notion of salvage to describe approaches to improving the lives of the elderly – see L. J. Martin and C. de Gruchy, *Salvaging Old Age* (New York: Macmillan, 1930).
53　N. Greeley-Smith, 'Now is the time for all women to train for the duties that war time may bring', *The Pittsburgh Press*, 10 April 1917, p. 20.
54　Mrs T. Parsons, *Brain Culture through Scientific Body Building* (Chicago: American School of Mental and Physical Development, 1912). Parsons later published an abridged version for 'use in homes, schools and colleges' – Mrs T. Parsons, *Making the Body Think* (New York: Kelmscott Press, 1926).
55　Greeley-Smith, 'Now is the time for all women'.
56　W. B. Pitkin, *Life Begins at Forty* (New York: McGraw-Hill, 1932).
57　J. Truslow Adams, *The Epic of America* (Boston, MA: Little, Brown, and Company, 1931), pp. 415–16.

58 S. Lewis, *Babbitt* (Leipzig: Bernhard Tauchnitz, 1922). The term 'Babbittry' became popular in America as a descriptor of narrow-minded materialism.
59 Pitkin, *Life Begins at Forty*, pp. 7, 24.
60 See Chapter 2 by Martin Moore for a discussion of contemporary commitments to emotional management in configuring health.
61 Pitkin, *Life Begins at Forty*, pp. 106–7. Pitkin stressed in particular the value of time: 'Time is neither a medium nor is it exchangeable', he wrote. 'It is the inmost stuff of life itself' – ibid., p. 86.
62 Ibid., p. 149.
63 Ibid., pp. 49, 107.
64 W. Pitkin Jr, *Life Begins at Fifty* (New York: Simon & Schuster, 1965), pp. 21–2.
65 S. Currell, 'Depression and recovery: self-help and America in the 1930s', in D. Bell and J. Hollows (eds), *Historicizing Lifestyle: Mediating Taste, Consumption and Identity from the 1900s to 1970s* (Aldershot: Ashgate, 2006), pp. 131–44.
66 E. Jacobson, *You Must Relax: A Practical Method of Reducing the Strains of Modern Living* (New York: McGraw-Hill, 1934); G. Hauser, *Look Younger, Live Longer* (London: Faber & Faber, 1950); N. Phelan and M. Volin, *Yoga Over Forty* (New York: Harper & Row, 1965); D. Dunne, *Yoga for Everyman: How to Have Long Life and Happiness* (London: Gerald Duckworth, 1951). On therapeutic relaxation in mid-twentieth-century Britain, see Chapter 6 by Ayesha Nathoo.
67 N. Brierley, *Relaxation for Men: Tension in Modern Living* (London: Ward Lock, 1965), p. 7.
68 E. J. Boome and M. A. Richardson, *Relaxation in Everyday Life* (London: Methuen, 1938), pp. 1, 99.
69 Hauser, *Look Younger, Live Longer*, pp. 188–97.
70 N. R. Kavinoky, 'A balanced life for mental health', *Marriage and Family Living*, 6 (1944), pp. 41–2, 58, 64. On the impact of these debates on regulating duty rosters in the airline industry, see Chapter 7 by Natasha Feiner.
71 Kavinoky, 'A balanced life for mental health'.
72 T. Lutz, '"Sweat or die": the hedonization of the work ethic in the 1920s', *American Literary History*, 8 (1996), 259–83.
73 F. Cooper, 'Medical feminism, working mothers, and the limits of home: finding a balance between self-care and other-care in cross-cultural debates about health and lifestyle, 1952–1956', *Palgrave Communications*, 2(2016), article 16042, available at www.nature.com/articles/palcomms201642, accessed 8 August 2017.

74 Pitkin, *Life Begins at Forty*, pp. 112–20.
75 Ibid. Pitkin's son also recognised the specific problems of middle-aged women: Pitkin Jr, *Life Begins at Fifty*, pp. 16, 211–13.
76 J. Malleson, *Change of Life: Facts and Fallacies of Middle Age* (London: Penguin, [1949] 1963), pp. 13–18. For Malleson's work on hormonal balance and menopause, see: J. Malleson, 'An endocrine factor in certain affective disorders', *Lancet*, 262 (25 July 1953), 158–64; J. Malleson, 'Climacteric stress: its empirical management', *British Medical Journal*, 2 (15 December 1956), 1422–5.
77 M. C. Stopes, *Change of Life in Men and Women* (London: Putnam, 1936), pp. 1–21. For an international study of 'disturbances of equilibrium' in mothers and housewives during the 'most difficult years' of the menopause, see Mrs O. van Andel-Ripke, 'Mother and housewife in the climacteric', in Medical Women's International Association, *The Menopause* (Rome: Edizioni Minerva Medica, 1954), pp. 93–8.
78 K. C. Hutchin, *The Change of Life* (London: W. & G. Foyle, 1963), pp. 67–9.
79 Houck, *Hot and Bothered*, pp. 114–32.
80 Beck and Beck-Gernsheim, *The Normal Chaos of Love*, p. 45.
81 Ibid., p. 68.
82 Ibid., pp. 66–7, 72.
83 Office of National Statistics, 'Vital statistics: population and health references tables', available at www.ons.gov.uk/peoplepopulationand community/populationandmigration/populationestimates/datasets/vitalstatisticspopulationandhealthreferencetables, accessed 12 September 2017.
84 'Address of Dr. Sidney E. Goldstein on the need of a White House conference on family', *Living*, 1 (1939), 13–14.
85 US Department of Health, Education and Welfare, *100 years of Marriage and Divorce Statistics: United States, 1867–1967*, HRA 74–1902 (Rockville, MD: Health Resource Administration, 1973); US Census Bureau, *Births, Deaths, Marriages, and Divorces* (Statistical Abstract of the United States, 2011), p. 96, available at www.cdc.gov/nchs/data/series/sr_21/sr21_024.pdf, accessed 15 April 2019.
86 In 1946, debates in the House of Lords drew attention to the 'flood of cases' of divorce among servicemen and women that were putting pressures on the legal system – 'Services divorce delays', *The Times*, 27 March 1946, p. 8. The personal and domestic challenges of returning home from war was a familiar trope in post-war fiction: see Wilson, *The Man in the Gray Flannel Suit*.

87 *Final Report of the Denning Committee on Procedure in Matrimonial Causes*, Cmd. 7024 (London: HMSO, 1946), cited in R. Cross, 'Final Report of the Denning Committee on Procedure in Matrimonial Causes', *Modern Law Review*, 10 (1947), 184–92.
88 *Report of the Royal Commission on Marriage and Divorce*, Cmd. 9678 (London: HMSO, 1956), cited in O. Kahn-Freund, 'Divorce Law Reform?', *Modern Law Review*, 19 (1956), 573–600, at p. 577.
89 O. R. McGregor, *Divorce in England: A Centenary Study* (London: William Heinemann, 1957), pp. 126, 152.
90 Cross, 'Final Report of the Denning Committee', p. 185.
91 A. T. M. Wilson, 'Some reflections and suggestions on the prevention and treatment of marital problems', *Human Relations*, 2 (1949), 233–52.
92 *Report of the Royal Commission on Marriage and Divorce*, pp. 7–8.
93 J. Lewis, *The End of Marriage? Individualism and Intimate Relations* (Cheltenham: Edward Elgar, 2001), p. 11. The term 'flight from commitment' is taken from B. Ehrenreich, *The Hearts of Men: American Dreams and the Flight from Commitment* (New York: Anchor Books, 1984).
94 For approaches to rebuilding life after the war, see Sir J. Marchant (ed.), *Rebuilding Family Life in the Post-War World: An Enquiry with Recommendations* (London: Odhams Press, 1945).
95 Mace, *Marriage Crisis*, p. 14.
96 Ibid., pp. 14–15. An organisation to promote family values 'for the advantage of the individual and the Nation State', the National Council on Family Relations was founded in America in 1938. The first issue of the Council's journal, *Living*, published in January 1939, focused largely on marriage.
97 Ibid., pp. 111, 131.
98 M. Stopes, *Enduring Passion*, 2nd edition (London: Putnam, 1929), pp. 1–11. This was a sequel to the widely popular *Married Love*, written primarily for couples during the early years of their marriage.
99 Stopes, *Enduring Passion*, pp. 151–2, 189–90. In both men and women, Stopes argued, disturbances of 'internal glandular balance' could be rectified with glandular extracts.
100 Stopes, *Change of Life in Men and Women*, p. 22.
101 Ibid., p. 1. In 1937, Macpherson Lawrie, a physician in psychological medicine at Queen Mary's Hospital in London, blamed modern transport for estranging husbands and wives and damaging 'domestic sentiment' – M. Lawrie, *Love, Marriage and Divorce* (London: Methuen, 1937), pp. 185–8. See also R. Overy, *The Morbid Age: Britain Between the Wars* (London: Allen Lane, 2009).

102 On decline narratives more generally, see Gullette, *Declining to Decline*.
103 W. Brown, *Psychological Methods of Healing: An Introduction to Psychotherapy* (London: University of London Press, 1938), pp. 158–60.
104 M. Macaulay, *The Art of Marriage* (London: Delisle, [1952] 1956), pp. 96–7. Macaulay placed the burden for maintaining marital fidelity largely on the wife: 'The husband who knows he will be warmly welcomed at home and warmly welcomed in the bed has no need to look elsewhere for reassurance that he is loved and appreciated.'
105 G. I. Manus, 'Marriage counseling: a technique in search of a theory', *Journal of Marriage and the Family*, 28 (1966), 449–53.
106 J. H. Wallis and H. S. Booker, *Marriage Counselling: A Description and Analysis of the Remedial Work of the National Marriage Guidance Council* (London: Routledge & Kegan Paul, 1958), p. 39.
107 Ibid., p. 92.
108 Ibid., pp. 125–66, *passim*. The result was unknown in 33 per cent of cases.
109 Ibid., pp. 167–202, *passim*.
110 Ibid., pp. 270–4.
111 J. H. Wallis, *The Challenge of Middle Age* (London: Routledge & Kegan Paul, 1962), p. vii.
112 Ibid., pp. 1–13.
113 Ibid., p. 89.
114 Ibid.
115 Ibid.
116 Studies of the drivers of marriage guidance in the mid-twentieth century include: J. Lewis, 'Public institution and private relationship: marriage and marriage guidance, 1920–1968', *Twentieth Century British History*, 1 (1990), 233–63; A. Harris, 'Love divine and love sublime: the Catholic Marriage Advisory Council, the marriage guidance movement and the state', in A. Harris and T. Jones (eds), *Love and Romance in Britain, 1918–1970* (Basingstoke: Palgrave Macmillan, 2015), pp. 188–224; T. Chettiar, '"More than a contract": the emergence of a state-supported marriage welfare service and the politics of emotional life in post-1945 Britain', *Journal of British Studies*, 55 (2016), 566–91.
117 Wallis and Booker, *Marriage Counselling*, Appendix B, p. 100.
118 *Report of the Royal Commission on Marriage and Divorce*, paras 45 and 46; Jaques, 'Death and the mid-life crisis', pp. 51–6.
119 K. Bannister, A. Lyons, L. Pincus, J. Robb, A. Shooter and J. Stephens, *Social Casework in Marital Problems: The Development of a Psychodynamic Approach* (London: Tavistock Publications, 1955), p. 28.
120 Ibid., pp. 7–8.

121 Conversion of the 'vicious circle' into a 'beneficent spiral' was achieved in the case of Mr and Mrs Rivaux – ibid., pp. 67–78, at p. 78. For reference to the 'primary family unit', which included children, see ibid., p. 145.
122 Dicks, *Marital Tensions*, pp. 1–2.
123 Ibid., p. 42.
124 H. V. Dicks, 'Clinical studies in marriage and the family: a symposium on methods', *British Journal of Medical Psychology*, 26 (1953), 181–96.
125 Dicks, *Marital Tensions*, pp. 236–53. On the novelty of Dicks's approach, see G. Gorer, 'Book Review', *International Journal of Psycho-Analysis*, 49 (1968), 107–9.
126 Dicks, 'Clinical studies in marriage and the family'.
127 Ibid., p. 195.
128 M. Hilliard, *A Woman Doctor Looks at Love and Life* (New York: Doubleday, 1957), pp. 106–7, 112, 146; Papers of Viola Klein, University of Reading, MS 1215/29/1/762. On Hilliard's popular advice literature, see K. Mendes, 'Reading *Chatelaine*: Dr Marion Hilliard and 1950s women's health advice', *Canadian Journal of Communication*, 35 (2010), 515–31.
129 Dicks, 'Clinical studies in marriage and the family', p. 195.
130 Dicks, *Marital Tensions*, p. 225.
131 Beck and Beck-Gernsheim, *The Normal Chaos of Love*, p. 67.
132 Ibid., p. 6.
133 Marriage guidance was shaped explicitly by the work of child guidance clinics, which had been established on both sides of the Atlantic during the interwar years and which regarded juvenile delinquency and other behavioural disorders as partly the product of domestic difficulties and broken homes.
134 Hauser, *Look Younger, Live Longer*, pp. 188–97.

10

Balancing contested meanings of creativity and pathology in Parkinson's Disease

Dorothy Porter

Introduction

Parkinson's Disease is one of the defining degenerative diseases of ageing populations. In 2005 there were an estimated 4.1 million sufferers worldwide, a figure projected to reach 8.7 million by 2030.[1] However, those statistical projections have already been dramatically revised. Current estimates are that 7 to 10 million people in the world are affected, with estimates that this will double within a decade as economically developing and developed populations expand, age and chronically sicken.[2] One million people live with Parkinson's in the United States, with a further 60,000 diagnosed each year;[3] in Britain, a new person is diagnosed every hour.[4] The disease is characterised by limb tremor and bradykinesia, along with signs such as fixed facial expression, lack of eye blinking, hoarse inaudible voice, shuffling gait, asymmetrical arm swinging and loss of physical balance not easily regained. Cognitive impairment can accompany progressive physiological decline, ending in frontal lobe dementia.[5]

A cure for Parkinson's still eludes us, even as hopes run high among the experimental scientific community.[6] However, there has been a remarkable clinical managerial tool available from the 1960s, one that leverages dopamine substitution in brains where massive dopaminergic neuron death has triggered symptoms.[7] The pharmacological breakthrough of L-DOPA transformed the experience of patients living with gradual decline in motor function, and assisted in reducing some of the behavioural distress that can accompany the disease. L-DOPA was able to lift the spirits of some patients who had experienced at least a decade of suffocating clinical depression prior to diagnosis. Other successful pharmacological innovations in Parkinson's Disease management have extended the clinical arsenal.[8] Among the most effective of these has been dopamine agonist therapeutics, which reduce the horribly disconcerting dyskinesias that can be produced by L-DOPA treatment and prevent uncontrollable jerky neck, arms and legs. Some of the medicines in the Parkinson's Disease apothecary's chest, however, have indeterminate consequences for behavioural transformations and thus therapeutic balance between motor improvement and emotional instability is key to the highly specialised therapeutic management of the disease in each case. Complex behavioural reactions to dopamine agonist treatments in particular have led to clinical caution regarding their use.[9]

This chapter investigates questions about balance in Parkinson's Disease by analysing historical shifts in debates about a predetermined behavioural model of a Parkinson's Disease personality, its relationship to artistic creativity and implications for therapeutic equilibrium in clinical management. The aim of the chapter is to demonstrate that focusing on balance merely in terms of therapeutic dosage plans ignores broader dimensions of balancing cultural conflict surrounding ontological and emergent meanings of the disease and the transcendent metaphysics of creativity. In this way it speaks directly to the central themes of this volume, which addresses the contingent scientific and clinical normativities of physiological and psychological balance and their relationship to models of the self.[10] Drawing out the historical determinants of contingently normative neo-humoralism threaded through the story of Parkinson's Disease – evident in other manifestations of neurology[11] – this chapter also explores an alternative, and equally ancient, narrative of balance about the dualism of creative genius. Roy Porter used William Blake's lament about the 'mind forg'd manacles' of the creative imagination to epitomise the eighteenth-century European Enlightenment's mirror of reason and madness.[12] My task here is to examine how balancing drug reception in the brain is bound to the legacy of Enlightenment normative contingencies concerning madness and reason, genius and lunacy, creativity and manic compulsion. Before demonstrating how the history of Parkinson's Disease offers an opportunity to investigate shifting cultural epistemologies of the self as an ontological and emergent category, and the ways in which notions of balance were folded into studies of creativity in terms of stimulation and inhibition, the following section presents a brief history of the discovery of the disease, its causes and the emergence of an idea of a Parkinson's personality.

From physical tremor to mental torpor

The London physician from Hoxton Square, James Parkinson, described the experiences of six patients who all exhibited the definitive symptoms of what he termed 'the shaking palsy' in 1817: 'Involuntary tremulous motion, with lessened muscular power, in parts not in action and even when supported; with a propensity to bend the trunk forwards, and to pass from a walking to a running pace: the senses and intellects being un-injured.'[13]

Parkinson did not include personality or behavioural characteristics in his analysis of etiology but attributed the cause to pathology of the spinal cord.[14] He described each patient as having a different life story, their ages ranging from their mid-fifties to early seventies. Parkinson included contrasting psychological profiles of his subjects, but did not offer cultural characterisations comparable to contemporary medical discourses on gout or tuberculosis.[15] One patient, he recounted, was a gardener who had led a life of 'remarkable temperance and sobriety'. By contrast, a retired attendant at the magistrate's court attributed his condition to the 'consequence of considerable irregularities in his mode of living, particularly of indulgence of spirituous liquors'.[16]

Parkinson's descriptions of impeded gait in all the patients he observed equally fascinated the founding father of modern neurology, Jean Martin Charcot, half a century later.[17] Charcot worked and taught for thirty-three years at Paris' vast charity hospital, the Salpêtrière,[18] where his lectures became public spectacles, most famously when he used hypnosis to illustrate his theories about the neurological character of hysteria.[19] Charcot defined the clinical characteristics of multiple sclerosis, motor neuron disease and muscular dystrophy, and significantly expanded the neurological understanding of the Shaking Palsy, which he renamed Parkinson's Disease.[20] He differentiated resting tremor in Parkinson's from active tremor in multiple sclerosis. He also identified that patients with resting tremor exhibited rigidity and impaired ability to adjust bodily position, and slow movement (bradykinesia), that they had soft spoken voices and that movement alleviated their tremor. Throughout 1888 he studied and presented a patient, referred to as Bachere, to demonstrate and discuss the posture, stance and retropulsive and propulsive gait pathologies of Parkinsonism.[21] Charcot pioneered the use of visual representation as a research and teaching tool and left sketches of Bachere's abnormal stance and gait along with observations of his fixed facial muscle 'mask'.[22] While Charcot's drawings constitute the first representation of the clinical symptoms of the disease, perhaps the most emblematic was sculpted by the artist anatomist Paul Richer, who was Charcot's assistant and head of the Salpêtrière laboratory from 1882–96, and who had sculpted a female patient because she represented 'the almost perfect clinical schema of Parkinson's Disease'.[23]

Charcot's students and assistants began trying to uncover the causes of Parkinson's by suggesting that lesions in a small area in the mid-brain known as the *substantia nigra compactica* might be involved in the loss of muscle control. But it was a visitor to the Salpêtrière from Russia, Konstantin Tretiakoff – together with one of Charcot's students, Gheorghe Marinesco – who definitively demonstrated that destruction of cells in the *substantia nigra* was related to the onset of Parkinson's Disease,[24] by dissecting the brains of patients who had died from a new form of encephalitis – known as Von Economo's encephalitis, after its discoverer – that appeared during the First World War.[25] Following the war, a group of von Economo's patients developed Parkinsonism, and it was in the brains of fifty of these patients that Tretiakoff discovered marked loss of the dark melanin-pigmented neuron cells in the *substantia nigra* and noted that the remaining cells were damaged with pathological deposits he referred to as Lewy bodies.[26]

While Tretiakoff had identified that neuronal death in the *substantia nigra* was involved in causing Parkinson's, he could not explain how or why that anatomical destruction led to motor system dysfunction. That required moving beyond anatomical analysis to an examination of the chemical functioning of the brain and the role of dopamine,[27] which was first synthesised at the Wellcome Laboratories in 1910.[28] At that time dopamine was believed to be a precursor of the catecholamine neurotransmitters responsible for chemically transmitting information between neurons in the brain. But the biological function of dopamine as a neurotransmitter itself was discovered by a Swedish pharmacologist, the Nobel Laureate Arvid Carlsson, in 1958.[29] Carlsson made the discovery as the result of reanimating rabbits with the amino acid DOPA, stimulating the production of dopamine in the basal ganglia structures in the mid-brain, where motor function is located. Following this discovery, Carlsson and his colleagues announced at an international pharmacological meeting in 1959 that Parkinsonism was induced by dopamine depletion, which could be reversed by L-DOPA,[30] and subsequently used new forms of fluorescence histo-chemistry to map dopamine pathways in the brain. Over the next three decades, Parkinson's research focused on refining the therapeutic application of L-DOPA and adjunct dopamine agonists to control motor symptoms of the disease.[31] Such approaches were not unusual in this period: reconstructing physiological balance using metabolic hormones had been popular in the management of chronic illnesses since the early twentieth century.[32]

Carlsson and his team had originally sedated rabbits into a catatonic state with a neuroleptic drug, resperine. Neuroleptics are a class of major tranquillisers that have been used since the Second World War to control psychotic states such as schizophrenia, leading to the hypothetical postulate that dopamine variability – or imbalances – played a significant role in the development of schizophrenia and perhaps other forms of behavioural change.[33] The dopamine hypothesis of schizophrenia and broader categories of psychopathology was contested throughout the latter half of the twentieth century, but the dopaminergic neurobiology of the brain became central to genomic research on cognitive and emotional variation from the 1990s.[34]

The discovery of dopamine in Parkinson's Disease not only provided an explanation of motor dysfunction, but also created an opportunity to examine psychological aspects of the disease and revived interest in the idea of a 'Parkinson's personality'. Carl Dudley Camp, Professor in Nervous Diseases at the University of Michigan, had first posited the idea of a Parkinson's personality in 1913. He had suggested on the basis of anecdotal observations that:

> It would seem that paralysis agitans affected mostly those persons whose lives had been devoted to hard work ... The people who take their work to bed with them and who never come under the inhibiting influences of tobacco or alcohol are the kind that are most frequently affected. In this respect, the disease may be almost regarded as a badge of respectable endeavor.[35]

Dudley Camp offered a psychological profile of Parkinson's patients as characteristically socially and personally responsible, in ways that echoed the associations made between gout and social elevation in the eighteenth century or between diabetes, class and social prominence from the late nineteenth century.[36] In the 1980s, a number of neurologists and psychiatrists, including Andrew Lees and G. M. Stearn at University College London, the London psychiatrist Cecil Todes (who had himself developed Parkinson's Disease at the age of 39) and the Austrian neurologist Werner Poewe, expanded the idea of a pre-morbid Parkinson's personality.[37] The classic description offered by Todes and Lees in 1985 was that Parkinson's patients exhibited an emotional and attitudinal inflexibility, a lack of affect and a predisposition to depressive illness, which could antecede the development of motor abnormalities by several decades.[38] Introspective, overcontrolled, anhedonic personality traits, together with suppressed aggression, were frequently found. However, it was unclear whether these behavioural patterns were relevant aetiological factors or prodromal symptoms of the disease.[39]

At the same time as observational accounts were positing a Parkinson's personality, experimental biopsychologists were developing new tools for identifying biologically determined personality characteristics and types.[40] In his 'unified biosocial theory of personality', in 1986, Claude Robert Cloninger, Kantian transcendentalist philosopher-professor of psychiatry at Washington University, developed a system of 'tridimensional psychobiological temperament' measurement of correlations of catecholamine activity with personality traits of novelty-seeking, harm avoidance and reward dependence.[41] The tridimensional temperament system provided a new methodological and epistemological framework for genomic correlation with personality and cognitive analysis. Cloninger first developed his methodologies for constructing predictive personality models when working in Sweden in the 1980s on alcohol dependence through 'separation studies' – that is, investigating cohorts of children separated from their biological parents at birth.[42] By the end of the decade, he had codified his psychobiological temperament model in a Tridimensional Personality Questionnaire (TPQ) and a Tridimensional Character Inventory (TCI), tools that provided the neurobiology of cognition and character with a new framework of investigation.[43]

Cloninger's biological hypothesis of character and temperament resonated with investigations into genomic influences on dopamine-dependent cognitive and emotional variation.[44] From the earliest studies with twins, discourses on the inheritability of cognitive ability were embedded in the psychobiology of intelligence. Since the completion of the human genome map, the role of the dopaminergic system and its genetic variations have reframed this investigation.[45] Since 2000, a number of candidate dopaminergic genes in cognitive variation have been explored, and D2 receptor polymorphisms have become central to genomic investigations of a subset of cognitive function, namely creativity.[46] Dopaminergic variation currently occupies the central focus of neuromolecular analyses of creativity, defined and measured in terms of novelty-seeking divergent thought. Mesolimbic, or reward pathway,[47] accounts of creativity have now gained sufficient confidence to begin claiming the capacity to be predictive. For example, Sapra, Beavin and Zak from Claremont Graduate University and Loma Linda Medical School in California recently claimed to have demonstrated what they believe is the gene combination that produces highly successful careers.[48]

Apart from facilitating the genomic investigation of cognitive creativity variation, Cloninger's tridimensional personality and character system has also been used in genetic investigations into emotional variation, especially psychobiological charting of dopaminergic pathways in personality trait characteristics of reward learning, novelty-seeking and pathological addiction, a development that influenced neuromolecular constructions of a pre-morbid Parkinson's patient personality.[49]

In line with modern preoccupations with 'personality types' as determinants of chronic disease, psychobiologists have characterised Parkinson's patients as possessing distinctive personality traits of industriousness, seriousness and inflexibility.[50] Cloninger's tridimensional character framework has rescripted this characterisation profoundly, as his TPQ and TCI have become major methodological tools for identifying and investigating a pre-morbid Parkinson's personality in terms, not only of the onset of motor dysfunction, but also of progressive cognitive and behavioural transformation. In 1993, Matthew Menza and colleagues, from the Robert Woods Johnson Medical School in New Jersey, identified dopamine-related personality traits in Parkinson's Disease using Cloninger's TPQ.[51] Menza et al. claimed that low novelty-seeking Parkinson's patients were reflective, stoic, slow-tempered, frugal, orderly and persistent, but by contrast high-scoring on Harm Avoidance. In 1995, the Menza team claimed to be able to explain this correlation by confirming – through PET (positron emission tomography) scans of Parkinson's Disease patients – that low 18 F-Dopa striatal uptake correlated with low novelty scores.[52]

Although subsequent studies have argued that Menza's results could simply be demonstrating the effects of long-term medication on advanced Parkinson's Disease patients, the neuromolecular pursuit of the predisposed low creative, high harm-avoiding personality continued. In 2011, Graham Pluck then at Sheffield University and Richard Brown from Kings College London attempted to extend the temperament model of predisposed Parkinson's personality through a study on cognitive attention capacity. Using Cloninger's framework, Pluck and Brown claimed to have demonstrated a characteristic apathy in Parkinson's Disease patients that was unrelated to the depression and anxiety often associated with the disease. They claimed instead that high apathy scores were correlated with the characteristic cognitive function of the pre-morbid Parkinson personality, legitimising their claims by suggesting that historical studies – stretching back to Charcot's description of low motivation in patients with Parkinson's Disease – confirmed the existence of a pre-morbid Parkinson's personality.[53]

Balancing cultures of creativity: pathological creativity

According to neuromolecular biopsychological theory, when genetically predisposed low novelty-seeking Parkinson's personalities demonstrate creativity it is a pathological symptom, an assumption that has been reinforced over the last two decades. In 2001, Anette Schrag and Michael Trimble from University College London reported what they believed to be the first case of poetic talent being 'unmasked' by dopamine agonist treatment for Parkinson's.[54] Their patient was aged 40 when he was first diagnosed with Parkinson's with a tremor in his left hand, dragging of left leg and dystonia of the left foot. As his symptoms increased, the patient started treatment with the dopamine agonist lisuride and L-DOPA at age 44. His symptoms significantly improved, and within the first month of treatment he began writing poetry for the first time in his life, completing ten poems in the first year of treatment. His poems achieved significant publishing success, and he won a prize in the annual contest of the International Association of Poets.[55]

The patient had always considered himself intellectually inferior to his siblings and family generally, never having achieved an equivalent level of academic success. He did, however, have a maternal grandfather who was a published poet, and he was related to a well-known Irish poet. No other changes occurred until, after twelve years of treatment, the patient began to show symptoms of depression, aggressive and volatile behaviour, along with grandiose ideas, paranoid delusions, extreme circumstantiality, over-talkativeness and pressured speech. After various therapeutic adjustments the patient returned to a stable emotional and cognitive state, with sustained control of motor symptoms. Throughout this period, and to the end of his life, the patient continued to write and publish his poetry. Schrag and Trimble explored a wide range of possible explanations for their 'poet unmasked', including contradictory implications of the classic 'pre-morbid PD personality theory', but found none sufficiently satisfactory. They finally speculated that 'the effect of dopaminergic and serotonergic drugs, either through cognitive enhancement, increased perception or a hypomanic syndrome in addition to selective fronto-cortical dysfunction, led to the release of previously inhibited creative power in this patient'.[56]

If Schrag and Trimble were only tentatively speculating that their patient's art was a form of hypomanic 'high', by the mid-2000s a more reductive neuropsychological explanation was being offered of visual art produced by patients with Parkinson's Disease. In 2005, Ruth Walker and colleagues at the Veterans Affairs Medical Center New York and NYU School of Medicine described a patient who had possessed pre-morbid undeveloped 'artistic tendencies' for sketching that dramatically changed seven years after beginning dopamine agonist therapy.[57] At this point he started producing several pastel drawings a week – sometimes two a day. After moving to an assisted living facility he had even more time to devote to his art, but at the same time began to show hypersexual disinhibition in what they describe as 'excessive flirting with women on the street and asking residents and staff of his assisted living facility to pose nude for his artwork'.[58] His disinhibition became controlled following what they describe as 'education', and his artwork began to be shown and sold in local galleries in the Bronx. In contrast to Schrag and Trimble, Walker et al. describe their patient's artistic productivity as a pathological symptom of compulsive disorder equivalent to the pathological gambling and hypersexuality associated with excessive dopamine stimulation. Thus, Walker's team identified their patient's creativity as the result of the overstimulation of the third dopaminergic pathway in the brain, which is responsible for reward learning, that can become pathologically transformed into compulsive addiction.[59] The clinical reduction of creativity to chemical imbalance, as we will see later, has been dramatically challenged by patients' accounts of their experience.[60]

In 2006, Anjan Chatterjee, Roy Hamilton and Prin X. Amorapanth from the University of Pennsylvania were far more reluctant than Walker to reduce their patient's art to the ravages of Parkinson's Disease, even after considering the benefits and challenges of defining it as a compulsive obsessive disorder.[61] CSD, the Chatterjee team's patient, was a 68 year-old graphic designer whose motor symptoms had progressed over fifteen years from 1992, while his agonist and L-DOPA medications had been adjusted to compensate. A psychologist encouraged CSD to start painting as a therapeutic activity to relieve his depression in 2002. While initially producing work derivative of Van Gogh, within a year he had begun producing uniquely original vibrant coloured pencil abstract works using fine regular lines. He used his right hand, in which his resting tremor was severe enough to significantly restrict his capacity to write. But his artistic work used large amplitude proximal movements – reaching rather than distal movements used in writing and grasping – that allowed him to feel 'a sense of bursting forth and tearing back walls'. CSD expressed an urgency to produce, and utilised the sleep disruption produced by Parkinson's Disease to wake early and work. His complete immersion into a visual image prevented him, he noted, from working on more than one painting at a time. While Chatterjee et al. note that CSD's preoccupation with his art could be interpreted as a compulsive obsessive disorder equivalent to addictive gambling, they allow his own words to express its meaning for him:

> The train has left the station and I have just been served a delicious dinner in the café car. The train is picking up speed so I have to eat fast so I can finish my meal before we get to the last stop and I have to get off.[62]

Using artistic creativity production as a measure of impulsive predisposition in Parkinson's patients has now become a standard clinical methodology. Although this has been challenged by the experience of patients themselves and patient advocacy organisations such as Parkinson's UK, which introduced the Mervyn Peake Awards for Parkinson's patients' artistic work in 2006,[63] artistic work redefined as a Cloninger novelty-seeking category has become regarded as an addiction symptom within the dopaminergic reward pathway. One component of addictive-proneness has been identified by Petra Schwingenschuh and her team at UCL and the Queen Square Institute, London, in a professional artist prior to the diagnosis of Parkinson's Disease. When pre-morbid Parkinson's Disease patients defy the Cloninger/Menza stereotypical low-creative, harm-avoiding profile, then they are likely to acquire 'dopamine dysregulation syndrome' during therapy – that is, self-overdosing and strategic deception to obtain more dopamine than they supposedly need. The Schwingenschuh team reported on four patients who had all been successful visual artists before diagnosis, and who developed dopamine addiction while being treated. 'Artists', they explained, 'require a certain stimulus and drive to produce new and creative work. In the cases described here, we suggest that the compulsive seeking of, and overdosing with, dopaminergic drugs may arise from the patients' need to fuel this drive and enhance their creativity.'[64]

Dopaminergic compulsion

Biological explanations for pathological creativity have focused on the indeterminate effects of *dopamine agonist* treatments on a second dopaminergic pathway in the brain, the mesolimbic pathway, which runs from the ventral tegmental area to the ventral striatum in the mid-brain. This pathway deals with reward learning, and if overstimulated can develop pathologies resulting in compulsive behaviour. Agonist drugs stimulate dopamine receptors in the brain to inhibit some of the dysfunctional side effects of treatment for Parkinson's with L-DOPA. They were developed in the 1970s after a decade of failed pharmacological attempts to compensate for L-DOPA's shortfalls and adverse side effects.[65]

L-DOPA was first developed by the Oxford-trained Viennese pharmacologist, Oleh Hornykiewicz. Following Carlsson's discovery of the true biological function of dopamine, Hornykiewicz and his research assistant H. Ehringer examined levels of dopamine in the post-mortem nigrostriatal systems of the brains of those who had suffered from Parkinson's Disease.[66] Having discovered the dramatic loss of nigrostriatal dopamine, Hornykiewicz persuaded Walter Birkmayer, an ex-SS officer who was now working at the Vienna Geriatric Hospital in Lainz, to administer L-DOPA to twenty Parkinson's Disease patients.[67] L-DOPA is the naturally occurring L-isomer of the amino acid D, L-dihydroxyphenylalanine. In 1938, Peter Holz had discovered that the enzyme L-amino acid decarboxylase (DOPA) converts the biologically inert L-DOPA into the biologically active catecholamine dopamine. The discovery of enzymes and metabolic hormones for rebalancing physiological systems became a dominant avenue of scientific research from the early twentieth century,[68] but Birkmayer was initially reluctant to use L-DOPA for Parkinson's Disease patients because he clung to his belief that reduction in hypothalamic serotonin was responsible for the condition. In 1961, however, Birkmayer agreed to intravenously administer 50 mg of L-DOPA to a single patient, who dramatically improved, and then agreed to administer 150 mg to twenty patients with moderate and severe Parkinson's Disease. Hornykiewicz and Birkmayer presented their results at the Viennese Medical Society in 1961, reporting that:

> The effect of a single intravenous injection of L-DOPA in Parkinson's Disease was, in short, a complete abolition or substantial relief of akinesia. Bedridden patients who were unable to sit up, patients who could not stand up from a sitting position, and patients who, when standing, could not start walking, performed all these activities after L-DOPA with ease. ... The voiceless, aphonic speech, blurred by palilalia and unclear articulation, became forceful and clear again as in a normal person.[69]

From the outset, adjunct therapies such as the administration of a monoamine oxidase inhibitor (MAOI) were tried to improve the effects of L-DOPA, especially to counteract the 'wearing off' period resulting from the short half-life of two hours of the dopamine precursor. While scepticism persisted about the efficacy of L-DOPA, in the late 1960s George Costzias demonstrated the emphatic anti-Parkinsonian impact of increasing dosage over a prolonged period of time. In 1969, Costzias began mixing L-DOPA with a peripheral dopa decarboxylase inhibitor (MK485) which diminished the dosage needed to control symptoms, and also reduced nausea and anorexia experienced by patients taking the drug.[70]

Further experiments with dopa decarboxylase inhibitors were pursued for the next decade in an attempt to improve the impact of L-DOPA, but the most serious side effects of motor fluctuations, uncontrollable jerking movements, dyskinesias and loss of drug efficacy in some patients persisted. These issues were not effectively addressed until the development of dopamine agonist drugs.

Apomorphine synthesised from morphine was first used in 1884 to treat Parkinsonism in patients with Sydenham's chorea and experimental efforts to treat Parkinson's Disease.[71] Although dopamine agonists synthesised from ergot were also experimented with to treat Parkinson's Disease from the end of the nineteenth century, it was in the 1960s that prolactin inhibitors, such as the ergot-derived bromocriptine, were shown to reduce dopamine turnover in hypothalamic and nigrostriatal dopaminergic neurons.[72] These discoveries led, in the 1970s, to the introduction of ergot-derived dopamine agonists to stimulate post-synaptic dopamine receptors in order to overcome the therapeutic shortfalls of L-DOPA and compensate for the loss of pre-synaptic pigmented neurons in the *substantia nigra*. By the mid-1970s, a range of dopamine agonists were developed that effectively prolonged dopamine receptor stimulation. By the early 1990s five dopamine receptors had been discovered,[73] and dopamine agonists such as bromocriptine, lisuride, pergolide and newer synthetic ergolines such as carboline were developed to produce prolonged stimulation as a monotherapy in early stage patients to provide a neuroprotective role. They were subsequently introduced as an adjunct therapy in increasingly advanced patients to overcome the adverse side effects of L-DOPA. Some non-ergoline-derived agonists, such as ropinirole and pramipexole, were further developed both as monotherapies in early stage patients and for compensating for L-DOPA shortfalls and side effects in patients with more advanced disease.[74]

However, problems emerged with dopamine receptor stimulation beyond the nigro-striatal dopaminergic pathway. As Chang and Grace note, patients 'with Parkinson's Disease who are treated with dopamine agonists to compensate for depletion in the motor systems often develop dysfunctions in reward-based learning, including impulse control disorders'.[75] These developments, they argued, 'were directly linked to pathological behaviors ultimately leading to definitional addictions, in recent years attention has been drawn to a complex group of impulse control disorders such as pathological gambling, hypersexuality, and compulsive eating or shopping.[76] 'These are usually triggered by dopamine agonist treatment and conceptualised as behavioral addictions associated with aberrant or excess stimulation of dopaminergic reward mechanisms.'[77]

Chang and Grace have posited that this may result from more rapid degeneration of some dopaminergic neurons than others. Motor loss results from dopamine degeneration in the dorsal tier of the *substantia nigra compactia* (SNC). However, the ventral tier of the SNC and the ventral tegmental area (VTA) may be affected less. Thus dopamine replacement therapies such as L-DOPA and agonist treatments may result in overstimulation where differential dopamine loss has been less marked, especially in the ventral tegmental area of the brain: 'because the medial SNC and VTA system are relatively spared', they argue, 'intact neurons could be over-stimulated as the dopamine agonist works across the entire system, with the consequence that pathologically high levels of dopamine receptor stimulation in limbic regions could occur. Such over-stimulation may increase the likelihood of Parkinson's Disease patients to develop impulse control disorders, such as pathological gambling, compulsive shopping, and hypersexuality.'[78]

In search of therapeutic balance

Clinical literature has increasingly emphasised the necessity of pursuing therapeutic balance in agonist treatment.[79] When considering the new prescription or increasing the dose of a dopamine agonist, expected benefits in motor nervous control must be balanced against the increased latent risk of impulse control disorders as well as other potential serious side effects. An extensive discussion in the clinical literature has explored staged therapeutics in which agonist drugs are used as the sole treatment for patients in the earliest stages of Parkinson's Disease, with the aim that their known neuroprotective function could delay the degeneration of motor function. In patients at later stages of the disease, agonists are subsequently recommended as adjunct treatment for the control of dyskenisias and to prevent or delay the development of dementia.[80] However, with regard to the control of the emergence of impulsive behavioural symptoms there is a lack of consensus other than the recommendation of 'fine-tuning':[81]

> It would seem pragmatic to be particularly watchful in the higher risk groups – especially younger males, those with prior mood disorders, obsessive-compulsive behavior, or drug, alcohol, or substance abuse history, and there is a clear need to be proactive in including a close family member or their prime carer in this advice.[82]

As several chapters in this volume show, families were often important conduits for medical advice and chronic disease management in the twentieth century. In literature on Parkinson's Disease, patients and families were warned that withdrawal of agonist drugs, or transfer from one to another, needed to be gradual and closely reviewed for adverse effects. However, all agreed that there was a significant lack of evidence on which to develop protocols for clinical practice.[83]

The clinical dilemma and search for therapeutic balance – and the interpretation of key moments of transition in management and experience of illness – is acutely illustrated in cases in which creativity has been diagnosed as a compulsive disorder resulting from the adverse effects of D2 receptor stimulation. A case reported by Jaime Kulisevsky and his group in 2009 exemplified the dilemmas faced in agonist therapeutic management where creativity in a Parkinson's patient is diagnosed as a pathological compulsion or addiction.[84] Noting earlier reports by Walker, Schrag and Chatterjee, Kulisevsky described a patient who was 47 years old; he was an amateur painter before being diagnosed with Parkinson's Disease, but his interest in art diminished after he was first medicated and became depressed with mild apathy. He retired from his employment, and nothing changed in his behavioural profile until two years later when the dopamine agonist cabergoline was added to his L-DOPA treatment. His motor symptoms significantly improved and he began painting again, but with a dramatically changed attitude towards his artistic endeavour. Prior to Parkinson's Disease he took months to complete a painting and his work was detailed and figurative, focusing on accurately depicting reality. Now he started to produce one painting a week, and his paintings grew more and more impressionistic, emphasising colour and light rather than detail. The patient explained the change as a need to 'express his refreshed inner emotions'.[85] Within

Creativity and pathology in Parkinson's Disease 301

nine months he painted every day and started showing and selling his work in local galleries. Kulisevsky et al. focused, however, on what they perceived to be degeneration into addiction as the patient began to continue painting through the night and his work pattern became disruptive to his family. They considered that his dysphoric response to suggestions that he should stop painting was a symptom of addiction to the activity. According to Kulisevsky, the patient regarded his artwork as 'positive for him as he was able to move more easily and he felt emotionally relieved', and no other behavioral changes occurred such as hypersexuality, dopamine dysregulation syndrome or other impulsive behaviours. Because the team considered the patient's artistic focus socially disruptive, cabergoline was withdrawn over a period of six weeks, during which the patient notably decreased his artwork and became increasingly apathetic and depressed.[86] They then increased L-DOPA, but the patient did not resume painting. Reinstituting cabergoline therapy at 4 mg per day led to the patient painting again with the same intensity; when cabergoline was reduced to 2 mg per day he stopped painting at night. The clinical team believed they had finally achieved the right therapeutic balance to manage what they interpreted as continuous dopaminergic stimulation through dopamine agonists producing 'a pathological usurpation of the neural mechanisms of creativity'.[87]

Balancing cultures of creativity: patients' meanings

In contrast to the neurobiological pathologisation of Parkinson's Disease patient art as a form of hectic compulsion, narrative accounts by patients themselves describe their creative work as establishing a sense of calm, release and transcendence equivalent to the experience of meditative Zen. Patients' narratives describe the relationship of their illness and creative work as an opportunity to experience new ways of what it means to be human. For Parkinson's patients, the impact of the illness on their creativity is accounted for in terms of humanistic meaning rather than biologically coded spirituality.

Johanne Vermette is a Parkinson's Disease patient who is a professional artist, a mother and a physician at Montreal University. Vermette was diagnosed with Parkinson's Disease in her late thirties and believed that her painting style became enhanced after her diagnosis: 'The new style is less precise but more vibrant ... I have a need to express myself more. I let myself go, sometimes painting with enraged fingers.'[88] Vermette is familiar with the theoretical view about the influence of her medication on her imagination, but she perceives her practice of painting through the night as a way to manage the chronic insomnia that accompanies Parkinson's and allows her undisturbed time while her children sleep. She sums up the experience of enhanced creativity as: 'When I paint I'm in the best place, because I am only doing that. There's no planning, no hierarchy of actions, but just the urgency of living.'[89] Urgency to paint for Vermette is not characterised as compulsive addiction, but rather as calming release.

Similarly, in contrast to creativity defined as pathologically hectic compulsion in the neuropsychomolecular paradigm, Parkinson's patient Gwendoline Spurll, a haemotologist at McGill University, argues that artistic expression has given her a new Zen-like quality in her life generally and in her clinical practice, which is often commented on by her patients.[90] Spurll began painting in 2003 prior to her Parkinson's Disease diagnosis, when she focused on expressing the desolation she had felt during a period of her life twenty years earlier while struggling with infertility. Following her diagnosis of Parkinson's Disease in 2005 she started to focus on the existential dialectics of the embodied perception of joy and dismay:[91] dismay that her Parkinson's would one day force her to end her clinical career and probably leave her home, but joy that she would at least be able to paint, probably throughout the duration of her degenerative condition.[92] 'Does painting affect my practice as a physician?', Spurll asks. 'I think so. My patients often describe my bedside manner as calm, even Zen.' Spurll accounts for this as a sort of transference of her own experience in sitting down with a blank canvas and starting to paint. For her it induces 'a calm state in my mind that removes me from the imperfections of my life – and it convinces me that patients can likewise accept whatever confronts them. Apparently this conviction is communicated to my patients through my calmness.'[93] Citing Sacks's discussion of the disruption of self-expression inhibition in neurological patients with lesions such as frontal lobe dementia, Spurll ponders whether this effect noted in Parkinson's patients was also happening to her.[94] 'What does this mean?', Spurll asks, 'I don't know.' What she does know is that painting 'induces a flow state, and removes from my consciousness the constant knowledge of my physical limitations. It is like a meditation. It is my Zen.'[95]

For another artist, Alan Babbitt, however, the relationship between his Parkinson's Disease and his creativity has nothing to do with therapeutics. For Babbitt, Parkinson's became an opportunity in much the same way as Henri Matisse described the impact of illness on his artistic life-world over a century ago:[96] Parkinson's Disease stimulated the creation of an entirely new artistic genre which he calls tremor enhanced photography.[97] Babbitt has been a locally renowned San Francisco Bay Area artist since the 1970s. His initial interest in photography stemmed from the transformative visual experience it gave him, having impaired vision from albinism, nystagmus, lazy eye and profound myopia.[98]

Babbitt makes fun of his 'addiction' to photography, admitting to becoming shamelessly 'high' on it, breaking trespass laws in order to feed his habit. When the movement disorders of Parkinson's began to appear for the first time in 2003, 'darkness filled my viewfinder'. He lost interest in photography, rarely venturing out to shoot, and was bored with the results. One night on the Las Vegas Strip – 'of all places', he says in disbelief – 'I began to see the light ... I began to let the tremor have its way as I clicked the shutter.'[99] The experience was 'Whoa!! ... The visual gumbo of flashing lights, multi-tinted neon and watery reflections became wonderful smears, blurs and streaks of color. Now THIS was fun!'[100] Beyond the sheer exuberance of the work, Babbitt describes an epistemological shift in understanding photography and Parkinson's Disease: 'Liberated from the photo dogma of "still"ness and sharpness, I've experienced a rush of creative freedom like never before. Rules? Who needs rules?'[101] Babbitt puts it this way: 'The damn disease has given me a terrific gift!'[102]

Conclusion

According to Aristotle, 'There is no great genius without a tincture of madness.'[103] The complex relationship between creativity and cultural representations of pathological mentalities has a long contested history, from theories about epilepsy in the ancient world to investigations of schizophrenia and bipolar disorder in the twentieth and twenty-first centuries.[104] In this chapter a new moment of that contested history between pathology and creativity – and the shifting balance between them in medical and patient understandings of illness – has been examined in the context of the artistic work of patients suffering from Parkinson's Disease.

Parkinson's Disease currently remains a neurodegenerative disease that has effective pharmacological management tools that relieve suffering, including L-DOPA and dopamine agonists. Elsewhere I have documented the experience of the disease in an era before L-DOPA, when acute suffering, decline and premature mortality resulted from disablements in motor function.[105] However, as scientific understanding of the disease developed throughout the late twentieth century, Parkinson's Disease became less a singular nosological entity defined by motor nervous dysfunction than a cascading process of multi-layered biological and behavioural transformation.[106] In a neuromolecular framework, the behavioural consequences of dopaminergic death, substitution and stimulation have increasingly preoccupied scientific and clinical discourses on pathology. Over the last four decades a neuropsychobiological model of a genetically predetermined Parkinson's personality emerged within these discourses, reinforced by biopsychological measurement tools such as Cloninger's tridimensional paradigm. The neuromolecularly predetermined Parkinson's Disease personality has been characterised as measurably low novelty-seeking, high harm-avoiding, inflexible and apathetic. When the genetically predisposed low-creativity paradigm of the Parkinson's personality is disrupted by artistic expression in patients, it is therefore frequently interpreted clinically as a pathological symptom of excessive stimulation of dopamine receptors in the reward–learning mesolimbic pathway, producing compulsive behaviour and addiction. Creativity is redefined in this context as an unintended pathological behavioural by-product of therapeutic intervention.

The search for evidence-based 'best practice' in dopamine agonist treatments has therefore preoccupied clinical literature since their introduction,[107] and has so far not moved beyond anecdotal protocols advocating flexibility or adaptive clinical management aimed at achieving a balance between motor function improvement and behavioural equilibrium.[108] Clinical debates concerning balance and the regulation of artistic self-expression do not, however, address how the fuller dimensions of balance might be considered and explored. As this chapter has shown, the notion of therapeutic balance needs to be considered within broader discussions of the clash between patient experiences, scientific knowledge and clinical understanding. Neuromolecular psychobiological characterisations of the relationship between creativity and Parkinson's Disease have generated a counter-culture represented in the narratives articulated by patients, according to which ontological stasis is replaced with emergence, changing the relationship between embodiment and becoming. As a result, sufferers have dispersed the materiality of disability by creating the meaning of shifting embodiments for themselves and others: for example by engaging, expressing and disseminating the contradictions of dread and subliminal exquisiteness through artistic work, thereby unfolding the consequences of the misfolding proteins that are causing their degenerative physical change. In Parkinson's patients' accounts of their experiences of creativity, Paul Longmore's vision of a new meaning of ability becomes a material possibility.[109] For Parkinson's patients engaged in creative artistic work, the essentialist concept of disability disappears into limitless opportunities for creating meaning, not out of being but out of incessantly becoming human.

Notes

1 University of California, San Francisco, 'Projected worldwide increase in prevalence of Parkinson's disease in 2005 and 2030 (in million patients)', Statista website (2018), available at www.statista.com/statistics/215459/projected-worldwide-increase-in-prevalence-of-parkinsons-diseas/, accessed 21 August 2019.
2 'Parkinson's Disease Statistics', *Parkinson's News Today* (2018), available at https://parkinsonsnewstoday.com/parkinsons-disease-statistics/, accessed 21 August 2019.
3 Parkinson Association of the Carolinas, *Statistics on Parkinson's Disease* (2018), available at www.parkinsonassociation.org/understanding-parkinsons/, accessed 21 August 2019.
4 Parkinson's UK, *The Incidence and Prevalence of Parkinson's Disease in the UK: Results from the Clinical Practice Research Datalink Summary Report* (December, 2017), available at www.parkinsons.org.uk/about-us/media-and-press-office, accessed 27 September 2019.
5 'Parkinson's disease', *The Free Dictionary* (2018), available at https://medical-dictionary.thefreedictionary.com/parkinson%27s+disease, accessed 21 August 2019.

6 D.-H. Choi et al., 'Therapeutic potential of induced neural stem cells for Parkinson's Disease', *International Journal of Molecular Sciences*, 18 (2017), 224.
7 O. Hornykiewcz, 'A brief history of L-DOPA', *Journal of Neurology*, 257 (2010) (Suppl 2), S249–52.
8 E. Tolossa et al., 'History of L-DOPA and dopamine agonists in Parkinson's Disease treatment', *Neurology*, 50 (1998) Suppl., S2–10; discussion S44–8.
9 S. Khanam and Y. H. Siddique, 'Dopamine: agonists and neurodegenerative disorders', *Current Drug Targets*, 19 (2018), 1599–1611; K. Radad et al., 'Short review on dopamine agonists: insight into clinical and research studies relevant to Parkinson's Disease', *Pharmacological Reports*, 57 (2005), 701–12.
10 See Chapters 2, 8 and 9 in this volume. On cultural normativity in biomedical discourse, see W. Ernst, *History of the Normal and the Abnormal: Social and Cultural Histories of Norms and Normativity* (London: Routledge, 2006).
11 S. Finger, *Origins of Neuroscience: A History of Explorations into Brain Function* (Oxford: Oxford University Press, 1994), p. 1. S. Jacyna and S. T. Casper (eds), *The Neurological Patient in History* (Rochester, NY: Rochester University Press, 2012).
12 R. Porter, *Mind Forg'd Manacles: A History of Madness in England from the Restoration to the Regency* (London: Penguin, 1990).
13 J. Parkinson, *An Essay on the Shaking Palsy* (London: Sherwood, Neely and Jones, 1817), p. 1.
14 Parkinson, *An Essay*, p. 19.
15 See R. Porter and G. S. Rousseau, *Gout: The Patrician Malady* (New Haven, CT: Yale University Press, 2001); R. Porter, 'Consumption: disease of the consumer society', in J. Brewer and R. Porter (eds), *Consumption and the World of Goods* (London: Routledge, 1994), pp. 58–84; S. Sontag, *Illness as a Metaphor* (New York: Farrar, Straus and Giroux, 1978); M. Jackson, *The Age of Stress: Science and the Search for Stability* (Oxford: Oxford University Press, 2013).
16 Parkinson, *An Essay*, pp. 9–19.
17 C. Goetz, 'Charcot on Parkinson's Disease', *Movement Disorders*, 1(1986), 27–32.
18 A. Hustvedt, *Medical Muses: Hysteria in Nineteenth Century Paris* (New York: W. W. Norton, 2011); M. Micale, 'The Salpêtrière in the age of Charcot: an institutional perspective on medical history in the late nineteenth century', *Journal of Contemporary History*, 20 (1985), 703–31.

19 C. Goetz et al., *Charcot: Constructing Neurology* (New York: Oxford University Press, 1995).
20 Goetz, 'Charcot on Parkinson's Disease'.
21 C. Goetz, 'The history of Parkinson's Disease: early clinical descriptions and neurological therapies', *Cold Spring Harbor Perspectives in Medicine*, 1 (2011), 1–15.
22 Ibid., p. 5.
23 N. Ruiz-Gómez, 'The "scientific artworks" of Doctor Paul Richer', *Medical Humanities*, 39 (2013), 4–10, at p. 8.
24 A. Lees et al., 'The black stuff and Konstantin Nikolaevich Tretiakoff', *Movement Disorders*, 23 (2008), 777–83.
25 L. C. Triarhou, 'Constantin von Economo (1876–1931)', *Journal of Neurology*, 254 (2007), 550–1; Y. Kaya et al., 'Constantin von Economo (1876–1931) and his legacy to neuroscience', *Child's Nervous System*, 32 (2016), 217–20.
26 A. M. Rodrigues et al., 'Who was the man who discovered the "Lewy bodies"?', *Movement Disorders*, 25 (2010), 1765–73.
27 On the emergence of physiology, neurophysiology and neurendocrinology in the redefinition of neurological pathology, see Jackson, *The Age of Stress*.
28 S. Fahn, 'The history of dopamine and L-DOPA in the treatment of Parkinson's Disease', *Movement Disorders*, 23 (2008) Suppl. 3, S497–S508; O. Hornykiewicz, 'Dopamine miracle: from brain homogenate to dopamine replacement', *Movement Disorders*, 17 (2002), 501–8; D. L. Roe, 'From DOPA to Parkinson's Disease: the early history of dopamine research', *Journal of the History of the Neurosciences: Basic and Clinical Perspectives*, 6 (1997), 291–301.
29 'Arvid Carlsson', in L. R. Squire, *A History of Neuroscience in Autobiography, Volume 2* (New York: Academic Press, 1998), pp. 95–134; A. Carlsson, 'A half-century of neurotransmitter research: impact on neurology and psychiatry. Nobel lecture', *Bioscience Reports*, 21 (2001), 691–790.
30 Ibid.
31 S. Ovallath and B. Sulthana, 'L-DOPA: history and therapeutic applications', *Annals of Indian Academy of Neurology*, 20 (2017), 185–9; Fahn, 'The history of dopamine and L-DOPA in the treatment of Parkinson's Disease'; Hornykiewicz, 'Dopamine miracle'; Roe, 'From DOPA to Parkinson's Disease'.
32 M. Bliss, *The Discovery of Insulin* (Chicago: Chicago University Press, 1982); and Jackson, *The Age of Stress*.
33 H. Y. Meltzer and S. M. Stahl, 'The dopamine hypothesis of schizophrenia: a review', *Schizophrenia Bulletin*, 2 (1976), 19–76.

34 D. Ball et al., 'Dopamine markers and general cognitive ability', *Neuroreport*, 9 (1998), 347–9; S. Nakajima et al., 'The potential role of D3 receptor neurotransmission in cognition', *European Neuropsychopharmacology*, 23 (2013), 799–813, doi: 10.1016/j.euroneuro.2013.05.006, epub 2013 Jun 20.
35 Quoted in C. D. Camp, 'Neurology', in W. B. Shaw, *The University of Michigan, an Encyclopedic Survey* (Michigan: University of Michigan Libraries, 1951), pp. 856–7.
36 Porter and Rousseau, *Gout*; D. Arnold, 'Diabetes in the tropics: race, place and class in India, 1880–1965', *Social History of Medicine*, 22 (2009), 245–61; Jackson, *The Age of Stress*.
37 A. J. Lees, 'The pre-morbid personality of patients with Parkinson's Disease', *Journal of Neurology, Neurosurgery and Psychiatry*, 48 (1985), 97–100; L. Ishihara and C. Brayne, 'What is the evidence for a pre-morbid Parkinson's personality: a review', *Movement Disorders*, 28 (2006), 1066–72; W. Poewe, 'The preclinical phase of Parkinson's Disease', in D. B. Calne, R. Horowski, Y. Mizuno, W. Poewe, P. Riederer and M. B. H. Youdim (eds), *Advances in Research on Neurodegeneration*, vol. 1 (New York: Birkhauser, 1993), pp. 43–5.
38 C. J. Todes and A. J. Lees, 'The pre-morbid personality of patients with Parkinson's Disease', *Journal of Neurology, Neurosurgery and Psychiatry*, 48 (1985), 97–100.
39 Ibid.
40 On biopsychosocial models of disease, see S. Nassir Ghaemi, *The Rise and Fall of the Biopsychosocial Model: Reconciling Art and Science in Psychiatry* (Baltimore: Johns Hopkins University Press, 2009); R. E. Thayer, *The Biopsychology of Mood and Arousal* (Oxford: Oxford University Press, 1989); and T. C. Schneirla, 'Problems in the biopsychology of social organisation', *Journal of Abnormal and Social Psychology*, 41 (1946), 385–402.
41 C. R. Cloninger, 'A unified biosocial theory of personality and its role in the development of anxiety states', *Psychiatric Developments* 4 (1986), 167–226.
42 E. J. Devor and R. C. Cloninger, 'Genetics of Alcholism', *Annual Review of Genetics*, 23 (1989), 19–36; G. Hellinga et al., 'Robert Cloninger', in G. Hellinga et al. (eds), *Personalities: Master Clinicians Confront the Treatment of Borderline Personality Disorder* (Northvale, NJ and London: Jason Aronson, 2001), pp. 99–120. For discussion of alcohol studies, see Chapter 3.
43 C. R. Cloninger et al., 'The Tridimensional Personality Questionnaire: US normative data', *Psychological Reports*, 69 (1991), 1047–57; C. R.

Cloninger et al., 'A psychobiological model of temperament and character', *Archives of General Psychiatry*, 50 (1993), 975–90; C. R. Cloninger et al., 'Psychometric properties of the temperament and character inventory – revised in a Belgian sample', *Journal of Personality Assessment*, 85 (2005), 1931–46.

44 P. Heiden, 'Pathological gambling in Parkinson's Disease: what are the risk factors and what is the role of impulsivity?', *European Journal of Neuroscience*, 45 (2017), 67–72; X. H. Castro-Martínez, 'Behavioral addictions in early-onset Parkinson disease are associated with DRD3 variants', Parkinsonism & Related Disorders, (2018). pii S1353–8020(18)30011–7.

45 M. Reuter et al., 'The influence of the dopaminergic system on cognitive functioning: a molecular genetic approach', *Behavioral Brain Research*, 164 (2005), 93–9.

46 M. Reuter et al., 'Identification of first candidate genes for creativity: a pilot study', *Brain Research*, 1069 (2006), 190–7; D. L. Zabelina, 'Dopamine and the creative mind: individual differences in creativity are predicted by interactions between dopamine genes DAT and COMT', *Plos One*, 19 January 2016, doi: 10.1371/journal.pone.0146768.

47 The mesolimbic dopaminergic pathway connects the ventral tegmental area in the mid-brain to the ventral striatum of the basal ganglia in the forebrain. The ventral striatum includes the nucleus accumbens and the olfactory tubercle.

48 S. Sapra, 'A combination of dopamine genes predicts success by professional Wall Street traders', *Plos One*, 7 (January 2012), 1–7, e30844.

49 T. Suhara, 'Dopamine D2 receptors in the insular cortex and the personality trait of novelty seeking', *Neuroimage*, 13 (2001), 891–5; L. K. Teh et al., 'Tridimensional personalities and polymorphism of dopamine D2 receptor among heroin addicts', *Biological Research for Nursing*, 14 (2012), 188–96, doi: 10.1177/1099800411405030, epub 2011 May 25; S. W. Savage et al., 'Regulation of novelty seeking by midbrain dopamine D2/D3 signaling and ghrelin is altered in obesity', *Obesity (Silver Spring)*, 22 (2014), 1452–7, doi: 10.1002/oby.20690.

50 See, for example, R. Tomer and J. Aharon-Peretz, 'Novelty seeking and harm avoidance in Parkinson's Disease: effects of asymmetric dopamine deficiency', *Journal of Neurology, Neurosurgery and Psychiatry*, 75 (2004), 972–5, doi: 10.1136/jnnp. 2003. 024885; V. Kaasinen et al., 'Personality traits and brain dopaminergic function in Parkinson's Disease', *Proceedings of the National Academy of Sciences of the USA*, 98 (2001), 13272–7, epub 2001 Oct 30. See also, for example, the popular book written by I. Briggs Myers with P. B. Myers, *Gifts Differing: Understanding Personality*

Types (Palo Alto, CA: Consulting Psychologists Press, 1980); see also Jackson, *The Age of Stress*.
51 M. A. Menza et al., 'Dopamine-related personality traits in Parkinson's Disease', *Neurology*, 43 (1993), 505–8; M. A. Menza et al., 'Personality correlates of [18F]dopa striatal uptake: results of positron-emission tomography in Parkinson's Disease', *Journal of Neuropsychiatry and Clinical Neurosciences*, 7 (1995), 176–9.
52 Ibid.
53 G. Pluck and R. G. Brown, 'Cognitive and affective correlates of temperament in Parkinson's Disease', *Depression Research and Treatment*, (2001), Article ID 893873, 8 pages, doi: 10.1155/2011/893873; G. C. Pluck and R. G. Brown, 'Apathy in Parkinson's Disease', *Journal of Neurology, Neurosurgery and Psychiatry*, 73 (2002), 636–42.
54 A. Schrag, 'Poetic talent unmasked by treatment of Parkinson's Disease', *Movement Disorders*, 16 (2001), 1175–6.
55 Ibid.
56 Ibid., p. 1176. For parallel discussions about bipolar patients and creativity, see F. K. Goodwin and K. R. Jamison, *Manic-Depressive Illness: Bipolar Disorders and Recurrent Depression* (Oxford: Oxford University Press, 2007).
57 R. Walker et al., 'Augmentation of artistic productivity in Parkinson's Disease', *Movement Disorders*, 21 (2006), 285–6.
58 Ibid., p. 285.
59 Ibid., p. 286.
60 For a critique of chemical imbalance theories of psychiatric disease, see J. Moncrieff, *The Myth of the Chemical Cure: A Critique of Psychiatric Drug Treatment* (London: Palgrave Macmillan, 2008).
61 A. Chatterjee et al., 'Art produced by a patient with Parkinson's Disease', *Behavioral Neurology*, 17 (2006), 105–8.
62 Ibid., p. 106.
63 Editors, 'Creative and living with Parkinson's? Showcase your work in the Mervyn Peake Awards', *Parkinson's Life. A Voice for the International Parkinson's Community*, 10 March 2016, available at http://parkinsonslife.eu/creative-and-living-with-parkinsons-showcase-your-work-in-the-mervyn-peake-awards/, accessed August 2019.
64 P. Schwingenschuh et al., 'Artistic profession: a potential risk factor for dopamine dysregulation syndrome in Parkinson's Disease?', *Movement Disorders*, 25 (2010), 493–6, at p. 493.
65 Tolossa et al., 'History of L-DOPA and dopamine agonists in Parkinson's Disease treatment'.

66 Hornykiewicz, 'A brief history of L-DOPA'; Tolossa et al., 'History of L-DOPA and dopamine agonists in Parkinson's Disease treatment'.
67 H. Czech and L. A. Zeidman, 'Walter Birkmayer, co-describer of L-DOPA and his Nazi connections. Victim or perpetrator?', *Journal of the History of the Neurosciences*, 23 (2014), 160-91.
68 See the biography of Edward C. Kendall for discussion of the discovery of levothyroxine, available at *Nobel Prizes*, www.nobelprize.org/nobel_prizes/medicine/laureates/1950/kendall-bio.html (2018), accessed August 2019; for work that preceded Kendall on organs of internal secretion by J. F. Gudernatch, see J. D. Furlow and E. S. Neff, 'A developmental switch induced by thyroid hormone: *Xenopus laevis* metamorphasis', *TRENDS in Endocrinology and Metabolism*, 17 (2006), 38-45; on insulin see Bliss, *The Discovery of Insulin*.
69 W. Birkmayer and O. Hornykiewicz, 'The effect of 1-3,4-dihydroxyphenylalanine (=DOPA) on akinesia in parkinsonism', *Parkinsonism and Related Disorders*, 4 (1998), 59-60, at p. 60, originally published in German in *Wiener Klinische Wochenschrift*, 73 (1961), 787-8.
70 Tolossa et al., 'History of L-DOPA and dopamine agonists in Parkinson's Disease treatment', S3.
71 Ibid.
72 R. Horowski, 'A history of dopamine agonists. From the physiology and pharmacology of dopamine to therapies for prolactinomas and Parkinson's Disease. A subjective view', *Journal of Neurotransmission*, 114 (2007), 127-34.
73 For the history of receptor theory see V. Quirke, 'Putting theory into practice. James Black, receptor theory and the development of beta-blockers at ICI, 1958-1978', *Medical History*, 50 (2006), 69-92.
74 Radad et al., 'Short review on dopamine agonists'.
75 C.-H. Chang and A. A. Grace, 'Some dopamine neurons may be more impulsive than others: why differences in receptors and transporters can affect dopamine function in Parkinson's Disease', *Movement Disorders*, 28 (2013), 1319-20.
76 For historical contextualisation of the emergence of definitions of addiction see V. Berridge, J. Walke and A. Mold, 'From inebriety to addiction: terminology and concepts in the UK 1860-1930', *Social History of Alcohol and Drugs*, 28 (2014), 88-105.
77 Ibid.
78 Ibid.
79 D. G. MacMahon and G. J. A. Macphee, 'Dopamine agonists and impulse control disorders in Parkinson's Disease', *Progress in Neurology and*

Psychiatry, 12 (2008), 5–9. For comparative discussion in diabetes, see Chapter 2.
80 P. Jenner, 'The rationale for the use of dopamine agonists in Parkinson's Disease', *Neurology*, 45 Suppl. 3 (1995), S6–S12; L. M. Shuman, 'How to succeed in using dopamine agonists in Parkinson's Disease', *European Journal of Neurology*, 7 Suppl. 1 (2000), 9–13.
81 Shuman, 'How to succeed', p. 13.
82 MacMahon and Macphee, 'Dopamine agonists and impulse control disorders in Parkinson's Disease', S8.
83 Ibid.
84 J. Kulisevsky et al., 'Changes in artistic style and behavior in Parkinson's disease: dopamine and creativity', *Journal of Neurology*, 256 (2009), 816–20.
85 Ibid., p. 817.
86 For parallel discussion of social as well as physiological considerations in chronic disease management, see M. Moore, 'Food as medicine: diet, diabetes management, and the patient in twentieth century Britain', *Journal of the History of Medicine and Allied Sciences*, 73 (2018), 150–67.
87 Kulisevsky et al., 'Changes in artistic style', p. 819.
88 S. Pinker, 'Art Movements', *CMAJ*, 166 (2002), 224, available at www.ncbi.nlm.nih.gov/pmc/articles/PMC99284/, accessed August 2019.
89 Ibid.
90 G. M. Spurll, 'Zen and the art of painting', *CMAJ/JAMC*, 181 (2009), 175–9.
91 Ibid. See also M. Merleau-Ponty, *Phenomenology of Perception* (London and New York: Routledge, 2012; 1st edition Paris: Gallimard, 1945).
92 Ibid.
93 Spurll, 'Zen and the art of painting', p. 178.
94 Ibid., p. 178; O. Sacks, *Musicophilia: Tales of Music and the Brain* (New York: Alfred Knopf, 2007), pp. 270–83.
95 Spurll, 'Zen and the art of painting', p. 90; see also Sacks, *Musicophilia*, pp. 270–83.
96 See T. Zausner, *When Walls Become Doorways: Creativity and the Transforming Illness* (New York: Harmony Books, 2006), pp. 21–5.
97 A. Babbitt, 'Movement disorder. Un-still photography', available at www.abproductions.com/movement_disorder/movement_disorder_ss.html, accessed August 2019.
98 A. Babbitt, 'The photographer with lousy vision. Confessions of a photo addict', available at www.abproductions.com/about/about.html, accessed August 2019.
99 Ibid.

100 Ibid.
101 Ibid.
102 Ibid.
103 Aristotle (384–322 BC), *Problemata*, 30.1. Attributed to Aristotle by Seneca the younger, 'On the tranquility of mind' (17.10).
104 See J. Derrida, 'Cogito and the history of madness', in J. Derrida, *Writing and Difference* (Chicago: University of Chicago Press, [1967] 1978), pp. 31–63.
105 D. Porter, 'Tremor: the experience of Parkinson's Disease from the shaking palsy to neurobiological compulsion', *Canadian Bulletin for the History of Medicine*, forthcoming.
106 B. Patoine, 'Facing up to the "New Face" of Parkinson's Disease. An interview with Anthony E. Lang', news release, *Dana Foundation* website (2012), 1–3 (no longer available).
107 D. Deleu et al., 'An evidence-based review of Dopamine receptor agonists in the treatment of Parkinson's disease', *Neurosciences*, 7 (2002), 221–31; MacMahon and Macphee, 'Dopamine agonists'; J. A. Borovac, 'Side effects of a dopamine agonist therapy for Parkinson's Disease: a mini-review of clinical pharmacology', *Yale Journal of Biology and Medicine*, 89 (2016), 37–47.
108 Deleu et al., 'An evidence-based review'; MacMahon and Macphee, 'Dopamine agonists'.
109 P. K. Longmore, *Why I Burned My Book and Other Essays on Disability* (Philadelphia: Temple University Press, 2003).

11

Conclusion: balance, malleability and anthropology: historical contexts

Chris Millard

Introduction

The conference that first incubated contributions to this collection was held at the University of Exeter over two days in June 2016 and coincided with the national referendum on Britain's membership of the European Union. On Friday morning, the irony of speaking about histories of 'balance' as the country proceeded to plumb some of the most polarised depths in recent memory did not pass unremarked. Some months previously, an invitation had been sent to potential speakers, giving some suggestions and guidance regarding the focus and structure of the contributions. The panel that I was on was intended to 'help set up many of the themes taken up in the rest of the conference', and panel members were encouraged to highlight 'the role of institutions and organisations in the construction of the balanced self' and to go beyond ideas of 'individual agency'. This was initially a welcome suggestion: charting the 'construction of the self' in various ways remains at the core of my research interests. The idea that human beings are embedded in structures of thought, institutions and practices – historical horizons of possibility – is one of my grounding assumptions in the history of medicine.

After some reflection, however, the request to provide a reflexive springboard or foundation for the rest of the conference, a role that I am usually pleased to perform, provoked some disquiet. What caused me to pause were the following questions: If this idea of a constructed

Conclusion: historical contexts 315

selfhood is to be a conceptual foundation, then what are *its* foundations? Where am I standing? More precisely, what am I standing on, or pushing off from? Where does the notion that the 'balanced self' is just one possible, historically and institutionally specific way of being human come from?

As the various contributions in this volume have shown, there are many kinds of balanced personhood. They relate to specific local conditions, specific authoritative discourses, prescribed or proscribed practices, institutions or ideas. But it is important to differentiate between these different conceptions of balance and a more basic set of assumptions that lies beneath them. I now want to look more broadly at the foundation we are standing on when speaking of different 'balanced selves' at all. This concluding chapter, then, deals with intellectual and conceptual foundations, but we must pay attention to the source basis – and its omissions – for understanding. One of the common threads here is that humans' selves are ripe for intervention and remaking, that they can be worked on, balanced, rebalanced and reconfigured. But there is another sense that I want to explore. All these accounts presume that the changing notions of balance correspond to the possibilities available in time, in culture, in context. They are based, in short, on an idea that human beings are malleable, and that this malleability is shaped in historically and culturally specific ways.

One source for the idea that one's human-ness is constructible and malleable is that it is related to environments, institutions and local, particular factors. It is on this malleable humanity that we draw when talking of constructing a historically, environmentally specific 'balanced human'. The term 'malleable humanity' comes from Margaret Mead's controversial anthropological classic, *Coming of Age in Samoa* (1928). This signposts the area that I want to explore. How far are the malleable, plastic humans that populate social constructivist studies rooted in a specific, flourishing moment in twentieth-century anthropology? My sources here are anthropological texts, created through extensive fieldwork, interviewing, transcription and translation of interviews – practices that are not neutral or free of power dynamics.[1] This anthropological moment is associated with three names above all: Margaret Mead, Bronisław Malinowski and Franz Boas. I want to explore the history of anthropology and its related assumptions about human plasticity. This will help reflections on how we might build and critique notions of balanced humans. Finally, I hope to lay out some of the politics of this and to historicise the discussion: Why is this happening now? Why, early in the twenty-first century, might malleable humanity become more visible? An awareness of the contingency and specificity of our methodological tools brings our own present into focus – a particular present in which we wield these tools, and which bounds the histories we are able to produce.

Plastic human nature and anthropology

'Culture' is the most important concept in anthropology. The meaning of this word – as used in anthropology – shifted around the turn of the twentieth century, from culture as a universal measurement of civilisation, to culture describing a specific local environment. Anthropologist Philippe Descola noted recently in his important book *Beyond Nature and Culture* that one of the most influential formulations of the word 'culture' comes from Edward B. Tylor in 1871 (an important Victorian anthropologist). Descola argues that Tylor's formulation is so influential that it is

> traditionally regarded, so to speak as the birth certificate of modern anthropology ... Here, culture is not distinguished from civilization ... This was the view adopted by the evolutionary anthropologists of the last third of the nineteenth century. It accepts the possibility and necessity of comparison between societies arranged in order of their cultural institutions, which are more or less elaborated expressions of a universal human tendency.[2]

Culture here functions as a measuring stick, a universal scale. In less technical prose, Anna Green and Kathleen Troup argue that, according to this notion: '[s]ocieties and cultures were slotted into appropriate stages along the path of human development'. Naturally enough, 'the institutions and values of Europe were the apotheosis'.[3] Thus culture operates as a scorecard for various societies, enabling anthropologists to position them on the road towards Western Europe – the final destination and the epitome of 'culture' in this sense. At the dawn of the twentieth century, however, this idea of culture began to be displaced by another concept under the same term. As Descola writes: 'The strictly anthropological concept of culture did not appear until later. It was only at the turn of the twentieth century, in the ethnographic work of Franz Boas, that there emerged the idea that each people constitutes a unique and coherent configuration of material and intellectual features.'[4] Culture as a universal measurement is replaced by a sense of culture as an autonomous, coherent whole, as something to be studied in its specificity.

Heinrich Rickert (1863–1936), a leading neo-Kantian philosopher of the late nineteenth and early twentieth centuries, is seen by Descola as a prominent source of this notion of 'culture', later to be taken up by Boas, Malinowski, Mead and others. Although Rickert did classify the study of 'primitive peoples' as belonging to the natural sciences, his broad conception of culture functioned to 'carve out the space in which twentieth century anthropology would be able to operate. It would be a study of cultural realities, rather than natural realities.' Culture and nature are divided here in 'an implacable epistemological separation' that is not innate or inherent, but powerful nevertheless.[5]

This separation endured until the late twentieth century. Anthropologist Bernard S. Cohn, surveying anthropological practice in 1980, argues that the earlier idea of 'culture' 'rests on assumed biological determinants of human culture and society'. Biology is clearly associated with the notion of culture-as-measuring-stick. He further claims that this idea 'throws out ... the one central fact that anthropology has discovered – people lead meaningful lives, and that these meanings can only be discovered within the context of those lives, it cannot be imputed to them on the basis of some previously established ideas about the biological or psychological makeup of people'.[6] The focus of this twentieth-century anthropological culture concept is on contextual meaning, without necessitating an overarching comparison. So how does this shift happen in anthropology, and how does this relate to history? Here I want to deal specifically with how this notion of context-specific 'malleable humanity' begins to influence historians – particularly 'social constructionist' historians.

Bronisław Malinowski's anthropological classic, *The Argonauts of the Western Pacific* (1922), is a watershed for anthropology. Malinowski's approach to fieldwork demands that the ethnographer is fully immersed in the 'life of the native' and not just working through paid informants and sitting on the verandah of the mission station. Thus, according to Vincent Debaene's lucid study of French anthropology, the anthropologist's aim is to 'immerse himself, to soak up another culture, to "live from the inside" the experience of the "native"'. Further, this constitutes a 'privileging of the personal, concrete and psychological aspects of field experiences'.[7] This immersive fieldwork technique is not to everyone's taste. As the prominent anatomist and Egyptologist Grafton Elliott Smith rather acidly observes, he cannot understand why 'the sole method of studying mankind is to sit on a Melanesian island for a couple of years and listen to the gossip of the villagers'.[8]

As well as bringing the notion of 'experience' to the fore (which will later provoke questions of whose experience is *able* to be foregrounded), this method allows Malinowski to sketch out the ways in which he believes culture impacts one's core personhood:

> their mental states receive a certain stamp, become stereotyped by the institutions in which they live, by the influence of tradition and folk-lore, by the very vehicle of thought, that is by language. The social and cultural environment in which they move forces them to think and feel in a definite manner. Thus, a man who lives in a polyandrous community cannot experience the same feelings of jealousy, as a strict monogynist, though he might have the elements of them.[9]

Here is an idea of a radically plastic selfhood (or perhaps 'pre-self'), which is rooted in a specific kind of twentieth-century anthropology, and grows out of a particular conceptual opposition between 'nature' and 'culture'. It is important to remember that the anthropological fieldwork method allows Malinowski to *ventriloquise* rather than reveal this experience of the man in the polyandrous community. It is Malinowski who has the (imperial) power of speech, argumentation, editing, publication and so on. It is *his* reading and writing of the situation that is privileged, even as he attempts to centre his subject. However, his metaphor of the 'stamp' here implies that there is some universal blank slate on which our personhood materialises; it also establishes and foregrounds a tight relationship between what it is possible to think, and the constraints and possibilities of language. Most importantly (for we shall deal with the history of the emotions a little later), Malinowski argues that although there might be elements of feelings that are common across cultures, one cannot experience emotions such as jealousy in the same way in different cultures.

Conclusion: historical contexts

Six years later, in 1928, Margaret Mead celebrated the manifold differences in the process of adolescence ('coming of age') between North America and Samoa. Mead writes that 'neither race nor common humanity can be held responsible for many of the forms which even such basic emotions as love and fear and anger take under different social conditions'. But straight from this disavowal of common humanity she deploys something universal, writing of 'babies who have as yet no civilization to shape their malleable humanity'.[10] In fact, a fuller quotation bears analysis:

> With such an attitude towards human nature the anthropologist listened to the current comment upon adolescence. He heard attitudes which seemed to him dependent upon social environment ... ascribed to a period of physical development. And on the basis of his knowledge of the determinism of culture, of the plasticity of human beings, he doubted.[11]

As Roger Smith has noted, 'Mead argued with her vivid example [Samoa fieldwork] that culture rather than fixed biological determinants control a child's development.' Indeed, Smith quotes Mead as arguing that 'human nature is almost unbelievably malleable, responding accurately and contrastingly to contrasting cultural conditions'.[12] The passage from Mead focuses on adolescence. This idea of particularly significant transitional periods in the human life course is present in other discussions in the early twentieth century around physiology, adaptation, evolution and stress. In these discussions, the transitions (whether menopause, adolescence or another time of physiological change) had the potential to impair future adaptability, future malleability.

It is clear that anthropological discussions of nature/culture are not the only place that visions of malleable personhood emerge. One link between evolutionary thought and anthropological discussion can be seen in the work of W. H. R. Rivers, a doctor trained in physiological and psychological medicine who embarked (on something of a whim) on the Cambridge Expedition to the Torres Strait; he later did ethnographic work in India and the Solomon Islands.[13] It is as psychiatrist to First World War poet Siegfried Sassoon that Rivers is best known, and Rivers's evidence to the War Office Committee of Enquiry into 'Shell-Shock' shows how his work is explicitly concerned with adaptation, specifically with the effects of being unable to adapt to circumstances.

He argues that 'Every animal has a natural reaction to danger ... and man's is manipulation of such a kind as to get him out of the dangerous situation ... If he cannot have that, or if it is restricted in any way, you have a prominent condition for the occurrence of neurosis.'[14] Rivers, both psychiatrist and anthropologist, explicitly roots the problem of war neurosis in the frustration of evolutionary urges to adapt to situations.

Mead is mentored in her anthropological endeavours by Franz Boas, who writes an appreciative foreword to *Coming of Age in Samoa*. He claims 'much of what we ascribe to human nature is no more than a reaction to the restraints put upon us by our civilization.'[15] Boas, like Malinowski and Mead, ascribes special significance to language, and the way it influences thought. In 1920, he argues that 'the categories of language compel us to see the world arranged in certain definite conceptual groups which ... impose themselves upon the form of our thoughts'.[16] This approach to language in Boas and Malinowski, drawing out its formative influence on thought, is characteristic of much social constructivist history. Boas is also clear that he tries to treat these cultures as independent and coherent, arguing that 'on the whole the unique historical character of cultural growth in each area stands out as a salient element in the history of cultural development'.[17]

I am not arguing that the malleability of human nature is simply or exclusively an anthropological invention. We find it in a number of places in the early to mid-twentieth century, from the above-mentioned discussions of adaptation and evolution, to the varied concepts of psychoanalysis, where early experiences are said to mould future character and pathology to an enormous extent. This emerges very clearly in child guidance.[18] It is also evident in some strands of sociology – even as part of those ideas that deploy concepts of culture as a measure of civilisation.[19]

What I am arguing instead, is that an important and influential strand of this idea comes out of anthropology, as well as psychoanalysis. The similarities were visible to authors at the time. For example, Boas explicitly tackles this similarity between his ideas and those of Freud:

> It is certainly true that the influence of impressions received during the first few years of life have been entirely underestimated and that the social behavior of man depends to a great extent upon the earliest habits which are established before time when connected memory begins, and that many so-called racial or hereditary traits are to be considered rather

as of early exposure to a certain form of social conditions. Most these habits do not rise into consciousness and are, therefore, broken with difficulty only. Much of the difference in the behavior of adult male and female may go back to this cause.[20]

The links between psychoanalysis and ethnology/anthropology are also legion. Rivers is another reference point here, heavily influenced by Freudian psychoanalysis and the practice of anthropology. At the end of his enormously influential history of European human sciences, *The Order of Things*, Michel Foucault argues that:

> we can understand why psychoanalysis and ethnology should have been constituted in confrontation, in a fundamental correlation: since [Freud's 1913 work] *Totem and Taboo*, the establishment of a common field for these two, the possibility of a discourse that could move from one to the other without discontinuity.[21]

So perhaps the roots of this malleability cannot fully be grasped without probing the depths of psychoanalysis and evolutionary stress theory too, although I can only deal with anthropology here. However, under the influence of the anthropological output of Malinowski, Boas and Mead, plasticity provides a significant intellectual platform, foregrounding a vision of human nature that is fundamentally moulded by circumstance.

I have written elsewhere about the relationship between another prominent Foucauldian philosopher (Ian Hacking), the history of the self and a particular twentieth-century flourishing of anthropology.[22] Vast numbers of historians have built on the idea that one's self is malleable, constructible and fundamentally related to material and intellectual conditions. But the idea that the self is malleable *at all* seems to escape investigation. This idea – which is progressive, inclusive and open – falls into the category that Hayden White calls 'precritical' when talking of historical works: 'they contain a deep structural content which is generally poetic, and specifically linguistic in nature, and which serves as a precritically accepted paradigm of what a distinctively "historical" explanation should be.'[23] Thus, in the same way, nineteenth-century anthropology is animated by the idea of culture as a yardstick of progress, and 'Boasian culturalism' (to use the sometimes pejorative shorthand) inverts the whole *idea* of this hierarchy. It does not invert the hierarchy itself (reversing the positions on the scale) but inverts the idea: from a vertical conception of difference to a horizontal one. This horizontal conception of culture, this cultural relativism is the 'deep structural content' of twentieth-century anthropology and poststructuralist history. Human nature here is malleable and the differences are non-hierarchical. Thus far I have only gestured at ways in which history has been influenced by anthropology. The following section puts flesh on those bones.

Anthropology and histories of balance

Simon Susen has written a useful if rather jargon-heavy survey of *The 'Postmodern Turn' in the Social Sciences*. He argues that according to this turn: '[i]f there is anything essential about culture, it is its normalising capacity to make human actors treat socially contingent parameters of validity as naturally given laws of facticity'. In other words: one of the things that culture seems to do in all cases is to present the various rules and regulations that constitute it as though they are natural givens. Susen notes that 'anthropology teaches us that there is no essence to the human condition, apart from people's dependence upon culturally variable arrangements, constellations and interpretations. In other words, social history constitutes an ensemble of constantly developing – and, thus, spatiotemporally contingent – life forms.'[24] There are two points to note. One is that the essential unifying principle of the concept of 'culture', according to 'anthropology', is that it is dis-unified and non-essential in every other way. The other point is the telling slippage from 'anthropology teaches us ...' to 'social history constitutes ....'. This link between social history and anthropology is precisely what I am trying to tease out.

In Stuart Sim's *Irony and Crisis: A Critical History of Postmodern Culture*, he locates an important battle within the discipline of history in an exchange in the influential historical journal *Past and Present* in the early 1990s. This debate begins with Lawrence Stone (social historian of the early modern family) penning an attack on what he calls 'postmodernism': he views it as an 'ever-narrowing trap' and wonders 'if history might be on the way to becoming an endangered species.'[25] Stone isolates three strands of this 'trap': Derridean linguistics and deconstruction, New Historicism and contextualism, and (usefully for this conclusion) what he calls 'cultural and symbolic anthropology'. Stone's disdain for deconstruction is obvious as he directs readers to an article that has performed a 'damaging exposure of the many logical flaws in this form of argument'. New Historicism fares slightly better: 'at first sight a welcome return to the study of the text in its ... context'; but it ultimately comes unstuck because, according to Stone, it 'treats political, institutional and social practices as "cultural scripts", or discursive sets of symbolic systems or codes'. Quite why this is so contemptible is not made explicit by Stone. However, when he comes to symbolic anthropology, he has some much kinder words, calling it:

> at first enormously liberating and finally rather threatening [it] comes from the influence of cultural and symbolic anthropology as developed by a brilliant group of scholars headed by Clifford Geertz, Victor Turner, Mary Douglas and others. Their work has influenced many of the best historians of the last decade.[26]

There is clearly something valuable that Stone discerns in this anthropology: a productive cross-pollination of ideas. It also shows how 'postmodernism' (at least in part) is seen to grow out of anthropology. Another, more extended rearguard action against 'postmodernism' comes from Richard J. Evans in his *In Defence of History* (1997). He glosses this *Past and Present* debate, and engages with Catriona Kelly's response to Stone, citing her argument that historians can adopt 'an aggressive attitude' to the sources, focusing on 'secondary layers of meaning' and 'reading against the grain'.[27]

Part of Evans's argument in *In Defence of History* is that historians already do 'read against the grain' (which has somehow become conflated with whatever it is 'postmodernists' do), and this reading practice comes from a now familiar source: 'The real question at issue here is *what enables us* to read a source "against the grain", and here theory does indeed come in.'[28] His first example is anthropological theory developed in the study of twentieth-century rural Africa, used by Keith Thomas to explore early modern European witchcraft.[29]

This does not, of course, make Keith Thomas a 'postmodernist'. However, it highlights the exchange between social history and anthropology more generally. It shows how practices that are seen as part of 'postmodernism' in the 1990s are influenced by practices lifted from anthropology in the 1980s. Bernard Cohn sees deep connections between history and anthropology – the former making difference over time intelligible, the latter doing the same for space. He argues that they 'have a common subject matter, "otherness" ... one field constructs and studies "otherness" in space, the other in time. Both fields have a concern with text and context. Both aim, whatever else they do, at explicating the meaning of actions of people rooted in one time and place, to persons in another.'[30] Clearly anthropological ideas have been influential more generally. Even harsh critics of 'Boasian culturalism', such as Derek Freeman, admit as much: Freeman quotes a historian of American anthropology, who characterised such 'culturalism' as 'fundamental to all of American social science' as long ago as 1973.[31]

The links between postmodernist history and anthropology are hopefully clear. One effect of this traffic between disciplines is to bring to the fore ideas of *selfhood* as radically malleable. As Cohn argues: 'the reconceptualization of culture, not as a set of social or economic elements, but as a "pattern" of *psychological* elements ... hence the concern with the relationship between culture and personality. What was authentically cultural was then psychological, rooted in personality.'[32] Here we see concerns with selfhood, personality, history, culture, ethnology and psychoanalysis all present. Malleable selfhood and anthropology (along with psychoanalysis) are distinctively twentieth-century phenomena in the humanities.

Elwin Hofman has recently laid out 'How to do the history of the self', and rightly cautions against assuming that a concept as broad as the self has only one meaning. Eight are mentioned, including, at number two in the list: 'the cultural conception of the individual'. Two of the three scholars referenced are Clifford Geertz and Marcel Mauss.[33] Hofman argues that a 'sense of a stable self has always been disrupted by discourses of flexibility and malleability.'[34] This may well be true, but here we are charting a particular instance of instability as a product of a particular resonance between history and anthropology at a certain time. In fact, in the early twentieth century, myriad stress researchers (the most famous of whom is Walter Cannon) were building a conception of human beings as balanced and stabilised through concepts of homeostasis and research into the autonomic nervous system.[35] At a particular point in time, stability and malleability circulate in different registers.

Hofman buttresses his claim by citing Stephen Greenblatt's work on *Renaissance Self-Fashioning*. Greenblatt's work, which I briefly discuss elsewhere,[36] does claim to find a malleable sense of self in the Renaissance. However, he explicitly builds this claim on the work of twentieth-century anthropologists: Paul Rabinow, Victor Turner, Clifford Geertz and Mary Douglas, among others; he explicitly wants to 'practice a more cultural or anthropological criticism.'[37] The fact that he reads malleable selfhood through Geertz, Turner et al. means that he risks projecting that selfhood onto the Renaissance as much as he is able to find it there.

Anthropology is not the *only* source of this idea of 'malleable humanity', but it is an influential one. Postmodern, post-structuralist cultural historians spend much time unpicking the assumptions and contexts of their actors, and often leave their own untouched – this is why I am trying to 'pick at' the way a particular form of anthropology is an unacknowledged foundation, part of a 'deep structural content', of constructivist history. There is a strong argument here that to be intellectually consistent, we must unpick our assumptions, just as we uncover those of people in the past.

Many of the contributions in this volume focus on an individualisation of the responsibility for balance. Three examples will illustrate the point tolerably – if not comprehensively. Jane Hand's work on obesity visualisation shows how 'balanced selves' are bound up with notions of self-regulating consumers. This has a sharp political dimension, as 'selves' correspond to dominant economic ideologies. Hand argues – persuasively – that the 'individualisation of risk in this period enabled the state to reframe individuals as a new type of health citizen incorporated into a balanced conception of rights and responsibilities ... persuading the individual to act as a self-conscious and self-regulated consumer ... establishing a new social contract with the state'. Ayesha Nathoo, in Chapter 6, carves out a space for 'assessment of the consequences of teaching individuals to cultivate relaxed, balanced selves'. Again, individualisation and self-cultivation are central. Political concerns emerge, but the politics of the methodological insight that enables us to see selfhood as adaptable are less visible. Layering this analysis with an awareness of *its own specificity* enriches the narrative further

– not simply that it is possible because of a particular set of methodological tools, used in the present, but that this analysis of obesity and public health is itself politically charged in the context of further welfare retrenchment, stigmatisation of claimants and a further retreat of the state from responsibility for health.

Nicos Kefalas's argument about the rise of self-care is similarly charged with contemporary relevance, and he talks explicitly about the embrace of 'the notion of self-reflective, self-governing individualism' and links it to ideas of 'efficiency'. The contemporary relevance of this – to us *now* in 2019 – is left largely unsaid. Awareness of the contingency of the methodological tools we wield in the present, in pursuit of present objectives, according to our present resources, capacities and privileges, can bring this to the forefront of our awareness. Different conceptions of balance are parsed through a historically specific idea of malleable humanity: this awareness prompts an acknowledgement that *we are using these particular tools in a particular present*. Many of the contributions focus on how 'balance' transforms through reference to a 'consumer'. The visibility of this frame of reference – humans as autonomous, self-regulating, competitive, market-driven beings – is part of an economic common sense that is creaking and breaking apart *as we write these histories*. Historians are always writing about their present context, even as they write about the past. The different conceptions of balance and different ideas of selfhood could be deepened and made richer by an acknowledgement that they are based in a particular reading of anthropology – a particular mixture of self-understandings, or changing self-understandings that also need to become reflexive. When we acknowledge the present that bounds us, it not only helps to uncover the gaps or blank spots in one's analytical frameworks, but makes clear the contemporary political freight carried by all histories.

There is another specific reason why we should nurture this awareness of our methodological tools. Broadly speaking, what might be called the 'culturalism' or 'malleable humanity' thesis has come under attack from those who wish to give biology a greater role as a motive force for culture and behaviour. This concern is not new, as one such biological argument shadows Mead's argument above. Mead sets her hypothetical anthropologist up as doubting the role of 'physical development' that is thought to provoke the behaviour of adolescents.

Conclusion: historical contexts

What I am instead arguing is that a certain strand of thinking about malleability becomes influential and intertwined with certain philosophical approaches in the history of medicine and wider medical humanities. Cohn describes a certain kind of anthropological history, reading it explicitly against ideas of 'nature':

> All culture is constructed. It is the product of human thought. This product may over time become fixed ways of doing things. It may also be changed. Since culture is always being constituted and constructed, so it is also always being transformed. Cultures and societies are not natural objects. It is only through culture that we construct nature, not the other way around.[38]

This is very much the language of the early 'postmodern' historians, speaking of the 'social construction' or 'cultural construction' of race or gender in the past.

Why now? The return of biology

Having established that a strand of 'postmodern' or 'post-structural' thinking draws on insights from twentieth-century anthropology, we might ask whether it remains legitimate to project these twentieth-century insights back further into the past. I have answered this question in the negative elsewhere: I do not think it particularly good history to assume that selfhood in the past is the same as selfhood in the twentieth century. This is for the same reasons that I do not think it legitimate to diagnose medieval saints as anorexic, or as experiencing migraines. These concepts and categories are the product of certain times and places, and a significant part of their reality concerns how people understood themselves in relation to these categories. If the categories did not exist, I do not see how the people in the past could meaningfully inhabit those diagnoses. Others have made this point eloquently, with varying degrees of forcefulness.[39] The projection of the categories of one period of time onto the humans of another period flattens and collapses how these people lived, acted and understood themselves. Thus we can say (of 'balance' specifically) that its meaning and political purchase is fundamentally variable, and to collapse into one the malleability of cultural anthropology, the dynamic balance of the autonomic nervous system or the balance of various neurotransmitters is to obscure much of their specific, contextual resonance and meaning.

My point here is to ask a different question: How is it that this anthropological foundation becomes apparent now? What is it about our contemporary world that makes this position possible? The answer might be summed up as 'the return of biology'[40] to the social sciences, although it never really went away. People throughout history have had varying understandings about the material of their bodies, and the ways in which their natures are essential, fixed, flexible, rigid or otherwise. What has changed in the early twenty-first century is that new understandings of biology have come roaring back into the academic humanities, bringing with them new opportunities, risks and consequences. This is why the anthropological, 'culturalist' basis of post-structuralism has been thrown into relief. The rest of this section is a brief sketch of one way this has happened, and why I want to defend the idea of malleable humanity. This defence, however, must be in full knowledge of where this malleability comes from, what its limits are and the kind of politics it enables.

The history of the self emerges more fully as part of social or cultural history in the 1980s and 1990s. Much of this builds on Michel Foucault's late ideas around 'technologies of the self'.[41] In 1991, Lynn Hunt criticised Foucault's approach as ahistorical, since '[al]though the forms of self-transformation vary over time in Foucault's analysis, the grounds of its psychic possibility do not'. Foucault's concept is, she argues, 'a distinctly modern or post-eighteenth-century formulation, in which individuals are figured as separate beings with separate selves who are able to act upon themselves and even transform themselves'.[42] Indeed, Hunt's analysis in the early 1990s has much in common with what is being pursued here, attempting to historicise the very idea that one's self might be malleable. She charges that Foucault 'cannot imagine a self other than the one newly deployed in the eighteenth century'.[43] There is much value to this critique, especially the way in which Foucault rashly 'extends this notion' of the self back to ancient Greece in his work on the history of sexuality.[44] However, elsewhere Foucault does write about the historically specific emergence of 'separate beings with separate selves' in his work on penology in *Discipline and Punish*. Here he argues that 'for a long time ordinary individuality – the everyday individuality of everybody – remained below the threshold of description'.[45]

Conclusion: historical contexts

In any case, Hunt is absolutely right that notions of selfhood ought to be historicised; it ought not to be just presumed that social and cultural context alter or 'stamp' or 'construct' malleable selves in the same way. Fast forward two decades and Hunt's views on selfhood have changed. In 'The self and its history' (2014) she argues that 'given the uncertainties about selfhood (what it is and how it is produced), it might seem that any history of the self is next to impossible'.[46] However, one way she attempts to resolve this difficulty is to borrow from a particular reading of neuroscience: 'Despite many reasons for caution, an ongoing dialogue with neuroscience offers the prospect of new approaches to such perennially vexed issues as agency, experience, action, and identity.' She cautions that '[n]euroscience does not provide a handy model' that historians can simply apply to their research. It functions more like psychoanalysis once did (and still does for some); as a field, it poses important questions and opens up new approaches to the mind, the self, and human behavior.'[47] The mention of psychoanalysis is telling here – given the links between malleable selfhood, psychoanalysis, anthropology, 'culturalism' and postmodernism. Neuroscience here supplants other frames of reference, and it does not look so flexible. Neuroscience – or at least one popularised version of it – becomes a frame of reference competing with anthropologically influenced culturalism.

Drawing on the popularising work of neuroscientist Antonio Damasio, Hunt argues that '[t]he self is a perspective rooted in a relatively stable, endlessly repeated biological state that gets its core from the structure and operation of the organism and then develops through slowly evolving biographical data.'[48] The core self is here fixed as an 'endlessly repeated biological state', and it is only later that 'biographical' (or social, or cultural) data have an effect. My problem with this is not that it is straightforwardly wrong – in a number of senses, it is not. The problem is that it establishes a more or less definite split between nature and culture, and privileges the former. It cannot see, much less accept, that the ways in which human beings conceptualise nature (or science, or reality, or whatever) is already indelibly cultural. Lorraine Daston and Peter Galison show authoritatively how even as core a scientific concept as 'objectivity' is itself subject to far-reaching changes over time.[49] Why then should the 'neuroscience' of the late twentieth and early twenty-first centuries form a reliable guide for historical selfhood? Additionally, as Ruth Leys has shown, many of the scholars who rely (directly or indirectly) on neuroscientific findings to buttress their work rely heavily on popularisers like Damasio, rather than the peer-reviewed scientific content.[50] One reason for this, as Martyn Pickersgill has shown in the case of epigenetics,[51] is that there is often no unproblematic sense of coherence about a science among many of its influential practitioners.

My point here is not to enter into a detailed critique of the ways some in the humanities are appropriating neuroscientific (and epigenetic) insights to buttress or structure their work. Surveys and analyses of this traffic between the humanities and neuroscience (and other life sciences) exist, from the trenchant critiques of Roger Cooter and Ruth Leys,[52] through the pessimistic cautions of Martyn Pickersgill, Jörg Niewöhner and Tim Newton,[53] to the cautious but more open stance of Felicity Callard, Des Fitzgerald, Nikolas Rose, Joelle Abi-Rached and Ilina Singh, among many others.[54] Instead, my point here is to show that this shift towards friendlier cooperation between the life sciences and the human sciences is exposing the foundations of the old regime. This constructivism is not a denial of biology, as Steven Pinker has argued in his influential work *The Blank Slate*.[55] As Chris Renwick notes, Pinker disregards the fact that many social scientists simply have a different notion of the kinds of things that are inherited: 'many social scientists, social reformers, and politicians were comfortable with hard heredity because its implication was that each generation started from scratch in biological terms'.[56] In fact, the 'standard social science model' is enabled by a bedrock of hard heredity, even as it sees itself as anti-biological.[57] This is about the kind of boundary that is drawn between nature and culture, not disregarding one or the other. It is where malleable humanity comes from: a particular field of interest, with a specific boundary drawn between nature and culture. This boundary is changing.

As my remarks imply, I believe that these collaborations are risky for the humanities, and the rewards are relatively slim. There are obviously a huge number of questions begged by even this brief account of the ways in which human and life sciences intertwine. As Renwick recently cautioned: 'I'm not the greatest enthusiast for the idea that there are lessons that can be derived from history but one thing that does seem quite clear is that we should beware anyone who thinks they've got an easy application of biology to society.' Renwick is open to ideas of collaboration, as well as investigating how the differences and

Conclusion: historical contexts   331

entanglements *between* these disciplines have been formed *historically*: 'taking the mid-twentieth-century programmes of forced sterilisation in the USA and the Nazi regime as the obvious and only consequences of earlier ideas and assuming that people like Galton envisaged them [is problematic]. The history is much more complicated than that and a starting point for unravelling it is highlighting how it is actually embedded into the political world we still inhabit.'[58]

But what has changed? One of the reasons is that developments in epigenetics once again allow conceptual space for the 'social setting' or 'cultural environment' to impact on the core of humanity, envisioned in more or less biological terms. The other is the rise of neuroscience, and its partial adoption by those interested in 'affect theory' and, more generally, by historians of the emotions. Neuroscience and epigenetics have reconnected with the humanities, throwing light on the roots of the old models as fields shift and new approaches come into focus. As new collaborations now seem possible, it is also important to defend the insights of the humanities as critical tools to open up the claims of these sciences to scrutiny.

It is necessary to recognise, as Renwick says, that the 'contours of the debate about biology look very different now to twenty years ago, when the Human Genome Project promised to be the capstone of one hundred years of genetic science. The result, of course, was more questions than answers.'[59] I have written elsewhere about the relationship between cultural anthropology, the new genetics and criticisms of Margaret Mead.[60] Renwick anticipates the thrust of the qualms expressed here about the return of biology:

> Historically speaking, one of the major concerns about closer relations between biology and sociology has been that the latter will end up being colonized by the former ... Criticisms [of sociobiology and evolutionary psychology] quite rightly focused on the naturalization of conservative and reactionary ideas about the origin of things like gender identities. Whether one is for or against opening dialogue with biology, it is possible to accept that biosocial science need not be shaped by those values.[61]

I am not against collaboration, but I am cautious of the very real power dynamics at play: genomics and neuroscience do not 'need' social sciences for financial support, or to make their case to society more broadly for their value. In fact the reverse is the case. Funding is important here. Renwick notes that there exist 'lots of resources available for carrying out [such collaborative] research ... In an era of declining budgets for social science research, funding councils will look favourably on work that intersects with biology, not only because it will make bold claims that, if history is any guide, will not be delivered, but also because it will promise the kind of scientific credibility that governments periodically suggest the social sciences lack.'[62] Fitzgerald and Callard make a similar point in their book on rethinking collaboration with the neurosciences.[63] In any case, Renwick and Fitzgerald and Callard see more to be gained than lost: in Renwick's words, 'it is essential social scientists help decide what form [collaboration] takes.'[64]

It is difficult to practise such collaboration while both: a) remaining credible about what social sciences can offer when placed in a collaborative relationship with the life sciences; and b) maintaining a critical and independent stance. One recent example of this is Fitzgerald, Rose and Singh's article, 'Revitalizing sociology', in the *British Journal of Sociology* (2016), which advocates for collaboration between epigenetic science and sociology. Another is Callard and Fitzgerald's short book, *Rethinking Interdisciplinarity* (2016), about the theory and practice of collaborating with neuroscientists.[65] I have chosen these examples because they represent the best of those seeking collaboration: thoughtful, critical, generous and clear-sighted. They anticipate – eloquently and assiduously – the problems mentioned here, even as they press forward in calling for collaboration. The only thing I cannot share with these pieces is their optimism.

Fitzgerald, Rose and Singh argue that: 'We are committed to the view that there is no role for sociology as an add-on, or a "service" discipline here. Precisely the opposite: the history that we have explored teaches us that it is precisely a sociological form of attention that can help to thicken and enliven the connections that clinicians, epidemiologists, and neurologists are tracking between mental health and the metropolis.'[66] There is a significant slippage between not being an add-on, and then being precisely that: what can it mean to 'thicken' and 'enliven' if not to be added later, to be non-essential to the processes at work, to be an optional extra? This is not to nitpick, but to show how difficult it is to write and collaborate in a way that is credible and conceivable in the current climate and that is not – in essence – subservient to the life sciences. Callard and Fitzgerald admit, in *Rethinking Interdisciplinarity*, that social sciences are now able to collaborate with the life sciences because of changes in the latter's approach that admit the former's insights as relevant: 'there has been a qualitative shift, from the direction of the biological sciences, in perceptions of the grip that social life is thought to exert on the biology of the body'.[67] The shift towards inclusion has come from the life sciences. Callard and Fitzgerald argue elsewhere that 'we know well that awkward questions remain about the epistemological politics at stake within these generous-looking invitations'.[68] Similarly, Fitzgerald, Rose and Singh are quite clear and precise about the risks, about the caution and about the danger. I do not dispute that part of their analysis at all – they tease out many of the possible risks. But I cannot agree that they add up to a risk worth taking. They argue:

> If such a position is not without risk for the epistemological space that social scientists have carved out, those risks are outweighed by imaginary, such that the social life of the city and the molecular life of the body do not compete for priority but become mutually entangled within a complex, thickly-textured landscape of empirical research into the distribution of suffering, restoration and care.[69]

The idea that 'those risks are outweighed' and that sociology and molecular biology 'do not compete for priority' seems optimistic. Callard and Fitzgerald anticipate these points too: 'we are not naïve about how unevenly epistemic and institutional authority is likely to be distributed across such entanglements, and we do not elide the unequal dynamics of power and prestige here ... We have no fantasy of parity here.'[70] But this is precisely my point – calling for engagement across a divide that is acknowledged as vastly uneven seems questionable, to say the least. We live in a world where the life sciences have relatively vast funding and the social sciences are dwindling, instrumentalised and offered a path back to relevance if they participate in this frame of reference.

Why should these boundaries evaporate because social scientists wish to collaborate in new ways? Life sciences succeed on their own terms, attract (comparatively) huge amounts of money, and are quite comfortable sorting out their ontological and epistemological debates internally, without reference to social scientists. They are unwilling (in general, as a group) to change substantially to suit collaboration with social science, and why should they? To bring another iteration of this volume's central concept into play, the balance of power is in their favour: they are part of an entrenched, stable status quo.

Conclusion

I am fully committed to this idea of human nature being fundamentally contextual, inseparable from the various techniques with which we measure it, and the ideas we use to structure and understand it. This collection has shown how different notions of balance correspond to the various contexts in which they have been mobilised. 'Balance' has the potential to be a description, metaphor or analogy (or all three). Of course, whether or not things 'balance' depends on where you place the pivot. Like the 'political centre ground' or 'moderate politicians', balance is entirely in the eye of the beholder. That is almost a truism. But we should not forget that for people to be differently constructed or 'made up' in relation to different kinds of 'balance' requires a deep plasticity, born of a specific reformulation of a colonial concept in early twentieth-century anthropology. If we want to be reflexive and self-aware, we need to reckon with the consequences of this. We must also be more explicitly aware that this plasticity is becoming more obvious now because it is being reformulated within epigenetic or neuroscientific frames of reference.

Those pushing neurological and neo-biological visions of selfhood are aware of the kind of ground on which they stand – prestigious, highly technical life science methods. Of course, how we appraise and validate 'biology' is itself culturally and historically specific; thus any attempt to position biology as a pre-cultural foundation stone is fraught with difficulty. For those invested in plastic, context-specific notions of humanity, the question of the 'foundations of our anti-foundationalism' is rather more complex. This is a euphemistic way of saying that it is based on practices hanging over from one of the most murderous enterprises in human history: imperialism. After all, selfhood, psychology, anthropology and imperial administration are heavily entangled.[71] This is deeply troubling – but we need to reckon with this history and come out fighting. One way that the history of medicine has sought to disrupt the hegemony of science involves the mobilisation of 'personal narratives' or 'patient perspectives'. But these too are the product of history and are structured and constrained by notions of 'experience', psychoanalytic 'catharsis' and significant freight from 1960s social history.[72] It seems unwise to risk ceding the humanities to the new biology (as friendly collaboration seems ill-placed to challenge the damaging frame of reference where the social sciences are second-class add-ons), or unthinkingly picking up tools forged in the service of colonialist administration and differentiation.

But regardless of the specific contexts, there is one key aspect to be emphasised: if we can contextualise and take responsibility for the tools that we use, and thus the present contexts in which we use them, the politics of our histories emerges – not as a tacked-on 'soapbox' conclusion, but as an integral part of a methodological process. In much of this collection, balance is tightly bound with individualism, self-regulation and self-care in many of the contexts analysed. As broader questions emerge about the legitimacy of these pillars of economic common sense, the histories that we write are already implicated and bound up in them. This explicit present context is largely absent in the collection as it stands. Methodological self-awareness is one route to a robust present-centred perspective. There are no easy solutions, but we should begin by appreciating the historical context of the tools that frame our questions, and the political context in which our answers emerge.

Notes

1 M. Silverstein, 'The fieldwork encounter and the colonized voice of indigeneity', *Representations*, 137:1 (2017), 23–43.
2 P. Descola, *Beyond Nature and Culture* (Chicago: University of Chicago Press, 2013), p. 72.
3 A. Green and K. Troup (eds), *The Houses of History: A Critical Reader in Twentieth-Century History and Theory* (Manchester: Manchester University Press, 1999), p. 172.
4 Descola, *Beyond Nature and Culture*, pp. 72–3.
5 Ibid., pp. 77–8.
6 B. S. Cohn, 'History and anthropology: the state of play', *Comparative Studies in Society and History*, 22:2 (1980), 201.
7 V. Debaene, *Far Afield: French Anthropology between Science and Literature* (Chicago: University of Chicago Press, 2014), pp. 38–9.

8 G. W. Stocking, *The Ethnographer's Magic and Other Essays in the History of Anthropology* (Madison: University of Wisconsin Press, 1992), p. 58.
9 B. Malinowski, *Argonauts of the Western Pacific: An Account of Native Enterprise and Adventure in the Archipelagoes of Melanesian New Guinea* (London: Routledge, [1922] 2002), p. 23.
10 M. Mead, *Coming of Age in Samoa: A Study of Adolescence and Sex in Primitive Societies* (London: Penguin, [1928] 1954), p. 11.
11 Ibid., p. 11.
12 R. Smith, *Between Mind and Nature: A History of Psychology* (London: Reaktion Books, 2013), pp. 121–2.
13 A. Young, 'W. H. R. Rivers and the war neuroses', *Journal of the History of the Behavioral Sciences*, 35:4 (1999), 361.
14 War Office Committee, *Report of the War Office Committee of Enquiry into 'Shell-Shock'* (London: HMSO, 1922), p. 57.
15 F. Boas in Mead, *Coming of Age in Samoa*, p. 6.
16 F. Boas, 'The methods of ethnology', *American Anthropologist*, 22:4 (1920), 320.
17 Ibid., p. 318.
18 Anon., 'Reports of societies: medical aspects of child guidance', *British Medical Journal*, 1 (1948), 896–7.
19 See, for example, N. Elias, *Power and Civility: The Civilizing Process*, vol. 2 (New York: Pantheon, [1939] 1982), p. 328.
20 Boas, 'Methods of ethnology', p. 320.
21 M. Foucault, *The Order of Things: An Archaeology of the Human Sciences* (Abingdon: Routledge Classics, [1970] 2002), p. 414.
22 C. Millard, 'Concepts, diagnosis and the history of medicine: historicising Ian Hacking and Munchausen Syndrome', *Social History of Medicine*, 30:3 (2017), 567–89.
23 H. White, *Metahistory: The Historical Imagination in Nineteenth-Century Europe* (Baltimore: Johns Hopkins University Press, 1973), p. ix.
24 S. Susen, *The 'Postmodern Turn' in the Social Sciences* (New York: Springer, 2015), p. 94.
25 L. Stone, 'History and post-modernism', *Past and Present*, 135:1 (1991), 218.
26 Ibid., p. 217.
27 C. Kelly, 'History and post-modernism', *Past and Present*, 133:1 (1991), 212.
28 R. J. Evans, *In Defence of History* (London: Granta Books, 2001), pp. 81, 83.
29 Evans, *In Defence of History*, p. 83.
30 Cohn, 'History and anthropology', p. 198.

31 D. Freeman, 'Margaret Mead's *Coming of Age in Samoa* and Boasian culturalism', *Politics and the Life Sciences*, 19:1 (2000), 101–3, at p. 101.
32 Cohn, 'History and anthropology', p. 203.
33 E. Hofman, 'How to do the history of the self', *History of the Human Sciences*, 29:3 (2016), 8–24.
34 Ibid., p. 14.
35 M. Jackson, *The Age of Stress: Science and the Search for Stability* (Oxford: Oxford University Press, 2013), pp. 70–5.
36 Millard, 'Concepts, diagnosis and the history of medicine', pp. 583–4.
37 S. Greenblatt, *Renaissance Self-Fashioning: From More to Shakespeare* (Chicago: University of Chicago Press, 1980), p. 4.
38 Cohn, 'History and anthropology', p. 217.
39 C. Walker Bynum, *Holy Feast and Holy Fast: The Religious Significance of Food to Medieval Women* (Berkeley: University of California Press, 1988); I. Hacking. *Rewriting the Soul* (Princeton, NJ: Princeton University Press, 1995), pp. 234–57; A. Wilson, 'On the history of disease-concepts: the case of pleurisy', *History of Science*, 38:3 (2000), 271–319; K. Foxhall, 'Making modern migraine medieval: men of science, Hildegard of Bingen and the life of a retrospective diagnosis', *Medical History*, 58:3 (2014), 354–74.
40 T. Newton, 'The return of biology', in M. Meloni, S. Johnson Williams and P. A. Martin (eds), *Biosocial Matters: Rethinking Sociology–Biology Relations in the Twenty-First Century* (Hoboken, NJ: Wiley-Blackwell, 2016).
41 L. H. Martin, H. Gutman and P. H. Hutton (eds), *Technologies of the Self: A Seminar with Michel Foucault* (Amherst: University of Massachusetts Press, 1988).
42 L. Hunt, 'Foucault's subject in the history of sexuality', in D. C. Stanton, *Discourses of Sexuality: From Aristotle to AIDS* (Ann Arbor, MI: University of Michigan Press, 1992), p. 85; see also Hofman, 'History of the self', p. 17.
43 Hunt, 'Foucault's subject', p. 87.
44 Ibid., pp. 84–5.
45 M. Foucualt, *Discipline and Punish: The Birth of the Prison*, trans. A. Sheridan (London: Vintage, 1979), p. 191.
46 L. Hunt, 'AHR roundtable: the self and its history', *American Historical Review*, 119:5 (2014), 1579; Hofman, 'History of the self', p. 9.
47 Hunt, 'Self and its history', p. 1576.
48 Ibid., p. 1581.
49 L. E. Daston and P. Galison, *Objectivity* (Cambridge, MA: Zone Books, 2005).
50 R. Leys, 'The turn to affect: a critique', *Critical Inquiry*, 37:3 (2011), 434–72.

51 M. Pickersgill, 'Epistemic modesty, ostentatiousness and the uncertainties of epigenetics: on the knowledge machinery of (social) science', *The Sociological Review Monographs*, 64:1 (2016), 186–202.
52 R. Cooter, 'Neural veils and the will to historical critique: why historians of science need to take the neuro-turn seriously', *Isis*, 105:1 (2014), 145–54; Leys, 'Turn to affect'.
53 Newton, 'The return of biology'; Pickersgill, 'Epistemic modesty'; J. Niewöhner, 'Epigenetics: embedded bodies and the molecularisation of biography and milieu', *BioSocieties*, 6:3 (2011), 279–98.
54 F. Callard and D. Fitzgerald, *Rethinking Interdisciplinarity across the Social Sciences and Neurosciences* (Basingstoke: Palgrave Macmillan, 2016); D. Fitzgerald, N. Rose and I. Singh, 'Revitalizing sociology: urban life and mental illness between history and the present', *British Journal of Sociology*, 67:1 (2016), 138–60; C. Renwick, 'New bottles for new wine: Julian Huxley, biology and sociology in Britain', in Meloni, Johnson Williams and Martin, *Biosocial Matters*, pp. 151–67.
55 S. Pinker, *The Blank Slate: The Modern Denial of Human Nature* (New York: Viking, 2002).
56 C. Renwick, 'The task of Sisyphus? Biological and social temporality in Maurizio Meloni's *Political Biology*', *History of the Human Sciences*, 31:1 (2017), 106.
57 M. Meloni, 'Political biology: in search of a new epistemic space between STS and biopolitical theory – a response', *History of the Human Sciences*, 31:1 (2017), 138.
58 D. Fitzgerald, '"We should beware anyone who thinks they've got an easy application of biology to society" – an interview with Chris Renwick', *History of the Human Sciences*, editorial, 5 December 2016, available at www.histhum.com/we-should-beware-anyone-who-thinks-theyve-got-an-easy-application-of-biology-to-society-an-interview-with-chris-renwick/, accessed 22 August 2019.
59 Renwick, 'New bottles for new wine', p. 163.
60 Millard, 'Concepts, diagnosis and the history of medicine', pp. 587–9.
61 Renwick, 'New bottles for new wine', p. 163.
62 Ibid., p. 164.
63 D. Fitzgerald and F. Callard, 'Social science and neuroscience beyond interdisciplinarity: experimental entanglements', *Theory, Culture & Society*, 32:1 (2015), 6.
64 Renwick, 'New bottles for new wine', p. 164.
65 Fitzgerald, Rose and Singh, 'Revitalizing sociology'; Callard and Fitzgerald, *Rethinking Interdisciplinarity*.
66 Fitzgerald, Rose and Singh, 'Revitalizing sociology', p. 19.

67 Callard and Fitzgerald, *Rethinking Interdisciplinarity*, p. 49.
68 Fitzgerald and Callard, 'Social science and neuroscience', p. 6.
69 Fitzgerald, Rose and Singh, 'Revitalizing sociology', p. 15.
70 Fitzgerald and Callard, 'Social science and neuroscience', p. 16.
71 E. Linstrum, *Ruling Minds: Psychology and the British Empire* (Cambridge, MA: Harvard University Press, 2016).
72 C. Millard, 'Using personal experience in the academic medical humanities: a genealogy', *Social Theory and Health*, (2019), online ahead of print available at https://link.springer.com/article/10.1057/s41285-019-00089-x, accessed 22 August 2019.

Index

A Way of Life (film) 106–10, 117–18
Abi-Rached, Joelle 330
Aboriginal people 236–7
Abrahams, Adolphe 193
adaptational studies 235–7, 240, 242
advice literature 17–19, 50, 97–100, 104, 106, 115, 118, 135–6, 143, 162–3, 263, 268, 274
Advisory Committee on Alcoholism (ACA) 80–5
age, consciousness of 253
ageing 254–7, 262, 274
ageing population 286
agency 13–14, 133, 142–3, 148, 167, 181, 229, 329
AIDS 106
air crashes, bad year for (1972) 200
Air Navigation Orders (ANOs) 192, 195, 199–200, 203, 206, 209
Air Operators' Certificate 203
airline pilots
　hours worked by 190–2, 195
　working practices of 192, 201
airline schedules, control and regulation of 193, 199–200, 209–10

Albala, Ken 132
alcohol consumption 17, 64–88, 115
　per capita reduction in 81
　setting limits to 76–7, 81–2, 86
　wider consequences of 76
Alcohol Education Centre 71
alcohol policy network 69
alcohol pricing 81–4, 87–8
Alcoholics Anonymous 179
alcoholism 68–9, 81
alternative therapies 6
altitude physiology 223–8, 232, 234
American Medical Association (AMA) 134, 141
amphetamines 230–1, 241
'Andean man' 220
Antarctica 220, 236, 239–40
anthropology 315–16, 319–28
antidepressants 6
Apple, Rima 132, 136
Armstrong, David 34
artistic work 295, 296, 302–5
astronauts, recruitment of and support for 220, 228
Atkins, Robert (and the Atkins diet) 131, 138–42, 146–9

Index

audio recordings 164–5
audio-visual forms of education 116–17
Australia 237
autonomic nervous system 166

Babbitt, Alan 303
Bader Committee 202–7
balance
  between the interests of the individual, the family and the state 11–12, 104, 275
  between public and private interests 87–8
  between safety and commercial concerns 210
  conceptions of 2–4, 8, 10, 13–16, 21–2, 34, 54, 110, 145–6, 149, 159, 241–2, 274, 315, 326, 334
  dietary 103, 115–16, 129, 132–3, 140–1, 146
  and fatigue 192
  in health education 64, 70, 77, 97, 104–6
  and homeostatic regulation 231
  in the human body 137
  individualisation of responsibility for 325
  link with relaxation and stress 159
  in medical treatments 4–7
  in *micro* and *macro* worlds 221
  of nature 8–9
  as the pathway to health 127–9, 150
  physiological and psychological 5, 6, 7–8, 13, 35–8, 40, 45, 48, 52–4, 149, 174, 251–2, 258–9, 276, 290
  pursuit of 10–11, 17–20
  research on 219–20, 235
  in research 229, 237–8
  of risk 118
  as a scientific calculation 103
  in terms of both diet and exercise 97, 117–18
  therapeutic 37, 299–300, 304–5
  within and between duty cycles 205–8
  for women 239–40, 263
Balance (journal) 5, 48
'balanced self' concept 314–15
Beck, Ulrich 129, 264, 267, 273
Beck-Gernsheim, Elisabeth 264, 267, 273
Bernard, Claude 222
Berridge, Virginia 40, 96
biofeedback technology 165–6, 177, 180
biology, new understandings of 328
Black Report (1980) 112
blood circulation 232
blood doping 227
blood packing and blood transfusions 231
Boas, Franz 23, 315, 317, 320–1, 324
body image 96
Bowhill Working Party 195–204
Bradford Hill, Austin 66
British Airline Pilots Association (BALPA) 197–9, 208
British Broadcasting Corporation (BBC) 163–4
British Diabetic Association (BDA) 17, 33, 38, 47–50, 53–4
British Medical Journal 113, 173–4
'burnout' 20, 193, 204

Canguilhem, Georges 7
Cannon, Walter 5, 10, 129, 159, 324
Carlsson, Arvid 289–90, 296–7
cassette tapes 165

Central Office of Information (COI) 106–9
Charcot, Jean Martin 288–9, 293
childhood as a key period 113–14
China 2
circadian rhythms 201–2, 205, 242
citizenship, social 104
Civil Aviation Authority (CAA) 200–1, 206–8
civil aviation industry 20, 191–3, 200–2, 206–7
  economic considerations in 196–9
class divisions 44, 52, 177–8
'climatic aggression' 234
cold, adaptation to 235–7, 240
collectivism 198, 209
commercialisation of the language of balance 6
Committee on Medical Aspects of Food Policy (COMA) 98–9, 107
commodification of health 146, 150
compensatory mechanisms of the body 232–3
Confidential Human Factors Incident Reporting Programme (CHIRP) 208–9
Conservative Party 111–12, 198
consumerism 96–7, 100, 128
coronary heart disease (CHD) 98–9, 107–8, 116
correspondence courses 169
creativity and creative artists 296, 300–4
culture
  anthropological concept of 316–17
  construction of 327
  and nature 329–30

Denning Committee (1946) 265–6
Department of Health and Social Security (DHSS) 78–86, 99, 106, 116
Department of Trade 84
determinants of ill-health 67–8, 76, 118
diabetes, its treatment and management 16, 33–40, 45–8, 51–3, 148
diet 97–100, 104, 107, 115–17, 237–8
Dimbleby, Jonathan 112–14
divorce 264–8
documentaries 97, 106–7, 110
Doll, Richard 66
dopamine treatments 286–304
drink driving 68

early childhood experiences 320–1
eating patterns 128
ecological stability 9–10
emotional balance 5, 22, 34, 49–54, 174, 182, 260, 262, 271, 294
emotional health 204
emotional stress 239
'empty nest syndrome' 257
environmental pressures 8–9, 221
epidemiology 69, 95–8, 115, 176
epigenetics 330–2
erectile dysfunction 73
Erikson, Erik 257
Everest (mountain) 225, 227, 240
expeditionary fieldwork 222, 229
expert committees 98–9
extreme environments 20–1, 219–20, 224–6, 229, 233, 237–42
extreme physiology 222, 225, 232–5, 238–40

Index   343

family relationships 264–7, 271–3
fatigue
   acute or cumulative 199–200,
      207, 210, 224
   affecting airline crew 190–7,
      202–5, 209
   assessment of 201–2
   definition of 192–3
   medication against 230
   responsibility for management of
      196–200, 209–10
   social consequences of 210
   at work 194–5
fats, saturated and unsaturated
   99–100
feminism 12, 252–3
film 97, 106–8, 117, 175
   see also *A Way of Life*;
   *Understanding Stresses and
   Strains*
flight time limitation 192, 195–210
Flight Time Limitations Board
   (FTLB) 206–7
Food and Drug Agency (FDA) 148
food preferences and beliefs 104
foodways 130
'forty-phobia' 255–6
Foucault, Michel 11, 14, 65, 142, 181,
   321, 328
Framingham Heart Study 98
Freud, Sigmund (and Freudian
   theory) 6, 13, 250, 320–1

Gaia hypothesis 9–10
Galen and Galenic tradition 64, 129,
   138
gendered constructions 43–4, 96–7,
   100, 108, 241, 253, 255, 257,
   262–3
genomics 331
geriatrics 251

governmentality 12–13, 132, 142,
   160–1
group relaxation classes 167, 177
Gullette, Margaret Morganroth 255,
   257

Hacking, Ian 14, 321
haemodilution 231
Haldane, J. S. and J. B. S. 230, 240
harmony 128
Hauser, Gaylord 131–5, 139, 144,
   147–9, 262, 274–5
The Health Divide (1987) 112
health education 64–71, 79–84, 87,
   95–100, 110–11, 116–18, 162–3,
   176–7
Health Education Council (HEC)
   17, 66, 70–3, 76, 79–80, 86,
   95–111, 112, 117–18
health education campaigns in
   North East England (1974–81)
   70–9
'Look After Your Heart' campaign
   (1987) 111, 114
'Look After Yourself' campaign
   (1978) 95, 99–110, 114, 117–18
health warnings on packaging 82–3
'healthism' 67
healthy eating and healthy living
   18–19, 97, 107, 127–8, 132–3,
   146–7, 177
Hippocratic tradition 8, 129
Hobsbawm, Eric 1–2, 128
homeostasis 3, 9, 10, 129, 145, 159,
   221–2, 226, 231–6
   research on 224, 229, 235
Human Genome Project 331
hunger 145

ideologies 97
imbalances and their impacts 16

immersive fieldwork 317–18
imperial hierarchies and imperialism 1, 11, 43–4, 229, 318, 334
individualism and individualisation 3, 106, 117, 149, 264, 267, 274, 325–6, 335
individuals' responsibility for their healthcare 7, 10–12, 18–19, 40, 41–3, 54, 65, 67, 96, 110, 114–18, 128, 141–4, 149, 167, 181, 198, 210, 241, 325–6
individuation, Jung's concept of 251
inequalities in health 110–15, 118
insulin and insulin therapy 36–41, 46, 49
International Physiological Expedition to Antarctica (INPHEXAN) 220, 236, 240
Inuit people 241–2
investigative journalism 110–11

Jacobson, Edmund 159, 165–7, 170, 177, 180
Japan 257–8
Jaques, Elliott 250–7, 264, 270–5
'jet lag' 205
Jung, Carl 251, 257
'junk food' 115

Kallang Airport crash (1954) 190–2
ketosis and ketonuria 34, 36, 38, 41, 57n.30, 139, 148–9

Labour Party 12
L-DOPA 286–304
Ledermann, Sully (and Ledermann thesis) 69, 80–2
'life begins at 40' 260–1
life expectancy 253, 255
liver cirrhosis 68–9

Lock, Margaret 255, 257
low-cost airlines 207–8

'McDonaldization of culture' 128
'malleable humanity' 23, 315–30
marathon running 221, 225
Marmot, Michael 174
marriage guidance 253, 258, 266–74
masculinity 43–5, 52, 104, 140, 198, 240
Mead, Margaret 23, 315–21, 326, 331
media techniques 96, 116–17
Medical Council on Alcoholism 71
Medical Officer of Health (MOH) 69
medication against fatigue 230
menopause 253, 257, 263–4, 268
mental illness 6–8
midlife crisis 21–2, 250–75
 as a *social* event 273
milieu intérieur and *milieu extérieur* 222–4, 242
Ministry of Agriculture, Fisheries and Food (MAFF) 80, 84, 144
mood disorders and mood stabilisers 6–7
Morris, Jerry 66–7
mortality rates 103, 108, 113–16

narcissism 269–70, 274
National Aeronautics and Space Administration (NASA), US 228
National Health Service (NHS), UK 40, 46, 69, 99, 111–12, 118, 173, 267
National Marriage Guidance Council, UK 268–71
Nationwide (television programme) 163
'natural laboratories' 224, 236, 242
Nazi concentration camps 228–9

Index 345

neo-liberalism 3, 15, 54, 142, 209
neuroscience 329–32
New Historicism 322–3
New Right 112, 200
nutrition and nutritional policy 97–100
'nutritionism' 133

obesity 18–19, 67, 95–100, 106–10, 117, 130–1, 143
  in childhood 113–14
  on film 106–7
overwork 194
oxygen deficiency 222–3, 230–1

Parkinson's Disease 14, 22, 286–305
'Parkinson's personality' 22, 290–3, 304
Pauling, Linus 131, 136–8, 144–9
performance-enhancing substances 230
physiological perspectives on clinical medicine 35, 38, 40, 45, 48, 52–4
  see also balance, physiological and psychological
Pitkin, Walter B. and Walter Jr 260–3
polycythaemia 226–7, 232
population growth 9
postmodernism 323–4
preventive medicine 99, 104, 107, 116
psychoanalysis and psychoanalytic theory 250–1, 320–1
psychological management 45–8, 51–4
public discussion, need for 82–6
public health policy 64–70, 87–8, 95–7, 100–1, 104–6, 115–17, 234
  population-level approaches to 96
public information films 97, 106, 117

race 12, 30n.72, 43–4, 233–7, 241–2, 247n.62, 255, 319, 320–1, 327
radio broadcasts 163
rational decision-making 13, 14, 30n.72, 67, 79, 81, 143–4, 145, 240
Redlands (advertising agency) 76, 78
regulation 7, 10, 13–14, 20
  in civil aviation 201, 204–10
relaxation
  role in achieving equanimity 262
  see also self-regulation
Relaxation for Living (charity) 165–72, 179
relaxation techniques 19–20, 158–69, 174, 177–8, 181–2
  differential 177
  for men 168
  wider benefits from 164–5
relaxation therapy 170, 172, 175
relaxation training 169–73, 176–82
  main aim of 180
  research into the efficacy of 173
'relaxometer' device 166–7
risk 18, 96–7, 103–6, 115–18, 129–30
Royal College of Physicians 99
Royal College of Psychiatrists 77, 86–7
Royal Commission on Marriage and Divorce (1956) 265–6, 271
Royal Geographical Society 238–9
Russia 182

Saatchi & Saatchi (advertising agency) 71–6, 101
schizophrenia 2, 290
self-care 33–5, 39–44, 48–9, 52–4, 148–9, 167, 326

self-experiments 239–40
self-help literature 8, 16–19, 127–33, 141–50, 164, 169, 175, 251, 253, 258–63, 270, 274
　in Russia 182
　societal benefits from 145
selfhood 11–16, 23, 66, 87–8, 96–7, 110, 118, 127, 130, 133, 149, 181, 324, 327–9, 334
　plastic 318
self-regulation 7, 11–12, 43, 87–8, 96, 99–100, 115–17, 129, 133, 166, 176, 241, 325, 335
　in civil aviation 200, 206, 209–10
Selye, Hans 10, 129, 159–60, 176, 221
'sensible drinker' policy 65–6, 77–9, 83–8
Sheffield 111–13
Sherpa people 221, 226, 229–30, 240–1
smoking 114–16
Sno-Cats 238
social construction 320, 327
social determinants of health 67–8, 76
Staines air crash (1972) 201
state, the
　intervention by 12, 54, 136, 176–7, 193, 194, 198, 208–10, 213n.42
　role and interests of 3, 7, 11–12, 12–13, 40, 67, 82, 96, 104–6, 117, 142
　welfare 7, 40, 43–4, 99, 111, 129, 141–2, 326
sterilisation, forced 331
Stopes, Marie 268–70
stress and stress management 7–8, 10, 145, 159–62, 168, 173, 176–7, 182, 204, 220–1, 228, 239

target groups 79
Tavistock Clinic 252, 267, 271–2
Tavistock Institute of Human Relations 250
taxation 69–70, 83–5
'technologies of the self' (Foucault) 11, 142, 181, 328
television 110, 163
temperance movement 68
thalidomide 174
Thatcher, Margaret 8, 88, 193
Thatcherism 111, 209
Thomson, Mathew 13
tranquillisers 174–5
Treasury, the 84
Truslow Adams, James 260
twentieth-century extremes 1, 3

Understanding Stresses and Strains (film) 158, 160, 176
United States 15, 19–22, 194–5, 239, 252, 265–6, 273–4, 286

vaccination 65
Valium 174, 180
visual images 71–6, 96–7, 100–5, 110, 113, 117, 158, 295, 303
vitamin C 136–8, 145–9

white adult male (taken as the norm) 43, 219–22, 226, 240–1
Woman's Hour (radio programme) 163
women
　denied access to extreme spaces 220
　extreme physiology 225–6
　participation in expeditions 239
　research on and by 239–41
work 38, 40, 45, 46, 48, 49, 112, 114, 177–8, 192–3, 194–5, 200, 204,

Index

234, 242, 253, 259, 261, 262, 263, 270, 273, 290
working days, length of 190–2, 198, 201
working hours, regulation of 194–5
work-life balance 3, 7, 203–4, 205, 254, 262
World Health Organization 67, 180

You and Yours (radio programme) 163–4

Zellweger, Renée 140
'zero balancing' 5–6

EU authorised representative for GPSR:
Easy Access System Europe, Mustamäe tee 50,
10621 Tallinn, Estonia
gpsr.requests@easproject.com